LAMBINO

D1399532

EMERGENCY RADIOLOGY
SECOND EDITION

EMERGENCY RADIOLOGY

SECOND EDITION

Theodore E. Keats, M.D.
Professor and Chairman
Department of Radiology
School of Medicine
University of Virginia
Charlottesville, Virginia

YEAR BOOK MEDICAL PUBLISHERS, INC.
CHICAGO • LONDON • BOCA RATON

Copyright © 1989 by Year Book Medical Publishers, Inc. All rights reserved. No part of this publication may be reproduced, stored in a retrieval system, or transmitted, in any form or by any means—electronic, mechanical, photocopying, recording, or otherwise—without prior written permission from the publisher. Printed in the United States of America.

1 2 3 4 5 6 7 8 9 0 KC 93 92 91 90 89

Library of Congress Cataloging-in-Publication Data

Emergency radiology / [edited by] Theodore E. Keats.—2nd ed.
    p.   cm.
  Includes bibliographies and index.
  ISBN 0-8151-5044-X
  1. Diagnosis, Radioscopic.   2. Radiology, Medical.
3. Medical emergencies.   I. Keats, Theodore E. (Theodore Eliot), 1924–
  [DNLM: 1. Emergencies—atlases.   2. Radiography—atlases.
WN 17 E53]
RC78.E573 1989   88-20830
616.07′572—dc19   CIP
DNLM/DLC
for Library of Congress

Sponsoring Editor: James D. Ryan
Assistant Director, Manuscript Services: Frances M. Perveiler
Production Manager, Text and Reference/Periodicals: Etta Worthington
Proofroom Manager: Shirley E. Taylor

Contributors

Peter Armstrong, M.D.
Professor and Vice Chairman
Department of Radiology
University of Virginia School of Medicine
Charlottesville, Virginia

Wayne S. Cail, M.D.
Associate Professor
Department of Radiology
University of Virginia School of Medicine
Charlottesville, Virginia

W. Gray Mason, M.D.
Radiologist-in-Chief
Wolfson Children's Hospital at Baptist Medical
    Center
Jacksonville, Florida

Kurt W. Mori, M.D.
Attending Radiologist (Interventional Radiology)
Baptist Medical Center and Memorial Hospital
Jacksonville, Florida

Paul A. Mori, M.D.
Chairman, Department of Radiology, Nuclear
    Medicine, and Ultrasound
Baptist Medical Center
Attending Radiologist
Memorial Hospital
Jacksonville, Florida

Thomas Lee Pope, Jr., M.D.
Associate Professor
Department of Radiology
University of Virginia School of Medicine
Charlottesville, Virginia

Hans O. Riddervold, M.D.
Professor of Radiology
Department of Radiology
University of Virginia School of Medicine
Charlottesville, Virginia

K. K. Wallace, Jr., M.D.
Associate Professor of Radiology
Eastern Virginia Medical School
Chairman, Department of Radiology
Virginia Beach (Va.) General Hospital
Virginia Beach, Virginia

Preface to the First Edition

Books delight us when prosperity sweetly smiles; they stay to comfort us when cloudy future frowns. They lend strength to human compacts and, without them, grave subjects may not be propounded.
Richard De Bury, *Philobiblon*,
Grolier Club ed., vol. ii, p. 22

The need for a text of this sort has been documented by eight years of experience of several of the authors in teaching a postgraduate course in radiology for emergency physicians. In their prescribed role, these physicians must be all things to all patients, particularly during the hours when they do not have access to a full staff of specialists for immediate assistance. This problem is particularly acute in radiology, since this modality is so important in attaining a diagnosis in the emergency setting.

This text is dedicated to the basic tenet of helping the emergency physician "get through the night." Its scope is, therefore, limited to the kinds of problems apt to be seen in the emergency department and is not intended to be a comprehensive treatment of the entire field of radiology. Consequently, emphasis is on the diagnosis of trauma and acute diseases, together with some of the normal variants which may be mistaken for disease. Recommended reading lists are provided for the physician who wishes to explore any subject in greater depth.

It is our hope that this volume will serve as a useful working companion for the emergency physician who must often rely on his own resources in interpreting roentgen images.

Theodore E. Keats, M.D.

Preface to the Second Edition

We were delighted with the response of our readers to the first edition of this work. It was a surprise to learn that it had attracted as much interest from radiologists as it had from emergency physicians, indicating that there was a need for a concise work dealing with radiology in the emergency milieu.

To increase the usefulness of this edition, we have expanded our format to include references to some of the nonconventional techniques, such as nuclear scanning, CT, ultrasound, and MRI. These diagnostic techniques are not usually thought of as emergency procedures, but their contribution to the critically ill patient are often so important that knowledge of their application and, hence, the need for prompt referral is essential information for emergency personnel. Other additions include a number of normal variants of the upper extremity and, most important, a new chapter on pediatric emergencies, which we believe the reader will find most useful. Pediatric emergencies are sufficiently different in their manifestations to warrant special consideration.

I wish to thank my secretary, Patricia West, and my editorial assistant, Carol Chowdhry, Ph.D., for their invaluable assistance in the preparation of the manuscript.

Theodore E. Keats, M.D.

Contents

Preface to the First Edition vii

Preface to the Second Edition ix

1 Skull *By Hans O. Riddervold and Thomas Lee Pope, Jr.* **1**
  Technique 4
  Anatomy 6
  Pathology 6
  Normal Variants 21

2 Face *By Wayne S. Cail* **45**
  Classification of Fractures 47
  Fractures of the Lower Third of the Face 47
  Fractures of the Middle Third of the Face 55
  Fractures of the Upper Third of the Face 73
  Computed Tomography in Facial Trauma 73
  Normal Variants 81

3 Spine *By Thomas Lee Pope, Jr., and Hans O. Riddervold* **89**
  The Cervical Spine 91
  The Thoracolumbar Spine 111
  Normal Variants 127

4 Chest *By Peter Armstrong* **149**
  Plain Chest Radiographs 151
  Additional Plain Films of the Chest 156
  Computed Tomography 156
  The Abnormal Plain Chest Radiograph 159
  Interpretation of Radiological Findings 163
  The Pleura 171
  The Diaphragm 177
  The Mediastinum 178
  Trauma to the Chest 181
  Pneumonia and Lung Abscess 186
  Specific Infections 191
  Pulmonary Edema, Adult Respiratory Distress Syndrome,
    and Circulatory Disorders 195
  Inhalation of Noxious Gases and Smoke 195
  Airway Obstruction 208
  Pharyngeal and Upper Esophageal Foreign Body 211
  Rupture of the Esophagus 211

Intrathoracic Manifestations of Abdominal Disease 211
Normal Variants 213

5 Abdomen *By Paul A. Mori and Kurt W. Mori* **241**
Anatomical Approach 244
The Acute Abdomen 249
Bowel Obstruction 250
The Nonspecific Abdomen 251
Mechanical Obstruction 253
Adynamic Ileus—The Mechanism of Gas Accumulation 257
Distal Colon Obstruction Versus Adynamic Ileus 257
Summary of Basic Concepts for Recognition of Simple, Classic
    Obstructions 260
Barium Versus Water-Soluble Contrast 260
Abdominal Masses 268
Intussusception 268
Free Air in the Peritoneum—Intestinal Perforation 268
Interposition 272
Appendicitis, Coproliths, Appendiceal Abscess, Perforation 277
Acute Pancreatitis and Cholecystitis 277
Pelvic Inflammatory Disease, Pelvic Mass, and Ectopic Pregnancy . . . 281
Gallstone Ileus 286
Acute Diverticulitis 286
Peritonitis 286
Volvulus 293
Mesenteric Ischemia 295
The Decision Tree (The Acute Abdomen) 296
Flank Pain (Ureteral Colic) 296
Testicular Torsion 301
The Pregnant Patient—Radiation Exposure During Pregnancy 301
References 309
Blunt Abdominal Trauma 309
Penetrating Trauma 329
Normal Variants, Calcifications, Oddities, and "Aunt Minnies" 336
Calcifications and Opacities 336
Normal Variants 345

6 Pelvis and Hips *By Hans O. Riddervold and Thomas Lee Pope, Jr.* **365**
Technique 367
Anatomy 369
Pathology 369
Normal Variants 391

7 Extremities *By K. K. Wallace, Jr.* **401**
Anatomical Considerations 403
Patterns of Bone Injury 403
Patterns of Bone Repair 406
Radiographic Technique 406
General Considerations 409
Shoulder 410
Scapula 413
Clavicle 413
Elbow 418
Forearm 421

Wrist 421
Hand 427
Knee 431
Leg 435
Ankle 435
Foot 435
Foreign Bodies 436
Fatigue Fractures 439
Nontraumatic Conditions 439
Osteomyelitis. 439
Arthritis 439
Neoplasms 443
Normal Variants 445

8 **The Pediatric Patient** *By W. Gray Mason, Jr.* **477**
Technical Problems 479
Skull 480
Spine 480
Airway 483
Chest 486
Abdomen 492
Pelvis and Hips. 495
Skeletal Emergencies in Children. 497
Child Abuse 503

Index. **505**

1
Skull

Hans O. Riddervold, M.D.
Thomas Lee Pope, Jr., M.D.

The skull, like the cervical spine, is one of the most intimidating anatomical regions to evaluate in emergency medicine. The seriousness of the potential injury, together with the difficulty often encountered in clinically assessing possible damage to the intracranial contents, makes proper evaluation of this area one of the most demanding tasks facing emergency room physicians. Therefore, it is imperative that they have a thorough knowledge of how the radiograph may help in certain situations and why it is to be requested.

In a patient with head trauma, the primary diagnostic tests are plain skull x-rays, unenhanced and enhanced computed tomography (CT), and magnetic resonance imaging (MRI). All of these are complementary studies with various strengths and weaknesses and, in many instances, a combination of more than one examination is necessary to obtain a complete work-up of the head injury patient. In the acute setting, however, the plain skull series will probably be the initial screening study. This chapter will deal primarily with acute cases and will stress the strengths and potential weaknesses of plain films. The appropriate use of CT will also be discussed. An in-depth discussion of head CT findings in the acute ER setting is available from other sources.

A wealth of literature has dealt with the indications for the efficacy of skull roentgenograms in assessing trauma cases.[1-3] The efficacy studies of Bell and Loop on 1,500 patients[1] in the early 1970s identified a set of 21 high-yield criteria that detected 92 skull fractures in 1,065 patients. On the other hand, a list of low-yield criteria only detected one fracture in 435 patients. Phillips[4] modified these criteria and found a significant increase in positive findings, as well as a 40% reduction in the number of examinations requested.

A multidisciplinary panel headed by Masters[5] studied 7,035 patients with head trauma at 31 hospital emergency rooms. They also divided patients into low, moderate, and high risk categories (Table 1–1). Omitting a skull series in the low risk group would not have caused any significant intracranial injury to be missed, but in the moderate and high risk groups a plain skull series was probably worthwhile. The panel concluded, therefore, that abiding by a management strategy such as this could appreciably reduce radiation and cost without compromising quality. However, slight modification of the strategy was necessary for the pediatric population because children manifest acute craniocerebral trauma differently from adults.[5, 6] The references should be consulted for these modifications.

It should be stressed that any recommendations for obtaining radiographs in the trauma setting are merely suggested guidelines and are not intended to replace meticulous history-taking and thorough physical examination. These two procedures still probably provide the most helpful information in evaluating the need for and the yield of skull radiographs in trauma.

Another less commonly discussed, yet nonetheless important, rationale for obtaining skull radiographs in the trauma setting is the threat of malpractice. A large proportion of medicolegal actions result from failure to diagnose a fracture or dislocation. A 7-year survey by St. Paul Fire and Marine Insurance Company showed that 25% of all claims were due to "failure to diagnose" and about 5% of all claims were due to failure to diagnose fractures or dislocations.[7] Therefore, malpractice considerations can be important reasons for obtaining radiographs, depending on the experience and expertise of the physician, the understanding of the patient, and the rapport between the two.

Of course, CT has revolutionized the radiographic

TABLE 1–1.

Management Strategy for Radiographic Imaging in Patients With Head Trauma*†

Low-Risk Group	Moderate-Risk Group	High-Risk Group
Possible findings	*Possible findings*	*Possible findings*
Asymptomatic	History of change of consciousness at the time of injury or subsequently	Depressed level of consciousness not clearly due to alcohol, drugs, or other cause (e.g., metabolic and seizure disorders)
Dizziness		
Scalp hematoma		
Scalp laceration	History of progressive headache	Focal neurologic signs
Scalp contusion or abrasion	Alcohol or drug intoxication	Decreasing level of consciousness
Absence of moderate-risk or high-risk criteria	Unreliable or inadequate history of injury	Penetrating skull injury or palpable depressed fracture
	Age less than 2 yr (unless injury very trivial)	
	Post-traumatic seizure	
	Vomiting	
	Post-traumatic amnesia	
	Multiple trauma	
	Serious facial injury	
	Signs of basilar fracture‡	
	Possible skull penetration or depressed fracture§	
	Suspected physical child abuse	
Recommendations	*Recommendations*	*Recommendations*
Observation alone; discharge patients with head-injury information sheet (listing subdural precautions) and a second person to observe them	Extended close observation (watch for signs of high-risk group)	Patient is a candidate for neurosurgical consultation or emergency CT examination or both
	Consider CT examination and neurological consultation	
	Skull series may (rarely) be helpful, if positive, but do not exclude intracranial injury, if normal	

*From Masters SJ, McClean PM, Arcause JS, et al: *N Engl J Med* 1987; 316:84. Used by permission.
†Physician assessment of the severity of injury may warrant reassignment to a higher-risk group. Any single criterion from a higher-risk group warrants assignment of the patient to the highest risk group applicable.
‡Signs of basilar fracture include drainage from ear, drainage of cerebrospinal fluid from nose, hematotympanum, Battle's sign and "raccoon eyes."
§Factors associated with open and depressed fracture include gunshot, missle, or shrapnel wounds; scalp injury from firm, pointed object (including animal teeth); penetrating injury of eyelid or globe; object stuck in the head; assault (definite or suspected) with any object; leakage of cerebrospinal fluid; and sign of basilar fracture.

evaluation of head trauma. CT accurately depicts the condition of the intracranial contents and, because of its excellent density differentiation, can give data on acute hemorrhage or contusion.[8–10] It has understandably become one of the mainstays of diagnosis in the trauma setting and should be performed on all patients with suspected significant intracranial injury. The emergency room physician will not commonly be called upon to interpret an emergency head CT. However, he or she should be aware of the situations in which CT is appropriate. Despite its well-known advantages, CT must sometimes be supplemented by plain films or linear tomography, especially since standard CT techniques may miss minimally dis-

placed fractures (see Pathology section in this chapter).

Magnetic resonance imaging has been used sparingly in acute cases of head trauma, but has proven valuable for subtle pathology not detected by CT. After the patient is stabilized, MRI can be an important tool in evaluating residual pathology in the follow-up of these patients.[11]

Technique

If one of the moderate- or high-risk criteria are present in the acute trauma setting in emergency cases, plain films of the skull are generally the initial radio-

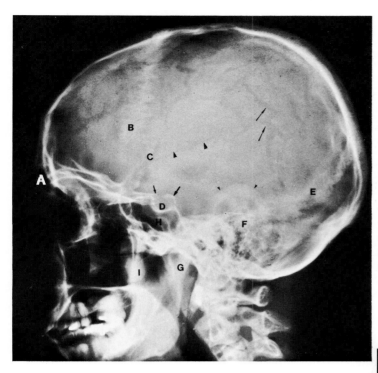

FIG 1–1.
Normal lateral skull. *A* = frontal sinus, *B* = coronal suture, *C* = groove for major branch of middle meningeal artery, *large arrowheads* = posterior branch of middle meningeal artery, *D* = sella turcica, *E* = lambdoidal suture, *F* = mastoid air cells, *G* = neck of mandible, *H* = sphenoid sinus, *I* = coronoid process of mandible, *large thin arrows* = intradiploic venous channels, *small arrowheads* = pinna of the ears, *large arrow* = posterior clinoid processes, *small short arrow* = anterior clinoid processes.

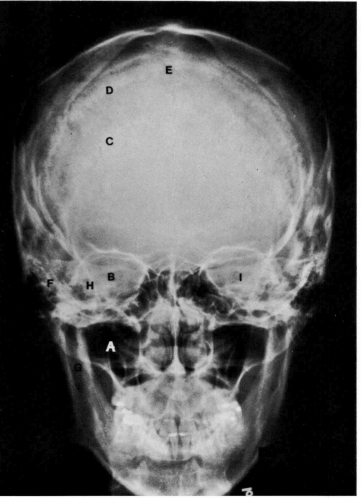

FIG 1–2.
Normal anteroposterior skull. *A* = maxillary antrum, *B* = orbit, *C* = lambdoidal suture, *D* = coronal suture, *E* = sagittal suture, *F* = mastoid air cells, *G* = mandibular ramus, *H* = greater wing of sphenoid (oblique orbital line), *I* = internal auditory canal.

logic test. We will stress the plain film signs of normal and pathologic anatomy.

Our routine "skull series" in the trauma setting consists of cross-table, brow-up lateral view, lateral view (with the opposite side of the patient's head against the cassette), anteroposterior (AP) view, Caldwell view, and Towne view. The most important view is probably the cross-table lateral because it may show air-fluid levels that suggest potentially serious intracranial injury. If depressed skull fractures are suspected, fluoroscopy or tangential views are often useful in delineating the exact anatomic location and the degree of depression of the injury. We rarely use tomography in the skull because of the availability of CT. Finally, of course, CT is the best way to detect serious intracranial pathology that plain roentgenograms do not disclose.

Anatomy

The anatomy of the skull (Figs 1–1 and 1–2) can be confusing and intimidating, and the emergency room doctor should be familiar with some of the more important landmarks. On the lateral view one should note the sphenoid sinus (checking for air-fluid levels), the sella turcica, the coronal and lambdoidal sutures, and the grooves for the anterior and posterior divisions of the middle meningeal artery. Also, other regions included on the film—particularly the facial structures and upper cervical spine—should be routinely evaluated. The pineal and any other calcified structures within the calvarium should also be found, if visible. Convolutional markings should not be confused with traumatic injury, and their normal state should be appreciated. Likewise, venous lakes, which are small or large irregular areas of decreased density situated in the diploë, should not be mistaken for pathology. On the Towne view, the pineal, if calcified and localized, should be measured to verify that it is within 2 mm of the midline.

As in any other anatomic area, normal variation in the skull may be confused with pathology. See the following section for common examples.

Pathology

Fractures of the skull are probably among the most important injuries to diagnose in the trauma setting because of the potentially serious consequences of overlooking them. Fractures are classified as closed or open and nondepressed or depressed. Closed fractures have no associated break in the overlying soft tissues, wheareas open fractures allow the subarachnoid space to communicate with the outside or with the sinuses. Both of these types of open fractures in-

volve a significant risk of meningitis (Fig 1–3). One exception to this general rule is a fracture that communicates only with the anterior wall of the frontal sinus. With this fracture, the posterior frontal sinus wall remains intact and protects the meninges from infection (Fig 1–4).

Nondepressed fractures have no significant displacement and can often be difficult to distinguish from sutural lines or vascular markings. A knowledge of the normal location of sutures and the common vascular pathways can help prevent errors. Also, appreciating the sharp margination and linearity of fractures as opposed to the often irregular, sclerotic margins of vascular and sutural lines can help to distinguish these two entities on plain films (Figs 1–5 and 1–6).

On CT examination, linear nondepressed skull fractures may be overlooked because the scanning angle does not cross the fracture at right angles or because the fracture is only minimally displaced. In these cases the plain film can be used as a complementary exam (Figs 1–7 and 1–8).

Another type of skull fracture, diastatic fracture, is a traumatic separation at suture lines. These may be difficult to appreciate without close scrutiny and good clinical correlation (Figs 1–9 and 1–10).

Depressed fractures are those in which bone has been displaced below the normal margin of the calvarium. Fluoroscopy or tangential plain views may be necessary to delineate the extent of these injuries and supplement physical examination, which should disclose the depressed area (Figs 1–11 to 1–14). These fractures are often associated with intracranial injury; hence CT should be performed in most patients with this finding (see Fig 1–14.)

Involvement of certain regions may prompt further evaluation regardless of the type of fracture. For instance, fractures of the temporal bone are often associated with epidural hematomas because of rupture of the middle meningeal artery (Fig 1–15). In these cases an ancillary finding on the plain films may be pineal shift. This shift should never be greater than 2 mm on either side of the midline. If it is greater than 2.5 mm, CT should probably be performed to exclude a potentially life-threatening cause (Fig 1–16).

Secondary signs of trauma in the sinuses may indicate significant intracranial pathology. Chief of these is the presence of an air-fluid level in the sphenoid sinus seen on the brow-up lateral film. This finding on plain films is sufficient reason for an emergency head CT because of the high percentage of intracranial injury, particularly basilar skull fractures in these patients.[12] In a basilar skull fracture, cerebrospinal fluid leaks into the sphenoid sinus, causing the air-

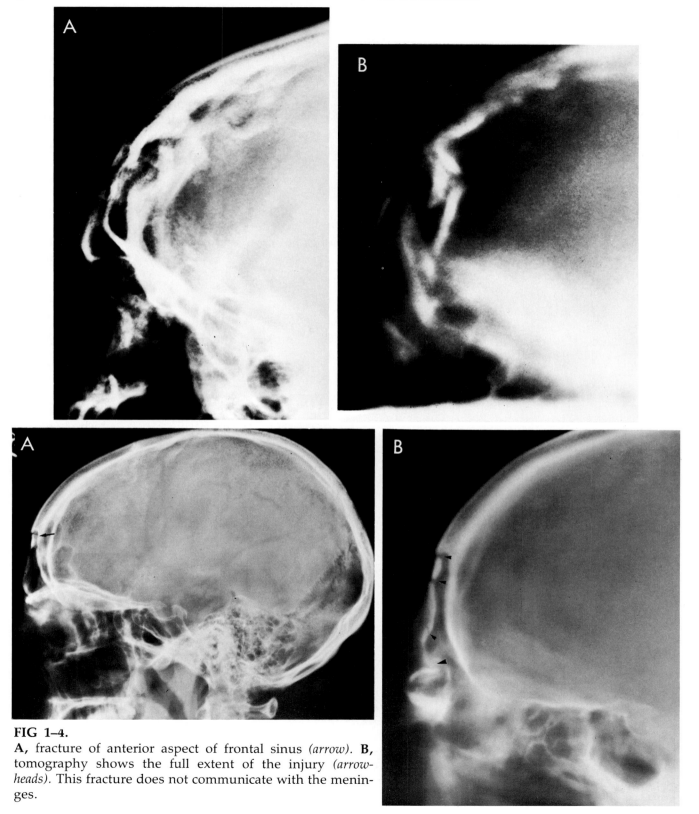

FIG 1–3.
A, close-up lateral view of 40-year-old patient following auto accident, interpreted initially as hyperostosis frontalis interna. **B,** tomography the next day showed depressed skull fracture involving the posterior wall of the frontal sinus.

FIG 1–4.
A, fracture of anterior aspect of frontal sinus *(arrow)*. **B,** tomography shows the full extent of the injury *(arrowheads)*. This fracture does not communicate with the meninges.

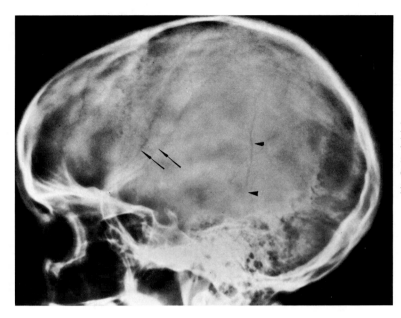

FIG 1–5.
Forty-year-old man with temporoparietal linear skull fracture *(arrowheads)* from auto accident. Grooves for middle meningeal arteries are designated by *arrows*.

FIG 1–6.
A, Towne view of 50-year-old man in motorcycle accident shows lucency projected over central portion of skull, which could be misinterpreted as metopic suture *(arrowheads).* **B,** accentuated Towne view shows line continuing down to the foramen magnum, indicating an occipital skull fracture *(arrow).* Note linearity and lack of sclerotic margins.

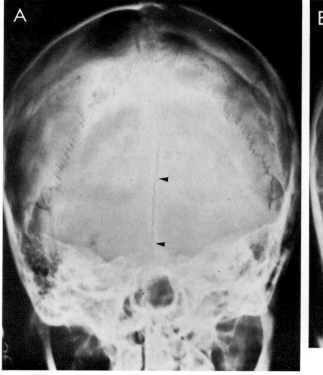 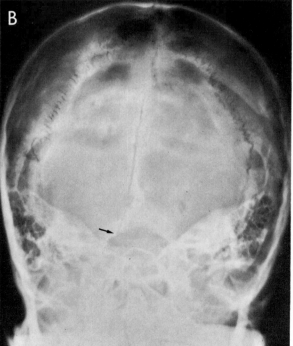

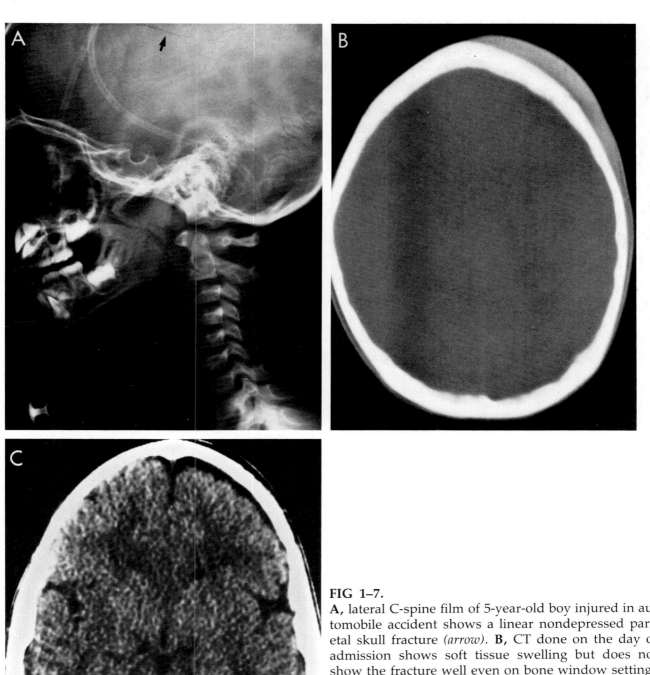

FIG 1–7.
A, lateral C-spine film of 5-year-old boy injured in automobile accident shows a linear nondepressed parietal skull fracture *(arrow)*. **B,** CT done on the day of admission shows soft tissue swelling but does not show the fracture well even on bone window settings because of the minimal displacement of the fracture. **C,** CT done ten days later shows cystic hygroma collection. Skull fracture is not demonstrated.

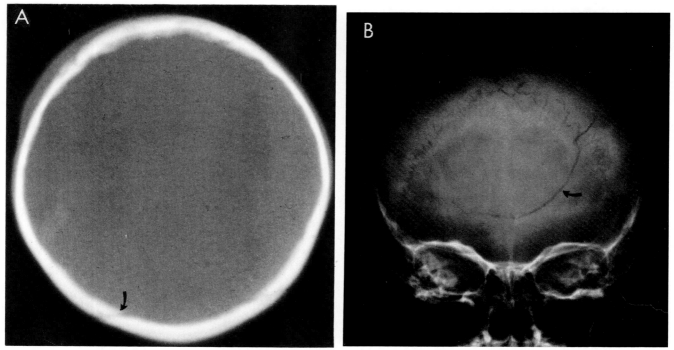

FIG 1–8.
A, unenhanced head CT on 27-year-old man performed prior to plain films shows linear nondisplaced occipital skull fracture *(arrow)*. **B,** Towne view from routine skull series shows fracture to a much better advantage *(arrow)*. In many situations, CT and plain films may be complementary (see text).

FIG 1–9.
Diastatic fracture of left lambdoidal suture. Note asymmetric widening *(arrowheads)*. Right lambdoidal suture shown by *arrow*.

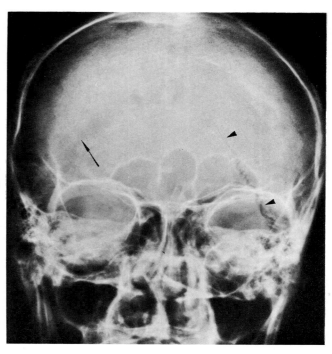

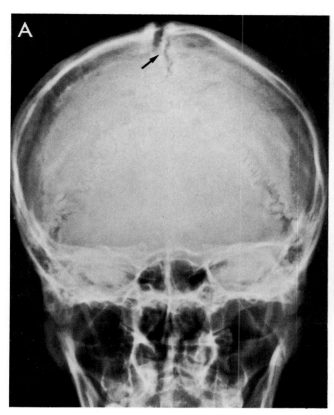

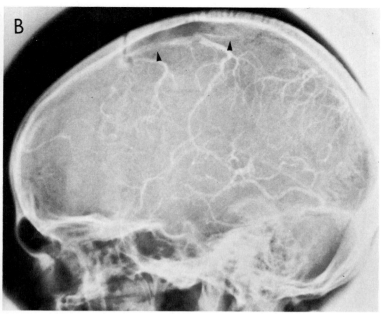

FIG 1–10.
A, diastatic fracture of sagittal suture *(arrow).* **B,** venous phase of angiogram on same patient, showing 9-mm separation of superior sagittal sinus from the inner table of the skull by an epidural mass, in this case, hematoma *(arrowheads).*

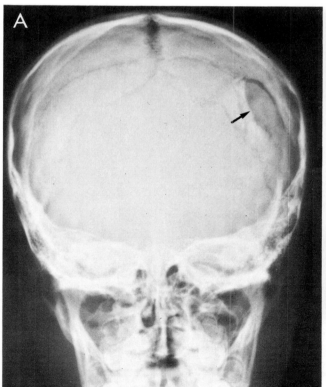

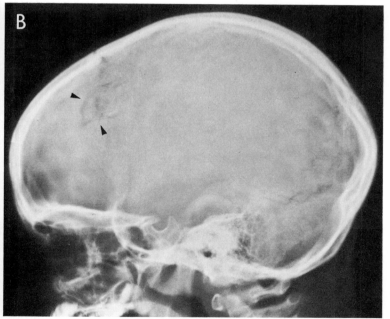

FIG 1–11.
A, depressed left frontoparietal skull fracture on anteroposterior (AP) view. **B,** lateral view confirms the fracture *(arrowheads).* All views in the skull series should be examined meticulously for such injuries.

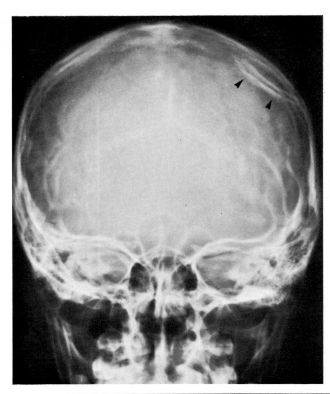

FIG 1–12.
Depressed fracture of left parietal region in person hit with a club *(arrowheads).* Fracture was not seen in lateral view.

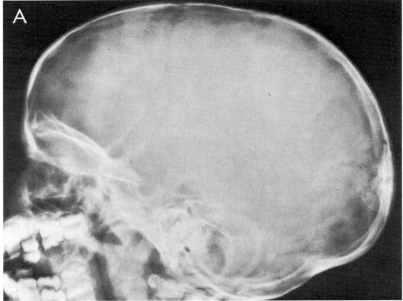
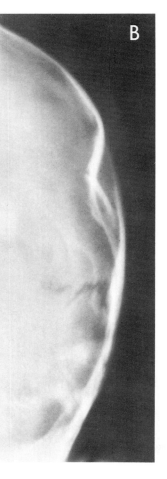

FIG 1–13.
A, lateral skull film of child hit in head shows no fracture. **B,** tangential view shows characteristic "ping-pong" skull fracture.

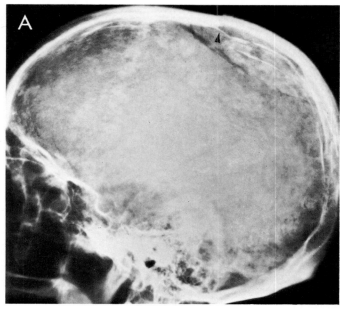

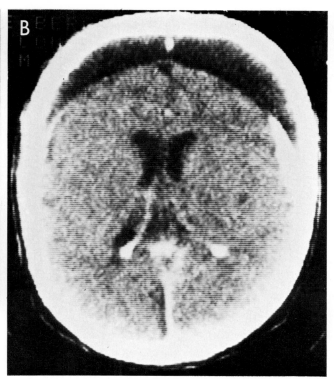

FIG 1–14.
A, lateral skull film showing depressed parietal skull fracture in a 61-year-old man after an automobile accident. **B,** CT scan showing large bilateral subdural fluid collection. Depressed skull fractures have a high association with intracranial injury.

FIG 1–15.
A, brow-up lateral skull film showing linear temporoparietal skull fracture *(large arrows),* as well as air-fluid levels in maxillary antrum *(double arrowheads)* and sphenoid sinus *(arrowhead).* **B,** CT scan showing large epidural hematoma *(arrowheads)* associated with marked edema and shift of the midline structures *(arrow).*

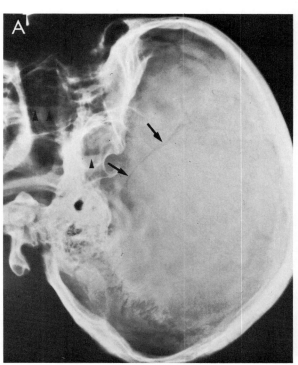

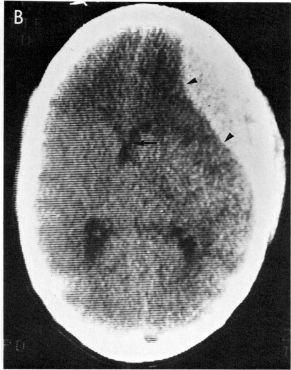

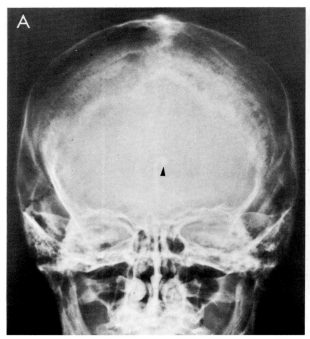

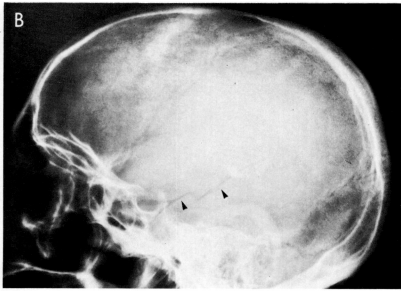

FIG 1–16.
A, anteroposterior (AP) skull view with calcified pineal shifted 5 mm from the midline *(arrowhead)*. **B,** lateral view of same patient showing temporoparietal skull fracture *(arrowheads)* with underlying epidural hematoma demonstrated on CT scan. The patient died on the operating table before the hematoma could be evacuated.

FIG 1–17.
A, brow-up lateral film of a 16-year-old patient involved in an automobile accident shows an air-fluid level in the maxillary sinus *(double arrows)* and sphenoid sinus *(single arrow)*. **B,** subsequent CT scan showed an intraventricular hemorrhage. Air-fluid levels in the sphenoid sinus may indicate serious intracranial injury.

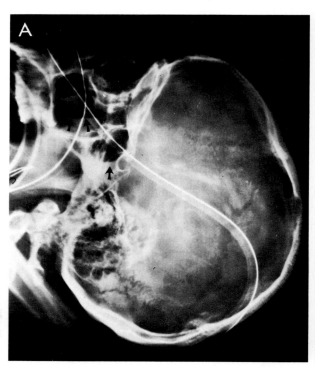

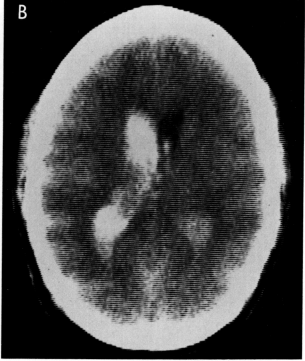

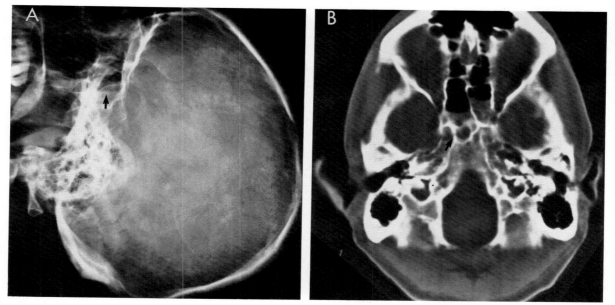

FIG 1–18.
A, brow-up lateral skull film on a 36-year-old man who fell from a ladder shows an air-fluid level in the sphenoid sinus *(arrow)*. **B,** head CT shows minimally displaced fracture *(arrow)*. This fracture would never have been visualized on plain films. An air-fluid level in the sphenoid sinus is sufficient indication for a head CT!

FIG 1–19.
Scalp laceration seen on Towne view of the skull may often mimic skull fractures *(arrowheads)*. This should be obvious clinically.

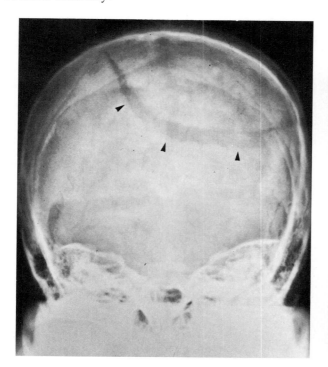

FIG 1–20.
Brow-up lateral skull film of a 45-year-old man injured in auto accident. *Arrow* points to air-fluid level in large scalp laceration.

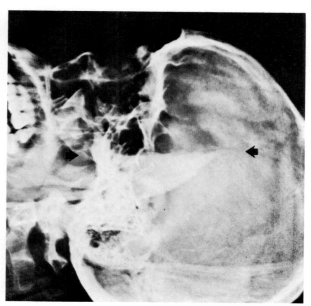

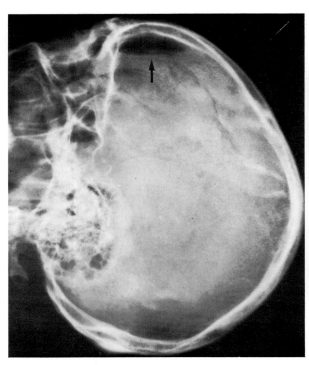

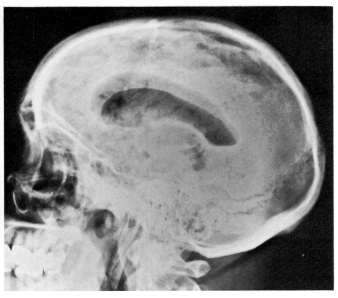

FIG 1–21 (top left).
Brow-up lateral skull x-ray of 45-year-old injured in automobile accident. Pneumocephalus is indicated by *arrow*. Pneumocephalus is always associated with an open fracture and often with severe intracranial injury.

FIG 1–22 (top right).
Lateral skull film of a 55-year-old man 4 days after bilateral nasal polypectomy and right ethmoidectomy. Marked intraventricular air secondary to this surgery is present.

FIG 1–23 (bottom left).
Lateral skull film of a 52-year-old woman showing multiple lytic defects. This represents multiple myeloma.

FIG 1–24 (bottom right).
Lateral skull film of 42-year-old woman with known breast cancer. Osteolytic lesions characteristic of metastatic breast carcinoma.

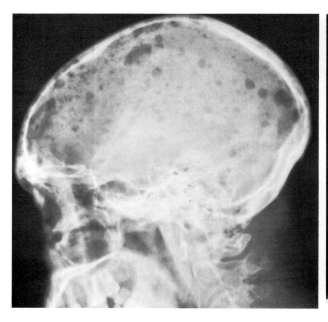

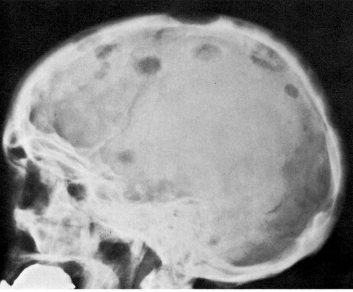

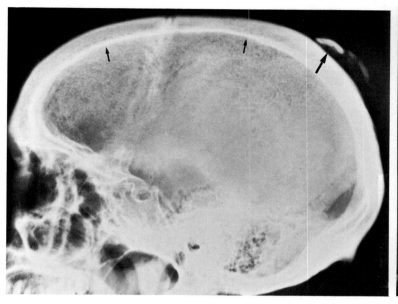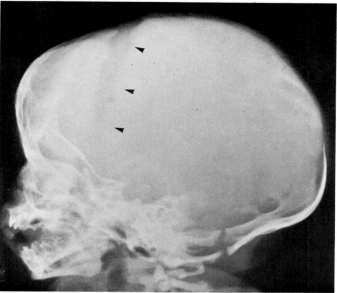

FIG 1–25.
Lateral skull view of 21-year-old man with severe seizure disorder who fell. Marked thickening of the skull secondary to Dilantin therapy *(small arrows)*. A calcified hematoma in the parietal region from repeated falls is also seen *(large arrow)*. CT scan on this patient was normal at the time of injury.

FIG 1–26.
Lateral skull film of newborn child shows marked widening of the coronal sutures *(arrowheads)* caused by hydrocephalus from an Arnold-Chiari malformation.

FIG 1–27.
A, lateral skull film of a 75-year-old man with head trauma and subdural hematoma. On this film, the possibility of a fractured odontoid *(arrowhead)* was raised. **B,** tomography confirmed the presence of an odontoid fracture *(arrowhead)*. The corners of the film may reveal important pathology.

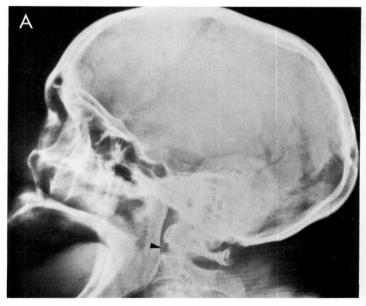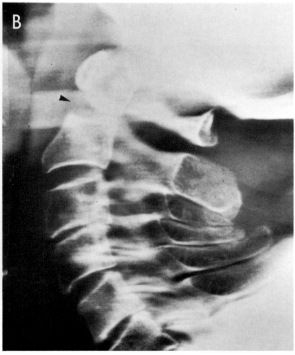

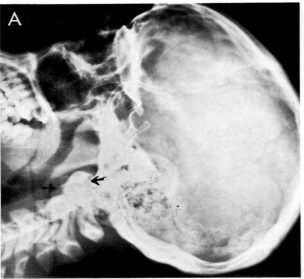

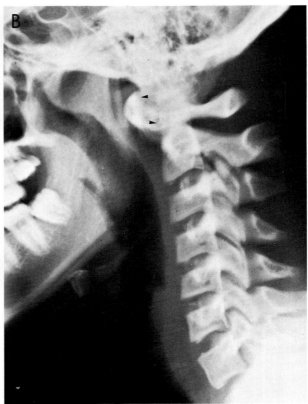

FIG 1–28.
A, brow-up lateral skull film of a 15-year-old boy injured playing football. Widening between the anterior arch of C-1 and the odontoid was noted on this study *(arrows)*. **B,** cervical spine film shows increased widening between the odontoid and anterior arch of C-1 *(arrowheads)*. This is an unstable situation caused by rupture of the transverse ligament.

FIG 1–29.
A, brow-up lateral film of a 24-year-old patient kicked in the face by a horse shows an air-fluid level in maxillary sinus *(arrow)* missed on the original films. **B,** exaggerated Towne (El Gammal) view of the skull shows fracture of the posterolateral wall of the left maxillary sinus *(arrow).*

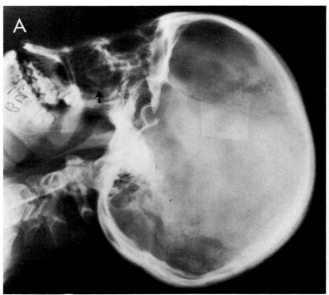

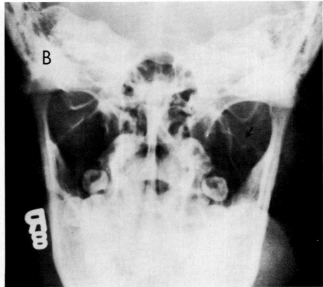

fluid level (Fig 1–17,A). These fractures are notoriously difficult to demonstrate by any modality, and a large percentage are never delineated. Therefore, it is important to recognize this secondary change and to order CT in those cases of suspected basilar skull fractures. CT serves two purposes. It may show the basilar skull fracture, but, even if it does not, it will often show associated intracranial injury (Figs 1–17,B and 1–18). As already mentioned, a skull fracture that communicates with the sphenoid, ethmoid, or posterior wall of the frontal sinuses is classified as "open" and needs antibiotic treatment to prevent possible infection.

Soft tissue changes may mimic more serious pathology. For instance, scalp lacerations, because of their configuration, are often misdiagnosed as linear nondepressed skull fractures. However, these lacerations are usually obvious clinically (Figs 1–19 and 1–20). Traumatic pneumocephalus, often signifying serious damage with communication between the subarachnoid space and the air outside or in the sinuses, is an ominous plain film sign and should not be missed (Fig 1–21). Of course, pneumocephalus may also be postoperative in origin and, if so, does not have the same serious significance as pneumocephalus occurring in the trauma setting (Fig 1–22). Systemic diseases not associated with trauma should not be confused with intracranial injury. Lytic metastases from myeloma or breast cancer may be seen first in the hematopoietic marrow of the calvarium and should not be misdiagnosed (Figs 1–23 and 1–24). The thickened calvarium resulting from treated hydrocephalus or phenytoin therapy may be mistakenly attributed to pathologic processes, but has a characteristic roentgen appearance (Fig 1–25). Further, the abnormally widened sutures in a child should not be disregarded, as they may represent increased intracranial pressure, metastatic disease (especially from neuroblastoma), or deprivational syndrome. Often, these findings may dictate immediate intervention (Fig 1–26).

Finally, the corners of all films should be scrutinized for pathology that may be hidden from the main field of view. We have termed these findings "corner clues" and have found that they are often overlooked unless a conscious effort is made to evaluate them. Unsuspected fractures or dislocations of the cervical spine may often become evident on the skull series, as may unsuspected air-fluid levels in the sinuses (Figs 1–27 to 1–29).

What we have attempted to do in this chapter is to introduce the reader to some of the commonly-encountered pathology on the routine skull series and suggest certain guidelines to be followed when requesting a skull series in the acute setting. Knowledge of the appropriate indications for skull films and of the normal skull anatomy is imperative for good emergency room practice. One should also realize that plain films, CT, and magnetic resonance imaging are all complementary tests and that each has inherent strengths and weaknesses. This awareness will help the emergency physician to avoid pitfalls.

References

1. Bell RS, Loop JW: The utility and futility of radiographic skull examination for trauma. *N Engl J Med* 1971; 284:236.
2. Masters SJ: Evaluation of head trauma: Efficacy of skull films. *AJR* 1980; 135:539.
3. Cummins RO: Clinicians' reasons for overuse of skull radiographs. *AJR* 1980; 135:549.
4. Phillips LA: A study of the effect of high yield criteria for emergency room skull radiography (FDA 78-8069). Washington, DC, Bureau of Radiological Health, US Public Health Service, Dept of Health, Education, and Welfare, 1978.
5. Masters SJ, McClean PM, Arcause JS, et al: Skull x-ray examinations after head trauma; recommendations by a multidisciplinary panel and validation study. *N Engl J Med* 1987; 316:84.
6. Thornburg JR, Masters SJ, Campbell JA: Imaging recommendations for head trauma: A new comprehensive strategy. *AJR* 1987; 149:781.
7. Claims analysis. *Malpractice Digest* 1980; 2:1.
8. Daves KR, Taveras JM, Roberson GH, et al: Computed tomography in head trauma. *Semin Roentgenol* 1977; 12:53.
9. Claussen CD, Lohcamp FW, Krastel A: Computed tomography of trauma involving the brain and facial skull. *J Comput Assist Tomogr* 1977; 1:472.
10. Allen JH: Computed tomographic scan findings in closed head trauma. *Comput Tomogr* 1977; 1:115.
11. Han JS, Kaufman B, Alfidi RJ, et al: Head trauma evaluated by magnetic resonance and computed tomography: A comparison. *Radiology* 1984; 150:71.
12. Quinn SF, Smathers RL: The diagnostic significance of post traumatic sphenoid sinus effusions: Correlation with head computed tomography. *CT: JCT* 1984; 8:61.

Suggested Reading

Williams AL, Haughton UM: *Cranial Computed Tomography. A Comprehensive Text.* St Louis, CV Mosby Co, 1985.

Rogers LF: *Radiology of Skeletal Trauma*, Vols 1 and 2. New York, Churchill Livingston, Inc, 1982.

Harris JH, Harris WH: *The Radiology of Emergency Medicine*, ed 2. Baltimore, Williams & Wilkins Co, 1981.

Siebert CE, Swanson WR, Debrase J: *Computed Tomography and Head Trauma.* Denver, Swedish Medical Center, 1976.

Normal Variants

Theodore E. Keats, M.D.

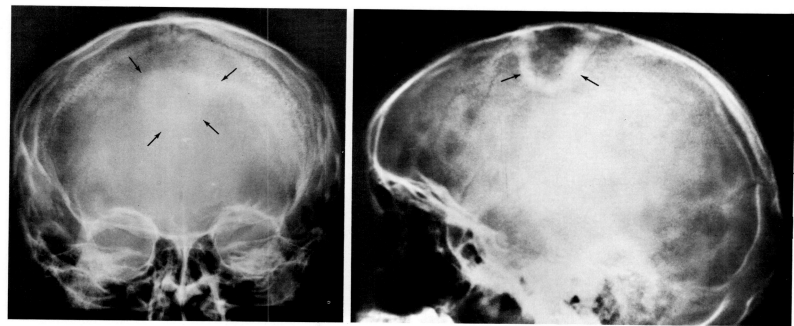

FIG 1–30 (top left).
Hair arrangements, in this case a pony tail, may produce unusual shadows.
FIG 1–31 (top right).
Hair braids producing an unusual shadow at vertex of skull.

FIG 1–32 (bottom left).
Hair braids with surrounding elastic bands simulating sclerotic lesions.
FIG 1–33 (bottom right).
Multiple small hair braids ("corn rows") producing unusual shadows in the frontal and parietal areas.

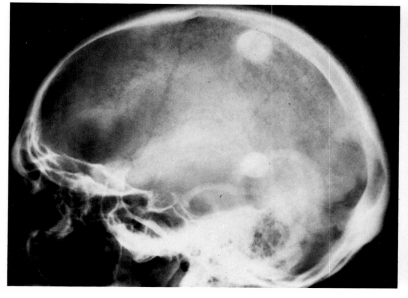
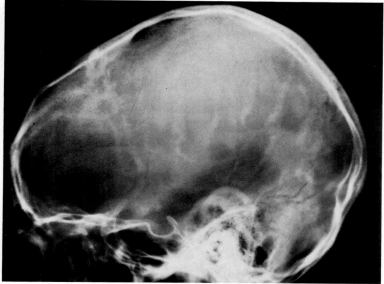

FIG 1–34.
Prominent digital markings. The prominence of calvarial digital markings varies widely, particularly between the 4th and 10th years. They do not, in themselves, necessarily reflect increased intracranial pressure. (Ref.: Macaulay D: Digital markings in the radiographs of children. *Brit J Radiol* 1951; 24:637.)

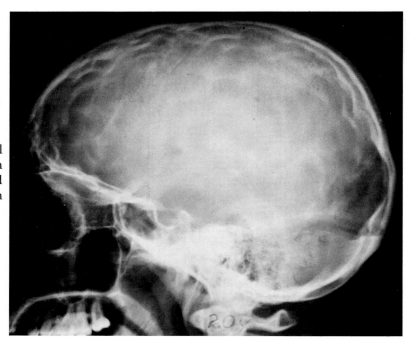

FIG 1–35 (bottom left).
Prominent diploic vascular pattern in a child.
FIG 1–36 (bottom right).
Vascular groove (sphenoparietal sinus) simulating fracture.

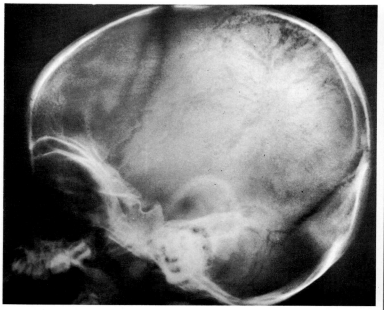

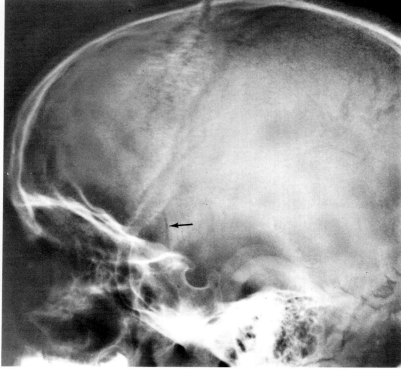

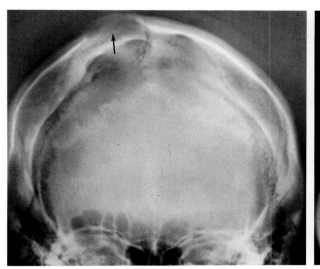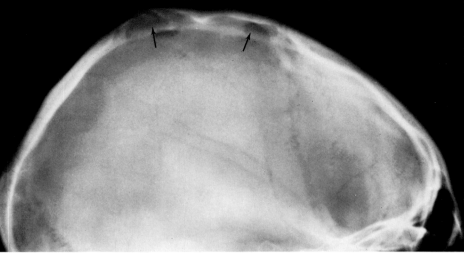

FIG 1–37.

Deep but typical pacchionian depressions. The external table of the calvarium is bowed, and the internal table is apparently absent. Failure to appreciate these features may lead to an erroneous diagnosis of erosion of the inner table of the skull.

FIG 1–38.
Anterior fontanel bone.

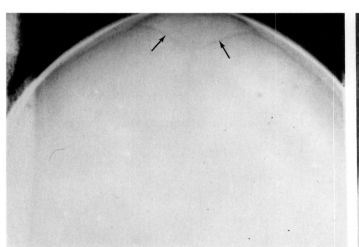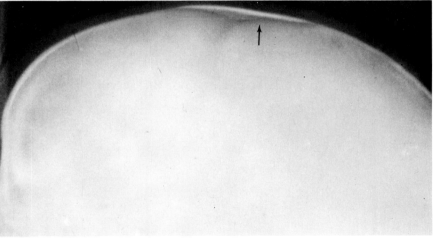

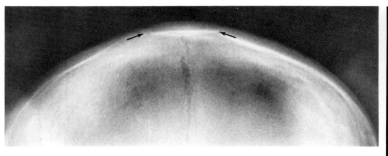
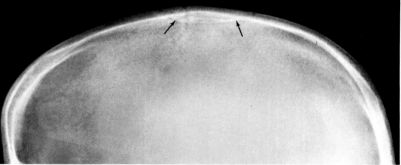

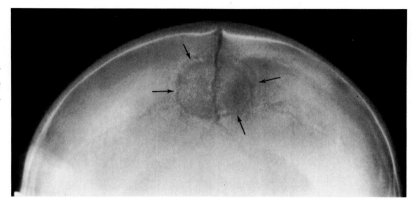

FIG 1–39.
Fusing anterior fontanel bone in a 3-year-old boy. This appearance may be confused with a depressed fracture in the lateral projection. (Ref: Girdany BR, Blank E: Anterior fontanel bones. *Am J Roentgenol* 1965; 95:148.)

FIG 1–40.
Wormian (sutural) bones in a 7-year-old child. These may be seen as a normal variant as well as in osteogenesis imperfecta and cleidocranial dysostosis.
FIG 1–41.
Normal frontal, temporal, and occipital lucencies seen in the aging calvarium.

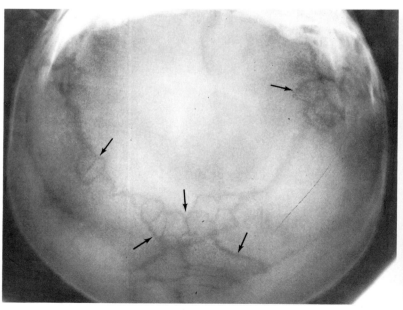
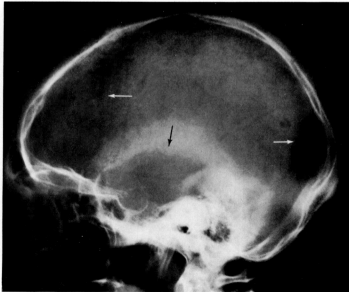

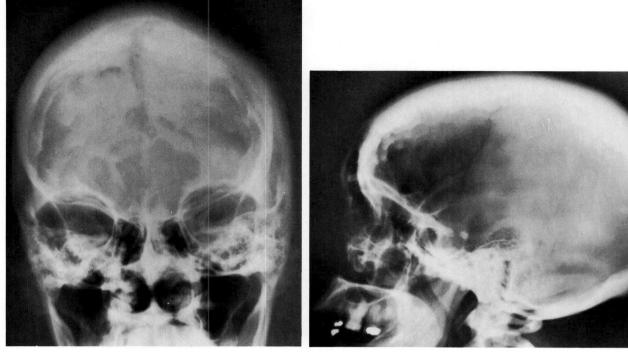

FIG 1–42.
Generalized and frontal benign cranial hyperostosis in a 38-year-old woman.

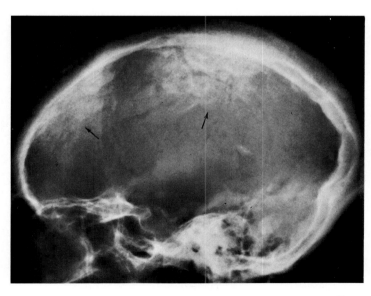

FIG 1–43.
Benign cranial hyperostosis in a 65-year-old woman. Diffuse thickening of the calvarium is present, as well as localized internal hyperostosis of the frontal and parietal bones.

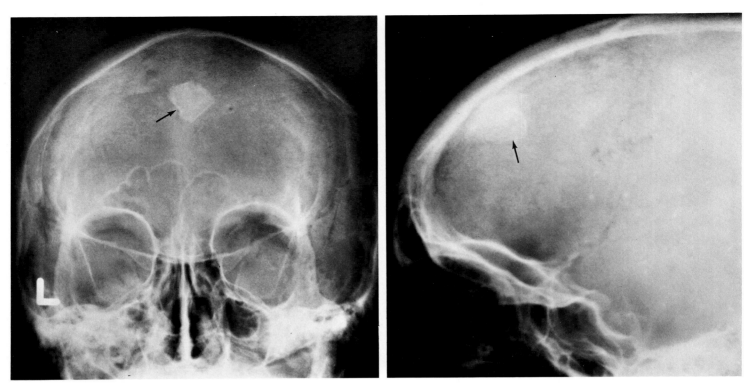

FIG 1–44.
Localized focal dural calcification in the frontal area.

FIG 1–45.
Heavy calcification of the falx cerebri.

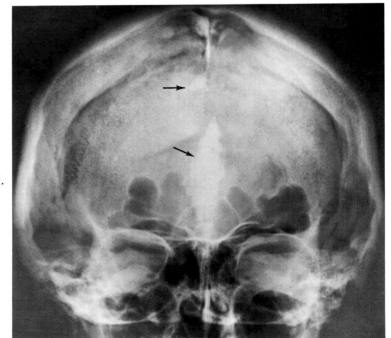

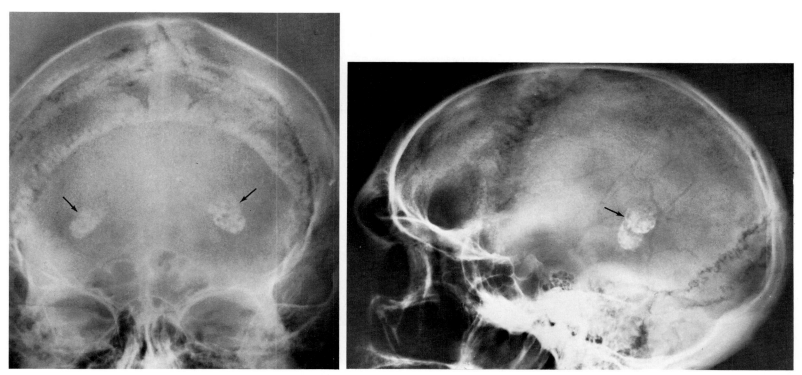

FIG 1–46.
Calcification in the glomus of the choroid plexus of each lateral ventricle.

FIG 1–47.
Normal asymmetry of the calcified glomera of the choroid plexus. These cannot be reliably used for evidence of intracranial abnormality.

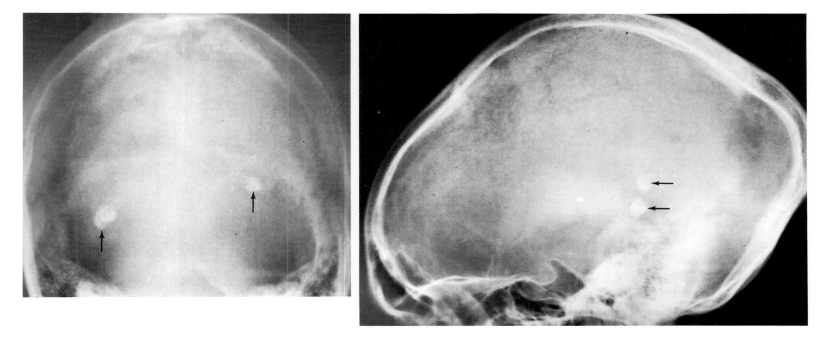

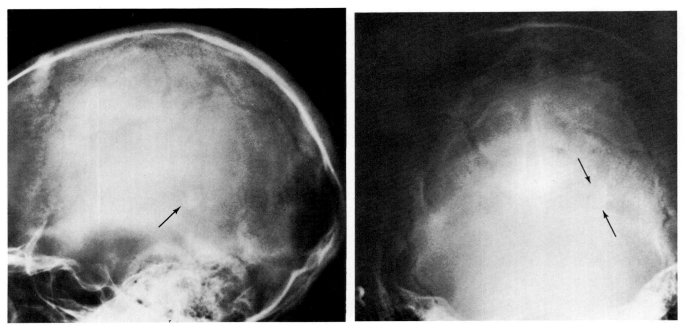

FIG 1–48.
Unilateral calcification of the glomus of the choroid plexus.

FIG 1–49 (bottom left).
Persistent metopic suture in a young adult. This suture may persist throughout life and be mistaken for a fracture.

FIG 1–50 (bottom right).
Prominent nasofrontal suture, not to be mistaken for fracture. This suture may persist into adult life.

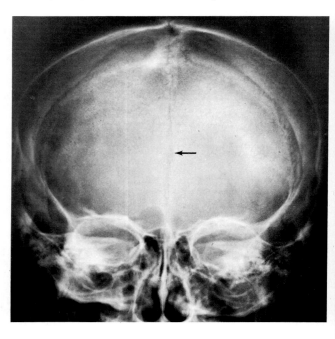

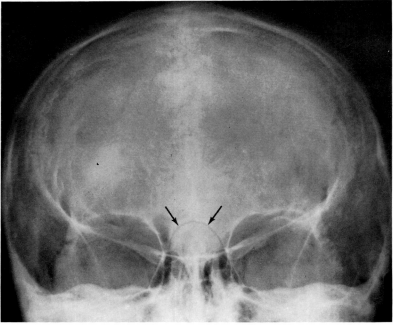

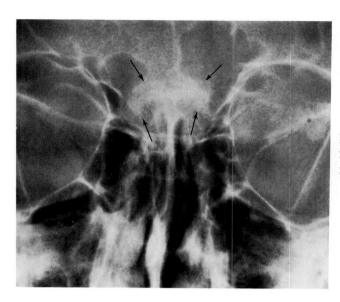

FIG 1–51.
Sclerosis of the nasofrontal suture, which might be mistaken for a meningioma of the anterior fossa.

FIG 1–52.
Vascular channel simulating skull fracture. (Ref: Schunk H, Maruyama Y: Two vascular grooves of the external table of the skull which simulate fractures. *Acta Radiol* [Stockh.] 1960; 54:186.)

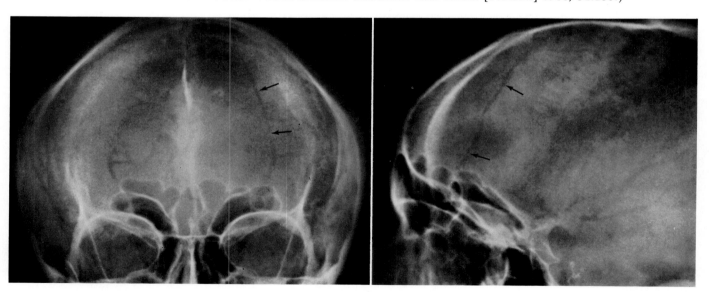

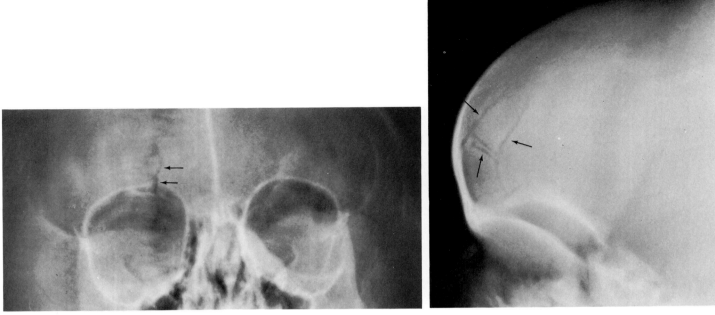

FIG 1–53.
Two additional examples of frontal bone vascular grooves which might be mistaken for fractures.

FIG 1–54.
Two neonates showing parietal fissures due to persistent strips of membranous bone matrix. These fissures disappear as the child matures and are often mistaken for fractures.

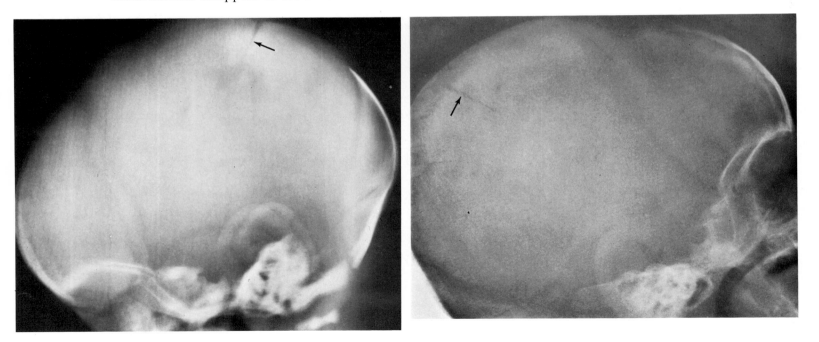

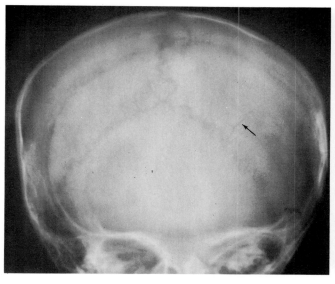
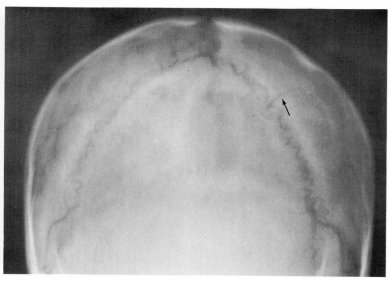
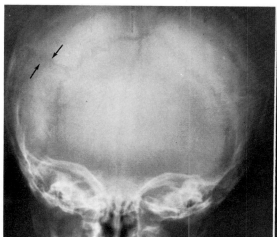
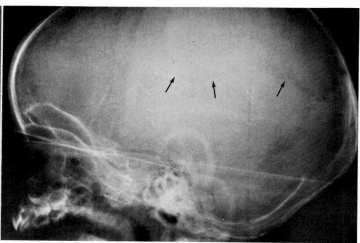
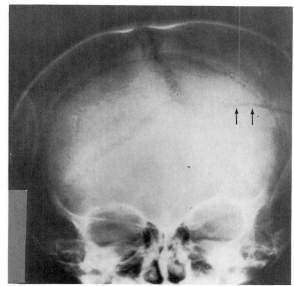

FIG 1–55 (top left and right).
Persistence of parietal fissure in a 1-year-old child simulating a fracture.

FIG 1–56 (middle left and right).
Unilateral intraparietal suture which divides the parietal bone into an upper and lower segment. This suture may also occur bilaterally and extends from the coronal to the lambdoid. (Ref: Shapiro R: Anomalous parietal sutures and the bipartite parietal bone. *Am J Roentgenol* 1972; 115:569)

FIG 1–57 (bottom left).
Unilateral intraparietal suture. When it is unilateral, the skull may be asymmetric with the side harboring the intraparietal suture being larger than that of the opposite side, as in this case.

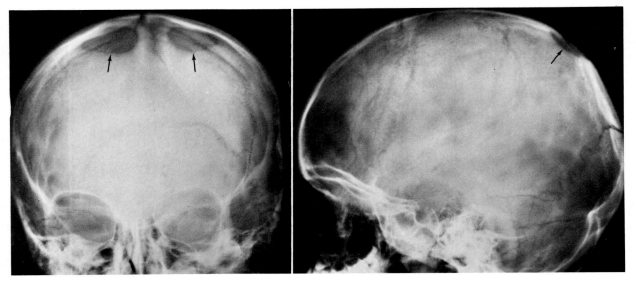

FIG 1–58.
Parietal foramina. These congenital defects vary in size, but they are consistent in location and often symmetric in size. They are not significant except in the differential diagnosis of cranial defects, including burr holes.

FIG 1–59.
Parietal foramina without central dividing strip in a 15-month-old child.

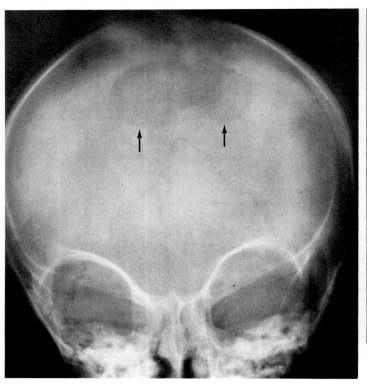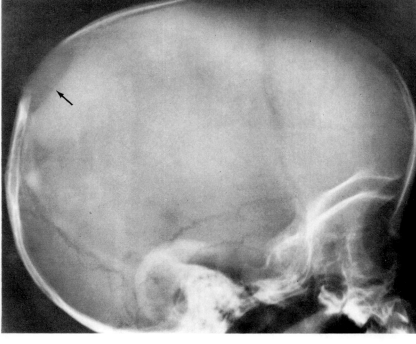

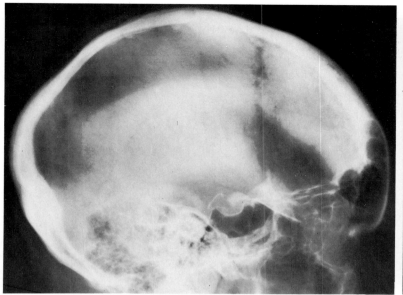

FIG 1–60.
Parietal thinning, a manifestation of postmenopausal osteoporosis. The outer table is lost with characteristic preservation of the inner table. Note also similar localized thinning of the frontal bone in the lateral projection. (Ref: Steinbach HL, Obata WG: The significance of thinning of the parietal bones. *Am J Roentgenol* 1957; 78:39.)

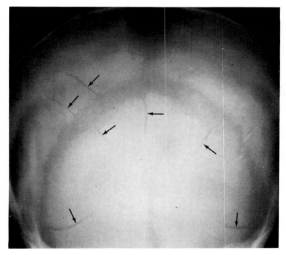

FIG 1–61.
Occipital and parietal fissures due to persistent strips of membranous bone, a common finding in infants which may simulate fracture. The mendosal sutures are evident *(arrows).*

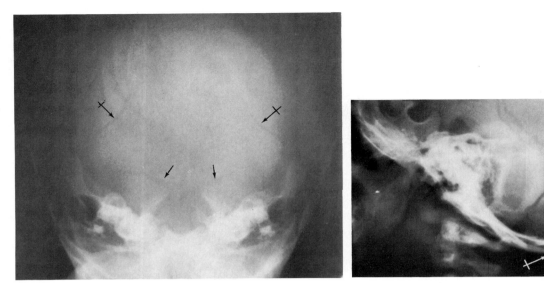

FIG 1–62.
The synchondroses between the supraoccipital and exoccipital portions of the occipital bone in a 6-week-old child (*arrows*). The mendosal sutures are also seen *(notched arrows)*.
FIG 1–63.
The mendosal suture *(arrow)* and synchondrosis between the supraoccipital and exoccipital portions of the occipital bone *(notched arrow)* in lateral projection in a 1-month-old child.

FIG 1–64.
Normal, large interparietal bone in a 3-month-old child in frontal and lateral projections.

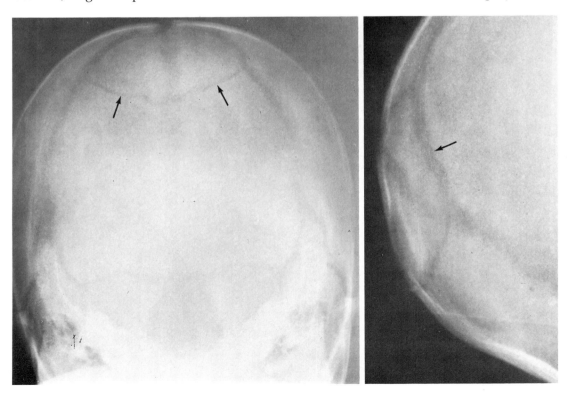

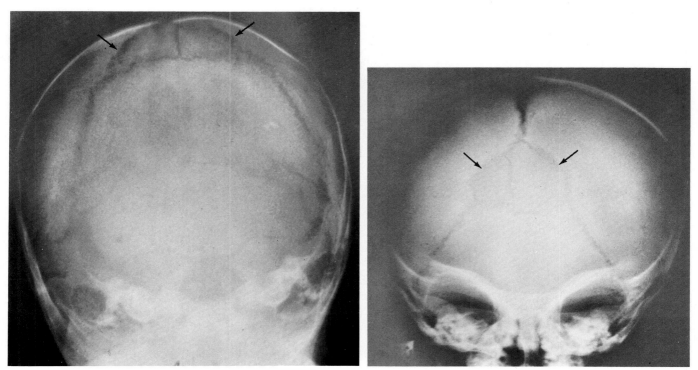

FIG 1–65.
Two examples of bifid interparietal bones (Inca bone). This should not be mistaken for a fracture. (Ref: Shapiro R, Robinson F: The os incae. *Am J Roentgenol* 1976; 127:469.)

FIG 1–66.
Two examples of how Inca bones may simulate fractures in the lateral projection.

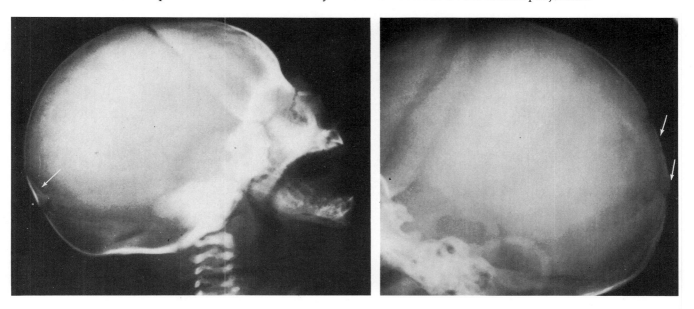

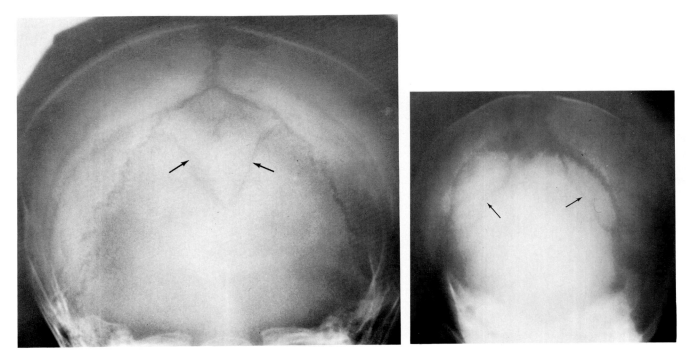

FIG 1–67.
Cone-shaped interparietal bone.

FIG 1–68.
Asymmetric closure of the synchondrosis between the supra- and exoccipital portions of the occipital bone in a 15-month-old infant. The open suture may be mistaken for fracture.

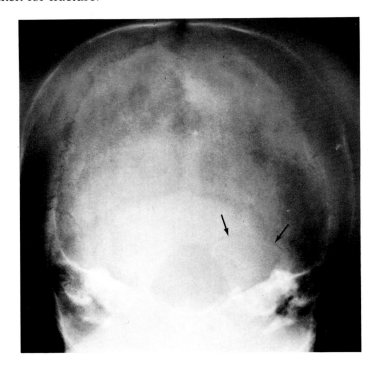

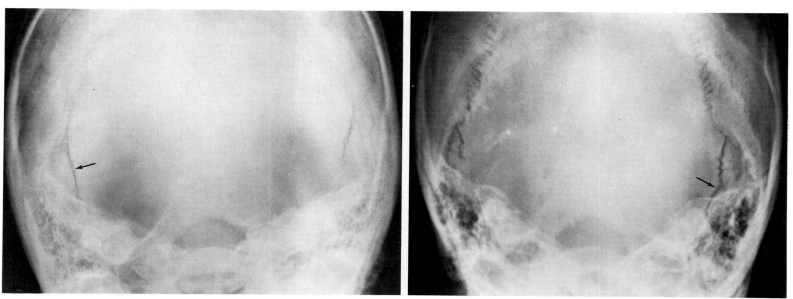

FIG 1–69.
Two examples of asymmetric prominence of one occipitomastoid suture, suggesting fracture.

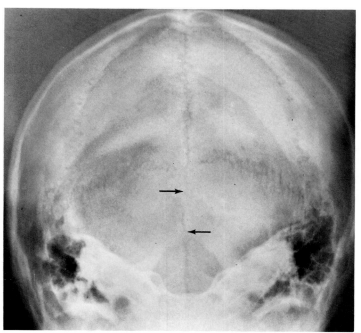

FIG 1–70.
The metopic suture may be seen in Towne's projection and confused with a fracture. Note its continuation across the outline of the foramen magnum.

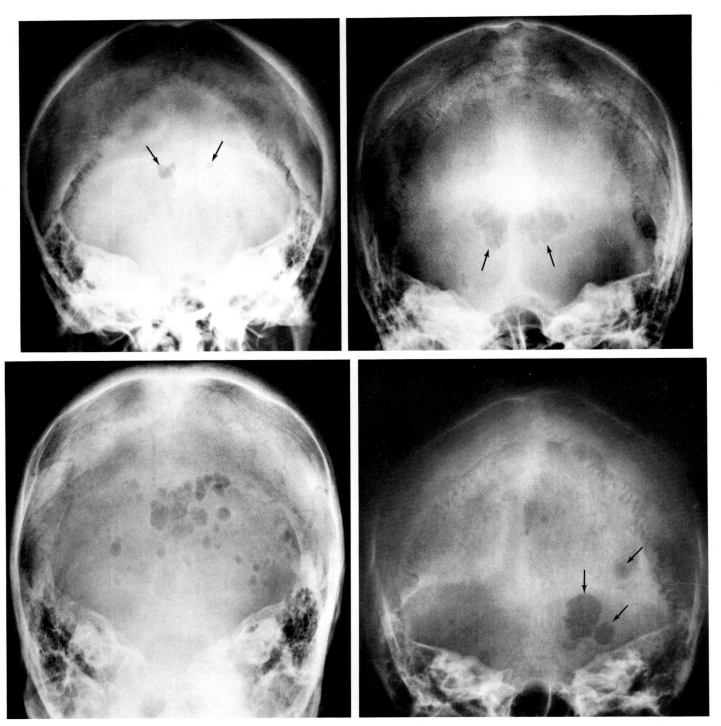

FIG 1–71.

Occipital venous lakes. These structures vary widely in number and appearance. They are usually seen near the midline of the occipital bone, most commonly in older individuals. These lakes lie in the diploic space and are of no clinical significance. (From Keats TE: Four normal anatomic variations of importance to radiologists. *Am J Roentgenol* 1957; 78:89. Reproduced by permission.) There is evidence that identical occipital radiolucencies may be the product of ectopic neural tissue. These are similarly without clinical significance. (Ref: Goldring S, et al.: Ectopic neural tissue of the occipital bone. *J Neurosurg* 1964; 21:479.)

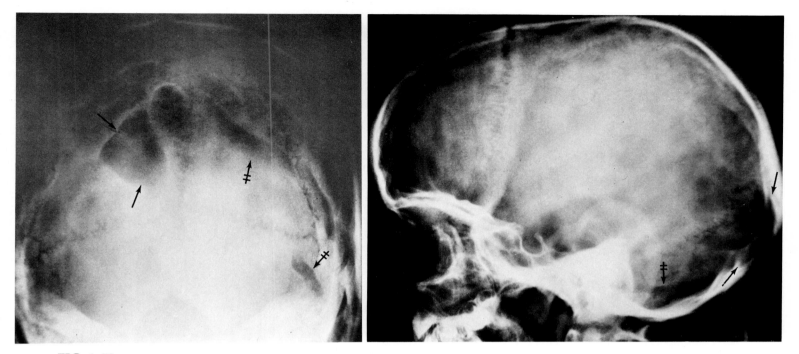

FIG 1–72.

The occipital bone may have a variety of symmetric or asymmetric areas of thinning near the midline which may simulate erosion of the inner table. Some of them relate to the configuration of the transverse venous sinuses. It is important that the innocence of these variants be recognized. The *notched arrows* indicate the venous sinuses.

FIG 1–73.

Additional examples of occipital thinning. Note similarity to changes of erosion of inner table.

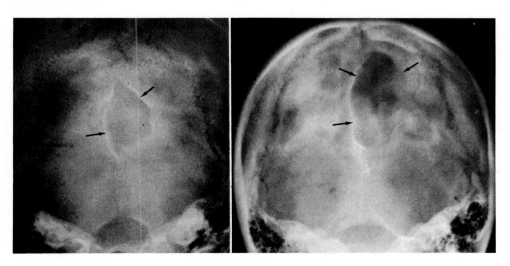

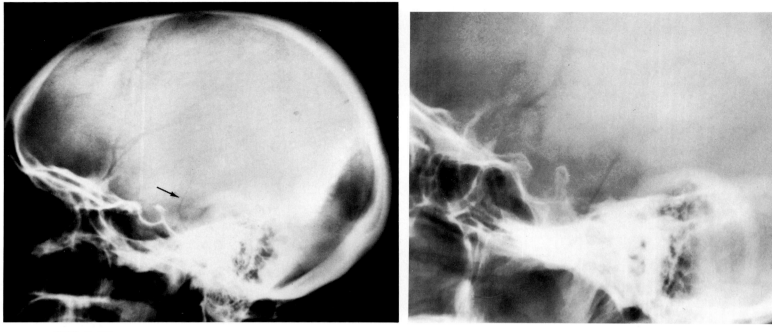

FIG 1–74.
Two examples of grooves for the middle temporal artery simulating fracture. (Ref: Schunk H, Maruyama Y: Two vascular grooves of the external table of the skull which simulate fractures. *Acta Radiol* [Stockh.] 1960; 54:186.)

FIG 1–75 (bottom left).
The coronal suture, seen in the base view, simulating a fracture.
FIG 1–76 (bottom right).
The sagittal suture, seen in the base view, simulating a fracture.

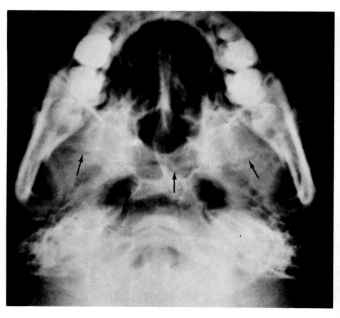
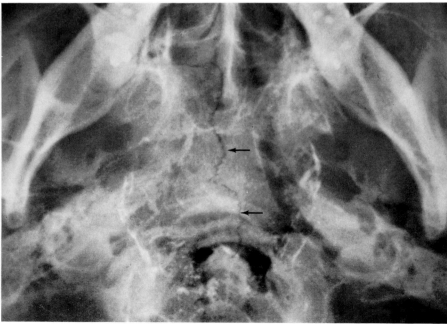

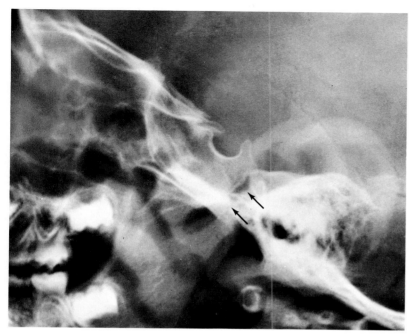

FIG 1–77.
The synchondrosis between the basisphenoid and basiocciput in a 2-year-old boy. This suture normally closes near puberty but may persist until the 20th year. It is at times mistaken for fracture.

FIG 1–78 (bottom left).
Shadow of the folded ear simulating suprasellar calcification.

FIG 1–79 (bottom right).
The intersphenoidal synchondrosis in a newborn. This entity should not be mistaken for a fracture, a persistent basipharyngeal canal, or the spheno-occipital synchondrosis. It has no pathologic significance and usually disappears by 3 years of age. (Ref: Shopfner CE, et al: The intersphenoid synchondrosis. *Am J Roentgenol* 1968; 104:184.)

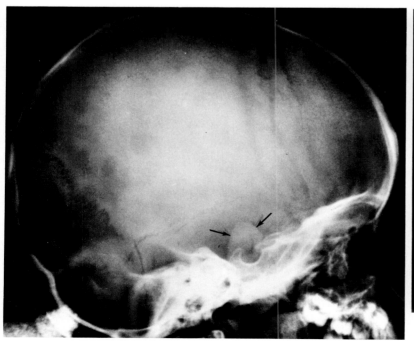

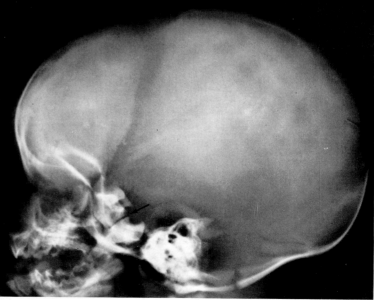

2
Face

Wayne S. Cail, M.D.

A major proportion of patients seen today with facial injuries have been involved in motor vehicle accidents. These patients are likely to have sustained serious associated injuries, commonly involving the cervical spine, skull, and intracranial structures. In the initial management of these patients, attention must first be directed to preservation and maintenance of an adequate airway, to control of bleeding and correction of shock, and to evaluation and treatment of associated injuries.

Evaluation of facial injuries then begins with systematic physical examination. Many facial fractures can be accurately diagnosed by observation and palpation alone. In these cases radiographs serve only to confirm and document the diagnosis. In other cases, however, radiographs are essential to accurately define the facial fractures. In any event, the patient's condition should not be jeopardized by the movements necessitated with most facial x-ray views. The x-ray examination therefore is obtained in the latter part of the emergency care and may even be deferred for several days.

Classification of Fractures

It is useful to group facial fractures according to their location in the lower, middle, and upper thirds of the face:

Lower third (mandible)
    Alveolar process
    Symphysis
    Body
    Angle
    Ramus
    Coronoid process
    Condyle
Middle third
    Nasal region
    Zygomatic arch
    Zygomaticomaxillary complex

    Orbital floor and medial wall (blow-out fracture)
    Maxilla (Le Fort fractures)
Upper third
    Superior orbital rim
    Frontal sinus
    Frontal bone

Fractures of the Lower Third of the Face

Mandibular Fractures

The mandible has a prominent and exposed position within the facial skeleton and is therefore very susceptible to direct trauma. Since the mandibular condyles articulate with the skull at the glenoid fossae, a blow to the chin will be transmitted to the skull base unless the force is absorbed by fracturing the mandible.

Disruption of the normal bony configuration may result in displacement of the mandible. The tongue and soft tissues of the floor of the mouth will also be displaced, compromising the airway. Soon after the injury, swelling of the tongue and soft tissues can threaten the airway even further.

Radiographic evaluation of the mandible begins with the lateral oblique views (Fig 2–1). The technique is designed to direct the x-rays through the floor of the mouth at such an angle that the side of the mandible nearest the x-ray tube is not superimposed on the side in contact with the film cassette. The view obtained extends from the neck of the condyle and the coronoid process to the second premolar tooth.

The lateral oblique view is most easily obtained with the patient upright. Filming can also be performed with the patient prone and the head turned into a true lateral position parallel to the cassette. Both techniques have the advantage of allowing the mandible to fall forward, protecting the airway. Alternatively, the patient can be placed supine with the head turned into the lateral position. Attempts to obtain a lateral oblique projection by angling the x-ray tube without rotation of the patient's head will meet obstruction by the patient's chest and shoulders.

The anteroposterior view images the mandible from a frontal direction (Fig 2–2). The patient lies prone with the neck flexed until the orbitomeatal line, joining the external canthus of the eye to the external auditory meatus, is perpendicular to the x-ray table. The x-ray beam is aimed vertically toward the skull base through the central incisor teeth. The anteroposterior view demonstrates the lower portion of the ramus, the angle, and the body on both sides of the mandible. However, the symphysis is difficult to evaluate on this view because of superimposition of the cervical vertebrae.

The symphysis is more clearly seen on a 15-degree mento-occipital view (Fig 2–3). While the patient remains prone, the neck is extended until the chin and nose are resting on the x-ray table. The x-ray beam is angled 15 degrees toward the feet and directed through the chin. This view also clearly demonstrates the coronoid processes of the mandible.

The best definition of the symphysis is provided by the occlusal view (Fig 2–4). This usually is obtained with the film held between the upper and lower incisor teeth and the neck fully extended. The x-rays are then directed at right angles to the film from below the mandible.

The standard anteroposterior view also obscures the condyle, coronoid process, and upper portion of the ramus on each side by superimposing the dense shadows of the petrous bone, mastoid process, and zygoma. This area is better visualized on the Towne view (Fig 2–5). The patient lies supine, with the orbitomeatal line perpendicular to the plane of the cassette while the x-ray beam is aimed 30 degrees toward the feet and through the condyles.

A panoramic view of the mandible can be obtained using a specialized x-ray unit (Fig 2–6). The patient must be able to sit upright while the x-ray table and film cassette rotate around the patient's head.

Except for the Towne and the occlusal views, which image only limited portions of the mandible, the views discussed thus far require considerable movement of the patient. If the patient must remain supine, a posteroanterior view must be accepted. Since the x-rays pass from the front of the skull posteriorly, the target-film distance is increased, reducing the definition of mandibular detail relative to that obtained on the posteroanterior view. A lateral view of the mandible may also be obtained with the patient supine without rotating the head (Fig 2–7). However, this "cross-table" lateral view superimposes the two sides of the mandible and especially obscures the coronoid processes.

Mandibular fractures are described by the location in which they occur (Fig 2–8). The alveolus is relatively weak and may be fractured independently of the main portion of the mandible. On the other hand, a direct force applied to one side of the mandible tends to also produce an indirect fracture on the opposite side. Bilateral fractures may occur in any combination, but the most frequent forms are bilateral fractures of the condyles, bilateral angle fractures, bilateral body fractures, and fractures of the body and the contralateral angle.

As the curve of the mandible is progressively distorted by trauma, the outer and inner compact layers tend to fracture independently. The fractures in the buccal and lingual surface of the mandible may be remote from each other and may be mistaken for a double fracture on radiographs, especially on the lateral oblique view.

Alveolar fractures occur most frequently in the incisor region, since this area is more directly exposed to direct trauma. They are frequently associated with avulsed and displaced teeth (Figs 2–9 and 2–10).

Fracture of the symphysis rarely occurs alone (Fig 2–11,A). When the fracture passes from the labial to the lingual surface in a sagittal plane, the fracture is relatively stable (Fig 2–11,B, C). More commonly, the fracture line has an oblique course, and the attached muscles will cause distraction and overlap of the fragments. When a symphysis fracture is associated with bilateral condyle, ramus, or angle fractures, the anterior portions of the mandible are pulled backward by the attached musculature (Fig 2–12). The associated internal rotation causes the angle of the mandible to protrude outward, giving a flared appearance on the anteroposterior view. The flared configuration indicates an unstable complex of multiple mandibular fractures, which can lead to complete airway obstruction.

A fracture in the body tends to occur in the region of the canine tooth, since this is the site of maximum convexity of the bony arch (Fig 2–13). When both mandibular bodies are fractured, the central fragment may be displaced inferiorly and posteriorly by the impacting force or by contraction of the attached muscles (Fig 2–14). Absence of the chin contour can be seen both clinically and radiographically. As the midsection of the mandible is displaced posteriorly, the tongue and soft tissues of the floor of the mouth prolapse into the pharynx and may obstruct the airway.

Attached to the ascending ramus of the mandible are three powerful muscles—the temporalis, medial pterygoid, and masseter—which tend to pull upward

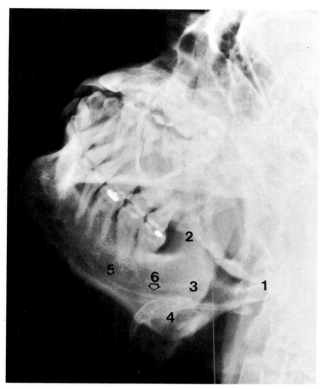

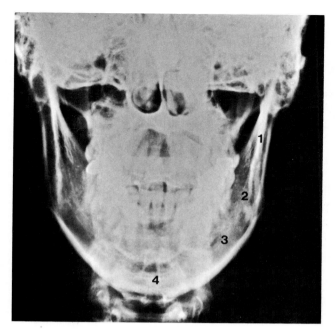

FIG 2–1.
Lateral oblique view of the mandible. *1,* condyle; *2,* coronoid process; *3,* ramus; *4,* angle; *5,* body; *6,* mandibular canal.

FIG 2–2.
Posteroanterior view of the mandible. *1,* ramus; *2,* angle; *3,* body; *4,* symphysis.

FIG 2–3.
Fifteen-degree mento-occipital view. *1,* symphysis; *2,* coronoid process.

FIG 2–4.
Occlusal view of symphysis.

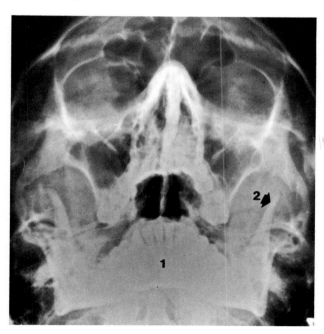

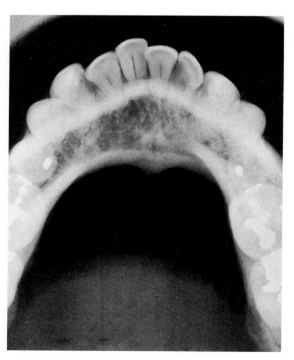

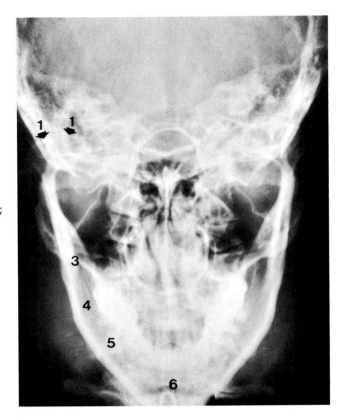

FIG 2–5.
Towne view. *1*, condyle; *2*, coronoid process; *3*, ramus; *4*, angle; *5*, body; *6*, symphysis.

FIG 2–6.
Panoramic view of the mandible. *1*, condyle; *2*, coronoid process; *3*, ramus; *4*, angle; *5*, body; *6*, symphysis; *7*, antegonial notch; *8*, mandibular canal; *9*, mental foramen.

FIG 2–7.
Lateral view of the mandible. *1*, condyle; *2*, coronoid process; *3*, ramus; *4*, angle; *5*, body.

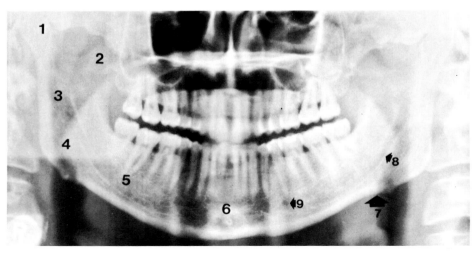

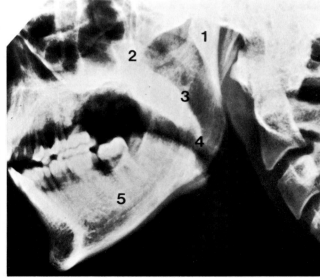

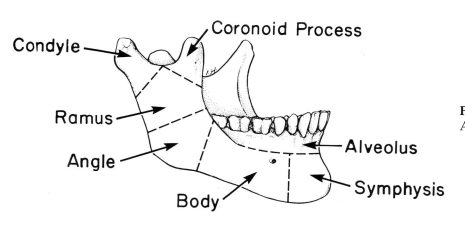

FIG 2–8.
Anatomical regions of the mandible.

Coronoid Process

Condyle

Ramus

Angle

Body

Alveolus

Symphysis

FIG 2–9.
Anteroposterior view of the mandible, showing avulsion of incisors.

FIG 2–10.
Panoramic view of the mandible, showing alveolar fracture *(1)* extending into the symphysis *(2)* with avulsion of teeth *(3)*.

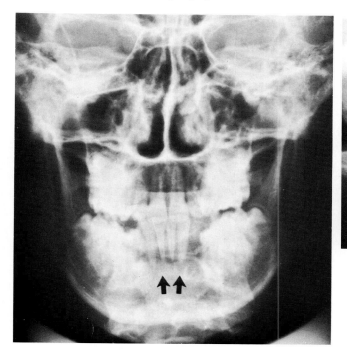

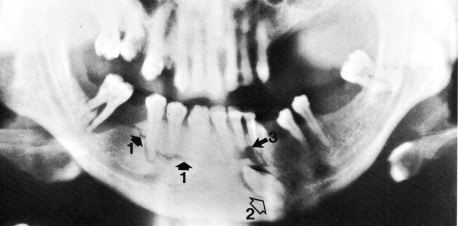

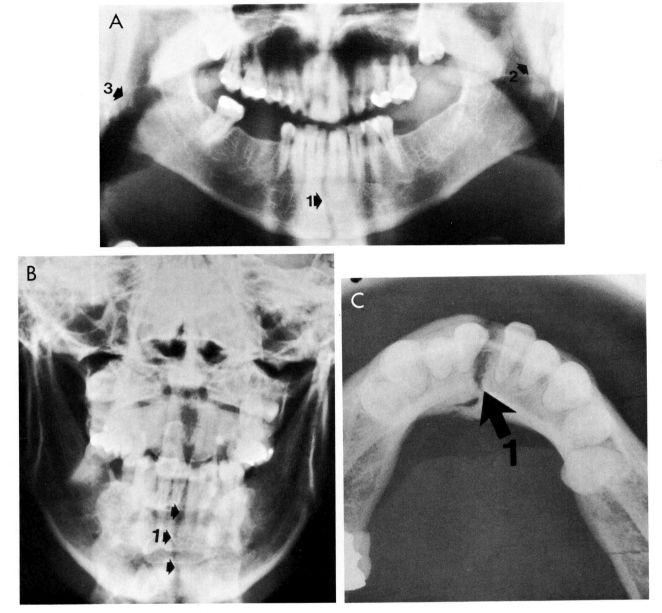

FIG 2–11.
A, panoramic view, showing symphysis fracture *(1)* and bilateral ramus fractures *(2 and 3)*. **B,** posteroanterior view of symphysis fracture *(1)*. **C,** occlusal view of symphysis fracture *(1)*.

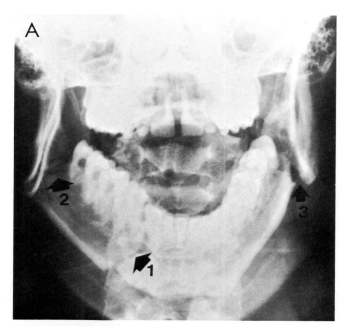

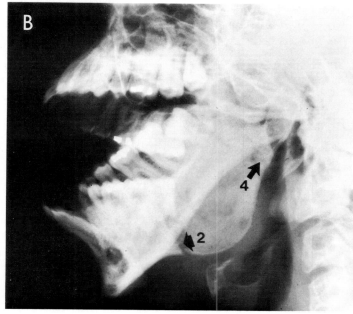

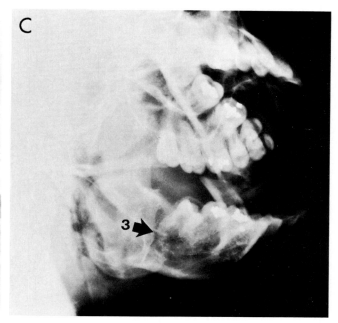

FIG 2–12.
A, anteroposterior view, showing oblique fracture of the body *(1)* and displaced fractures of both angles *(2* and *3).* The mandible has a "flared" appearance. **B,** lateral oblique view of the right side shows the angle fracture *(2)* and a subcondylar fracture *(4).* **C,** lateral oblique view of the left side shows the angle fracture *(3)* with overlap of the fragments.

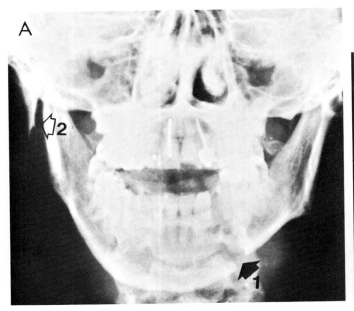

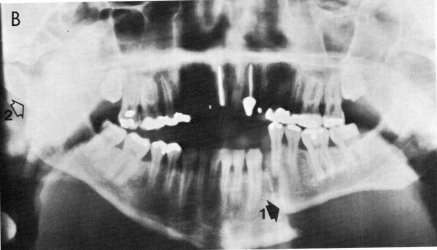

FIG 2–13.
A, posteroanterior view, showing fractures of the body *(1)* and right condylar neck. The condyle fragment is displaced lateral to the ramus. **B,** panoramic view shows extension of the body fracture *(1)* into the root of the first cuspid. Anterior angulation of the condylar neck is also shown *(2)*.

FIG 2–14.
Lateral oblique view of edentulous mandible with bilateral body fractures. The central fragment is displaced downward and backward.

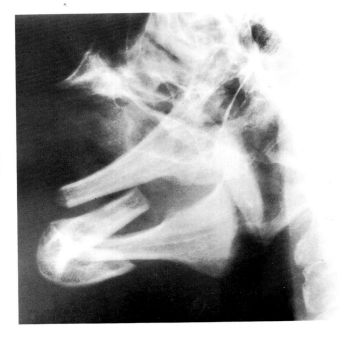

and medially. When a fracture of the angle passes downward and backward from the alveolar margin, the posterior fragment is pulled upward and the fracture is said to be horizontally unfavorable (Fig 2–15). This upward movement may be limited by the retention of a third molar in the posterior fragment that comes into occlusion with a corresponding tooth in the maxilla. The posterior fragment may also be displaced medially due to the pull of these muscles.

Ramus fractures will be easily detected on lateral oblique views (Fig 2–16). Displacement of the fragments is usually minimal, due to the splinting action of the internal pterygoid and masseter muscles. The fracture line may therefore be poorly seen on the anteroposterior view.

Fracture of the coronoid process is an unusual injury. Displacement of the fragment is usually limited by the temporalis muscle. When the muscle insertion on the ramus is also ruptured, the coronoid process will be displaced superiorly. This fracture is best seen on the lateral oblique view (Fig 2–17).

Fracture of the mandibular condyle most commonly occurs below the attachment of the temporomandibular joint capsule. This extracapsular fracture, also called subcondylar fracture, passes backward from the mandibular notch (Fig 2–18). When the periosteum and ligaments remain intact, there will be no displacement of the condylar head from the glenoid fossa, and the condylar neck will maintain a normal relationship to the ramus. More frequently, there will be anterior and/or medial angulation of the condylar neck relative to the ramus (Fig 2–19). When the fragments overlap, the condylar fragment will usually lie lateral to the ramus (see Fig 2–13,A). A subcondylar fracture associated with disruption of the temporomandibular joint capsule and ligament will allow dislocation of the condylar head from the glenoid fossa due to the medial and anterior pull of the lateral pterygoid muscle (Fig 2–20).

A fracture of the condyle may also occur above the attachment of the temporomandibular joint capsule (Fig 2–21,A). This intracapsular fracture usually does not involve the articular surface. Frequently, the condylar head is dislocated medially and anteriorly from the glenoid fossa (Fig 2–21,B).

Fractures of the Middle Third of the Face

Fractures of the Nasal Region

Trauma to the central portion of the midface may produce isolated fractures of the nasal bones (Fig 2–22,A and B). However, the majority of fractures also involve the frontal processes of the maxillae. The sep-

tal cartilage is frequently detached from its articulation with the vomer, and the bony nasal septum is fractured. In severe injuries, the fracture of the nasal septum extends into the cribiform plate, while the nasomaxillary fractures extend to include the lacrimal bones and the orbital plate of the ethmoid bone.

Fractures of the nasal region in adults are easily recognized. The deformity caused by displaced fractures is apparent on physical examination, especially if seen before significant swelling has developed. Radiographs serve mainly to confirm and document the clinical diagnosis. On the other hand, edema and ecchymosis may develop rapidly and obscure the true nature of the fracture on physical examination. Radiographs then become more important in diagnosis. Nevertheless, the degree of displacement of the fracture may not be accurately depicted by the radiographs, and the need for reduction remains a clinical decision.

Radiographic examination of the nasal region begins with a lateral view (Fig 2–23). With proper technique, the soft tissues and a portion of the upper lateral nasal cartilage will be shown, in addition to the bony profile.

The Waters view (Fig 2–24) is obtained by placing the patient prone, with the nose and chin in contact with the top of the table. The extension of the head is adjusted so that the orbitomeatal line forms an angle of approximately 37 degrees with the plane of the film. The x-ray beam is then directed perpendicular to the film, through the root of the nose. This projects the petrous ridges over the lower borders of the maxillae. The Waters view shows the bony arch of the nose and the nasal septum.

Displacement of the nasal bones may be well demonstrated with an axial view (Fig 2–25). This projection is most easily obtained with the patient supine and holding an occlusal film packet between the teeth. The x-ray beam is directed from above the head downward at the film. This view shows that portion of the nasal bones which extends beyond the glabella and the maxillary alveolus.

Lateral impact on the nasal region will detach the frontal process from the remainder of the maxilla on the affected side. The nasal bone and frontal process of the maxilla are then separated from the frontal bone close to their sutures (Fig 2–26).

The force may carry the frontal process of the maxilla on the side of the injury toward the midline while fracturing the opposite nasal bone and frontal process (Fig 2–27). Some rotation occurs, hinging on the area of separation from the frontal bone (Fig 2–28). An associated comminuted fracture of the nasal septum is often present.

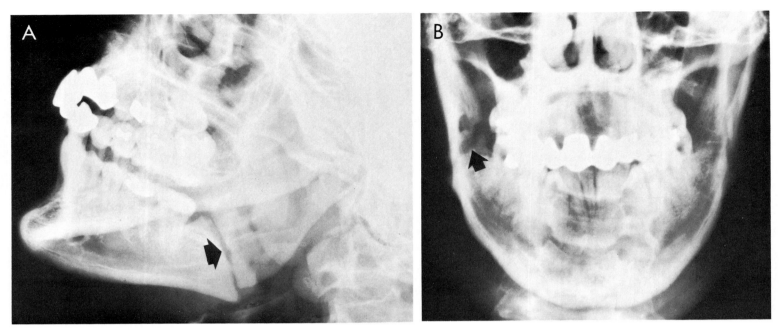

FIG 2–15.
A, lateral oblique view of horizontally unfavorable angle fracture. **B,** posteroanterior view of angle fracture.

FIG 2–16.
A, lateral oblique view of ramus fracture. **B,** posteroanterior view.

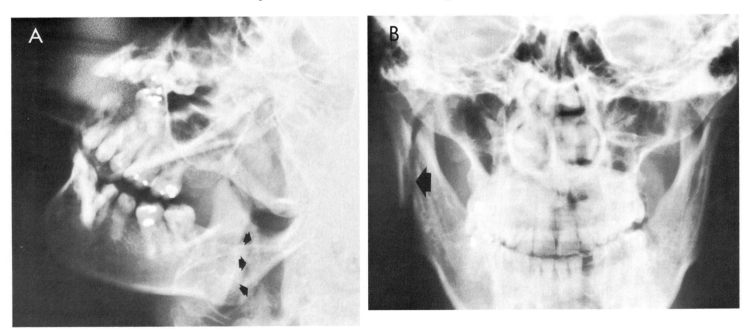

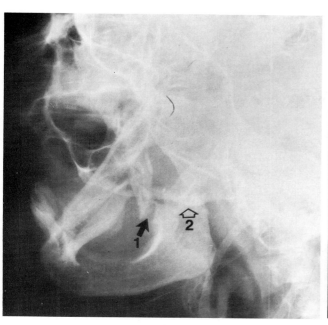

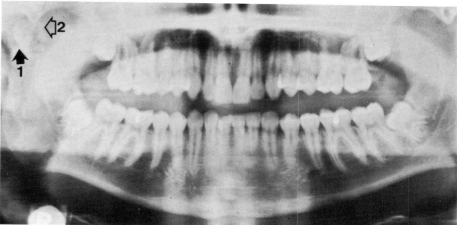

FIG 2–17 (top left).
Lateral oblique view, showing coronoid process *(1)* and subcondylar *(2)* fractures.

FIG 2–18 (top right).
Panoramic view, showing right-side subcondylar fracture *(1)*. The condyle *(2)* is rotated and displaced anteriorly out of the glenoid fossa.

FIG 2–19 (bottom left).
Towne view of subcondylar fracture *(1)* with medial angulation of the condyle fragment *(2)* relative to the ramus *(3)*.

FIG 2–20 (bottom right).
Lateral oblique view of subcondylar fracture *(1)*. The condyle *(2)* is dislocated anteriorly from the glenoid fossa *(3)*.

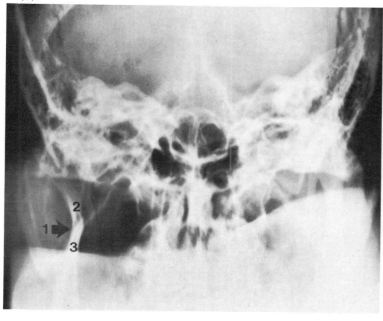

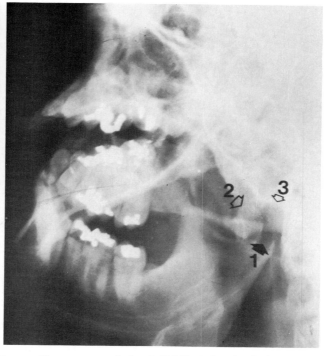

Face—Fractures of the Middle Third of the Face / **57**

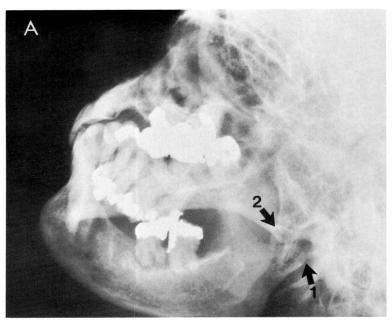
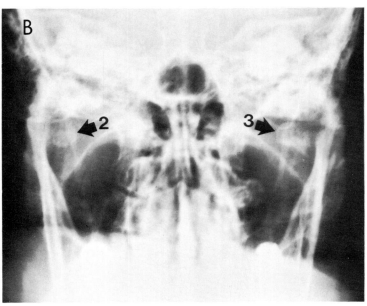

FIG 2–21.
A, lateral oblique view of condyle fracture *(1)*. The condyle *(2)* is displaced anteriorly. **B,** Towne view shows that the condyle is also displaced medially *(2)*. There was also a fracture of the left condyle with similar displacement *(3)*.

FIG 2–22.
A, external structures of the nose. **B,** nasal septum.

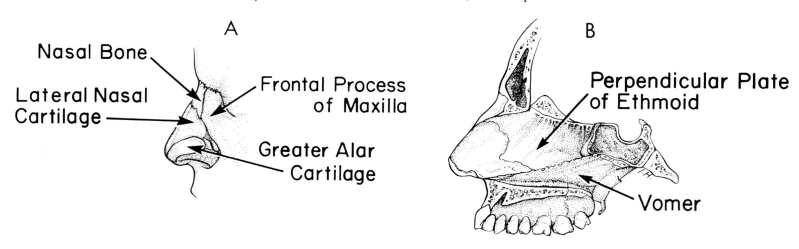

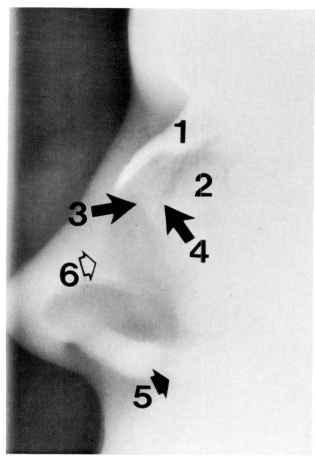

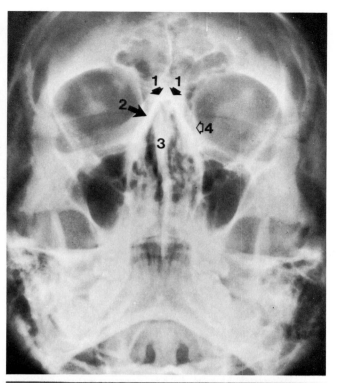

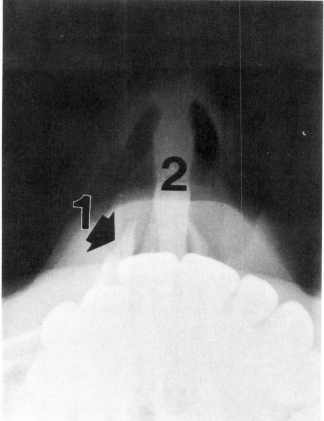

FIG 2–23 (top left).
Lateral view of the nose. *1*, nasal bone; *2*, frontal process of maxilla; *3*, edge of nasal bone; *4*, nasomaxillary suture; *5*, anterior nasal spine; *6*, upper nasal cartilage.

FIG 2–24 (top right).
Normal Waters view. *1*, nasal bones; *2*, frontal process of maxilla; *3*, nasal septum; *4*, anterior portion of the orbital plate of the ethmoid.

FIG 2–25 (bottom right).
Axial view of the nose. *1*, nasomaxillary suture; *2*, septal cartilage.

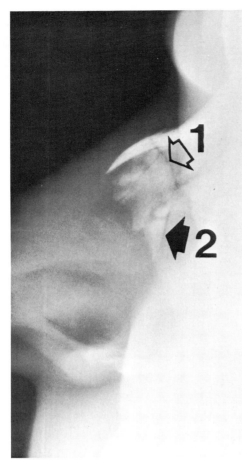

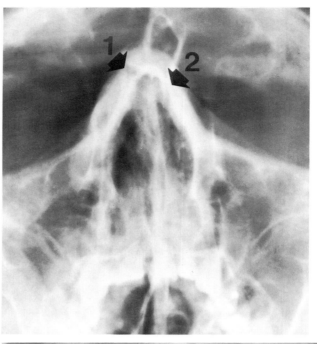

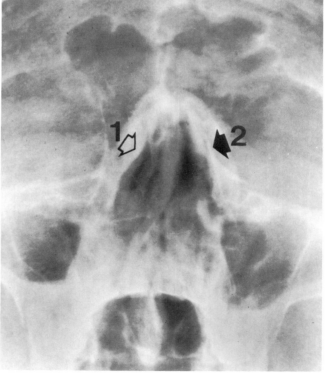

FIG 2–26 (top left).
Lateral view, showing fracture of the nasal bones *(1)* extending into the frontal process of the maxilla *(2)*.

FIG 2–27 (top right).
Waters view, showing lateral displacement of the right nasal bone and frontal process of maxilla *(1)* with medial displacement of the left nasal bone *(2)*.

FIG 2–28 (bottom right).
Waters view, showing displacement of the nasal bones from right to left with depression of the right frontal process of the maxilla *(1)* and lateral displacement of the left frontal process *(2)*.

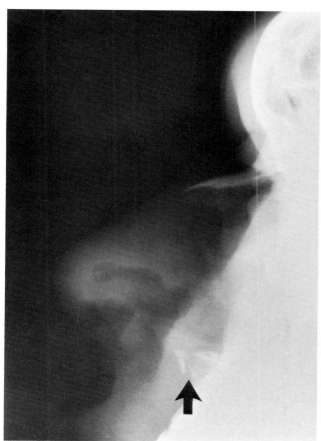

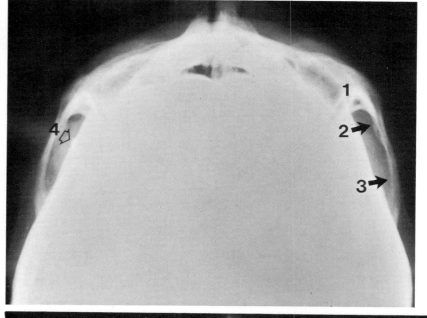

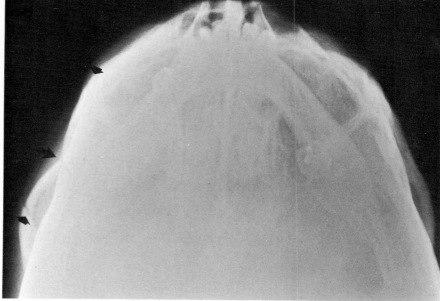

FIG 2–29 (bottom left).
Lateral view, showing isolated fracture of the anterior nasal spine of the maxilla.

FIG 2–30 (top right).
Modified base view. *1*, body of the zygoma; *2*, temporal process of the zygoma; *3*, zygomatic process of the temporal bone; *4*, coronoid process of the mandible lying medial to the zygomatic arch.

FIG 2–31 (bottom right).
Base view, showing fractures of the zygomatic arch with V-shaped depression of the fragments.

When the force comes from an anterior direction, the nasal bones are separated from their articulation with the frontal bone and driven backward into the nasal cavity. The frontal processes of the maxilla are fractured and splayed outward. Comminution of the bony external framework usually occurs. The bony septum may be comminuted as well.

In severe injuries, the lacrimal bones and the orbital surfaces of the ethmoid bone are involved. This permits lateral displacement of the medial canthal ligaments producing an illusion of increased separation between the eyes.

Fracture of the anterior nasal spine of the maxilla is commonly associated with a nasal fracture but may occur as an isolated lesion (Fig 2–29). The anterior nasal spine fracture may produce marked tenderness in the midline of the upper lips at its junction with the nose.

Fractures of the Zygomatic Arch

A direct blow to the side of the face may produce an isolated fracture of the zygomatic arch, formed by slender projections of the zygoma and temporal bones.

Fractures of the zygomatic arch may be seen on the Waters view. However, they are best seen on a modified base view (Fig 2–30). To obtain this projection, the patient lies supine and extends the neck as far as possible in order to bring the orbitomeatal line parallel to the film plane. This position is very uncomfortable and may not be possible for patients with associated injuries. The radiographic exposure is adjusted to outline the zygomatic arches and will therefore be inadequate to demonstrate structures in the skull base.

The fragments of the zygomatic arch are usually displaced inward (Fig 2–31). When the arch completely collapses, it commonly fractures in three places and assumes a V-shaped configuration. Since the coronoid process of the mandible, with its attached temporalis muscle tendon, lies medial to the zygomatic arch, impingement by the collapsed arch may restrict mandibular motion.

Fractures of the Zygomaticomaxillary Complex

Trauma to the malar region commonly produces a more extensive injury than an isolated fracture of the zygomatic arch. In addition to the slender temporal process, the zygoma has processes articulating with the sphenoid bone, the frontal bone, and the maxillary bone. The orbital process of the zygoma joins the greater wing of the sphenoid to form the lateral wall of the orbit. The frontal process forms the lateral orbital rim, while the maxillary process contributes to the inferior rim and floor of the orbit. Thickness and strength are apparent at the zygomaticomaxillary suture. However, medial to this interface, the anterolateral wall of the antrum consists of relatively weak bone.

A blow to the malar region is unlikely to fracture the maxillary process of the zygoma (Fig 2–32). Instead, the fracture occurs medial to the zygomaticomaxillary suture, coursing upward from the buttress of the maxilla, across the anterolateral wall of the antrum near the infraorbital foramen, over the inferior orbital rim, and backward across the orbital floor to the inferior orbital fissure. This fracture line completes a circle by coursing downward across the posterolateral wall of the antrum to the buttress. A fracture also occurs through the zygomaticofrontal suture and extends downward between the orbital process and the greater wing of the sphenoid to the inferior orbital fissure. Finally, the zygomatic arch fractures about 1 cm posterior to the zygomaticotemporal suture.

Radiographic evaluation of the patient who has sustained trauma to the malar region begins with the Waters view (Fig 2–33). Fractures of the zygomaticomaxillary complex produce a discontinuity at the buttress of the maxilla, and the fracture line may be seen passing upward to the infraorbital foramen. The maxillary antrum is usually opacified by hemorrhage or mucosal edema.

In the Waters view, the floor of the orbit produces two parallel lines (Fig 2–34). The upper line represents the palpable inferior rim of the orbit. The lower line is the floor of the orbit about 1 cm posterior to the rim and is interrupted by the margins of the infraorbital groove. The Waters view may therefore show discontinuity in both these lines as the fracture extends over the rim and across the floor of the orbit.

Separation at the zygomaticofrontal suture may also be seen on the Waters view (Fig 2–35,A) but is better defined in the Caldwell view (Fig 2–35,B). The patient is placed prone, and the head is positioned with the forehead against the cassette so that the orbitomeatal line is perpendicular to the film plane. The x-ray beam is angled toward the feet approximately 28 degrees and aimed through the glabella. This technique projects the petrous ridges just below the floor of the orbit. In addition to the zygomaticofrontal suture separation, this view shows the separation of the orbital process from the greater wing of sphenoid extending downward to the inferior orbital fissure.

While fracture of the zygomatic arch may also be detected on the Waters view, it is still best defined by the modified base view. Similar to the isolated fracture of the zygomatic arch, inward displacement of the zygomaticomaxillary complex may restrict mandibular motion. Furthermore, because of the greater force involved, the mandible may also be fractured (Fig 2–36).

When the traumatic force is inflicted by an object with a small cross-sectional area, the fracture may involve only a portion of the zygomaticomaxillary complex. This fracture usually involves segments of the orbital rim, such as midline displacement of the frontal process of the zygoma or fracture limited to the inferior orbital rim (Figs 2–37 and 2–38).

Orbital Blow-out Fractures

Trauma to the orbit may leave the rim intact while fracturing the floor. The posterior half of the orbital floor is formed by the thin orbital process of the maxilla (Fig 2–39). This thin portion of bone separating the orbital cavity from the maxillary antrum is further weakened by the infraorbital groove. The medial orbital wall is also relatively weak in the region of the orbital plate of the ethmoid.

The mechanism of blow-out fracture is somewhat controversial. Most commonly, it is postulated that a blow to the eye from a convex object of greater diameter than the orbit produces a sudden increase in intraocular pressure. The pressure is transmitted to the incompressible surrounding fat and bony walls, with resulting "blow-out" into the adjacent sinuses. This mechanism has been confirmed in cadaver experiments. However, the same fracture has also been produced in a dried skull by force restricted to the inferior orbital rim.

Diplopia is a common symptom at the time of initial presentation. The early explanation for the limitation of eye movement was entrapment of the inferior rectus muscle. It was postulated that, at the time of the impact, orbital contents herniate through the floor defect. As the force is dissipated, the fracture fragments tend to return to their normal position, trapping the inferior rectus muscle. However, it has now been shown that fixation of the muscles by the bony defect is rare. The fat pads lying between the inferior rectus and inferior oblique muscles may play a more important role. They contain fibrous bands connecting the muscle sheaths and the periosteum of the orbital floor. Increased tension on the fibrous bands by edema, hemorrhage, or entrapment of the fat pads may be the cause of limited ocular motility. Alternatively, it has also been suggested that the motility disorder results from direct injury to muscles or nerves at the time of impact.

Enophthalmos at the time of the initial presentation results from prolapse of orbital contents into the adjacent sinuses. Delayed development of enophthalmos may also occur due to gradual prolapse of orbital contents through a bony defect. It may also result from scarring and retraction of orbital contents without prolapse. Enophthalmos appears to correlate with the size of the orbital floor fracture. Large medial wall fractures with prolapse of the orbital contents into the ethmoid labyrinth may also be important.

Radiographic evaluation of possible orbital blow-out fracture begins with the Waters view (Fig 2–40). The inferior orbital rim appears intact, while the line of the posterior floor may be disrupted and displaced. Presumptive signs of a soft tissue density in the roof of the antrum (Fig 2–41), an antral air-fluid level, or orbital emphysema (Fig 2–42) will be well demonstrated.

The Caldwell view better demonstrates the floor and medial wall of the orbit (Fig 2–43). The floor is represented by two lines. In contrast to the Waters view, the inferior rim of the orbit is projected below the posterior portion of the floor. The upper line, representing the orbital plate of the maxilla, extends from the inferior orbital fissure to the medial wall of the orbit and is interrupted by the posterior portion of the infraorbital groove. The orbital plate of the ethmoid bone, forming the major portion of the medial orbital wall, is demonstrated by a line projected just lateral to the medial orbital rim.

The Caldwell view may demonstrate the orbital floor blow-out fracture as a step-off or depression of the orbital plate of the maxilla. In some cases, a portion or all of the orbital plate may appear to be absent. This view may also demonstrate a soft tissue density projecting into the antrum, as well as the presence of orbital emphysema (Fig 2–44).

Medial wall fractures occur in a high percentage of blow-out fractures produced experimentally. Most of these fractures are small and may only be evidenced by unilateral ethmoid clouding. Large defects may show medial displacement of the orbital plate of the ethmoid in the Caldwell view.

Most surgeons now agree that a blow-out fracture is not a surgical emergency. The presence of a fracture alone does not constitute an indication for operative intervention. Assessment of the need for surgery is delayed to allow resolution of edema and hemorrhage and is based upon the persistence of diplopia or enophthalmos. Therefore, radiographic evaluation is not urgent and should be delayed until the patient can tolerate the positioning required for the Waters and Caldwell views. Visualization of the orbit with a "reversed-Waters" or "reversed-Caldwell" pro-

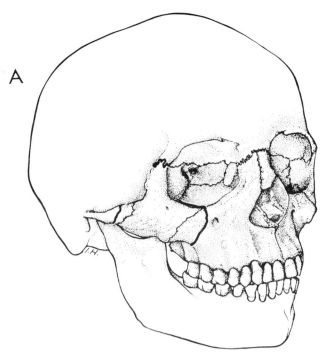

A

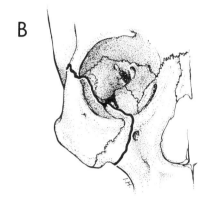

B

FIG 2–32.
A and **B,** schematic drawings of zygoma-ticomaxillary complex fracture.

FIG 2–33.
Waters view of zygomaticomaxillary fracture. The fracture passes from the lateral wall of the maxilla *(1)* to the inferior orbital rim *(2)*. Separation at the zygo-maticofrontal suture *(3)* extends across the orbital pro-cess of the zygoma *(4)* to the inferior orbital fissure. The zygomatic arch fracture *(5)* is evident as the com-plex is rotated and displaced medially.

FIG 2–34.
Waters view, showing the normal inferior orbital rim *(1)* and posterior floor *(2)* on the right. A zygomati-comaxillary complex fracture on the left passes from the buttress of the maxilla *(3),* through the inferior or-bital rim *(4)* to involve the floor of the orbit *(5).* The fracture at the zygomaticofrontal suture appears as a lucency *(6),* while the zygomatic arch fracture appears as a density due to superimposition of fragments *(7).*

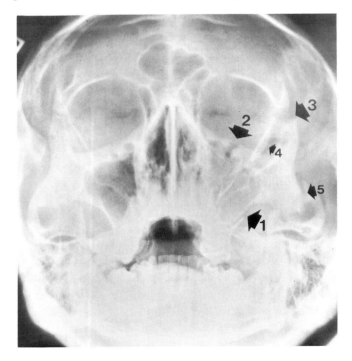

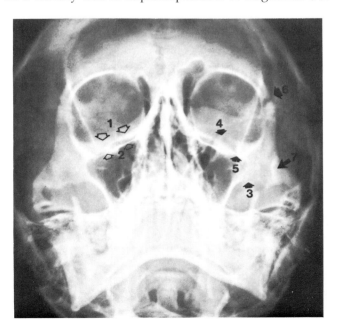

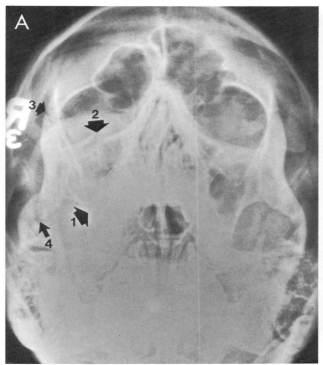

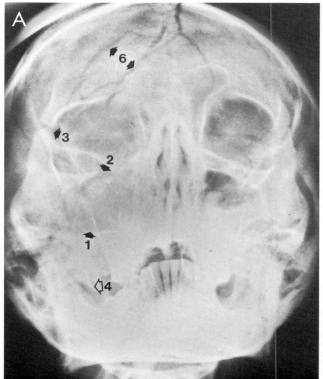

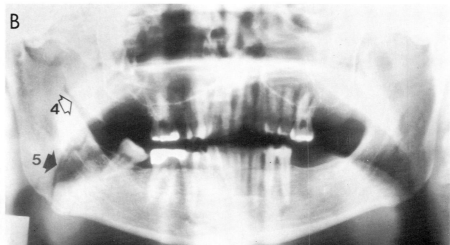

FIG 2–35.
A, Waters view of right zygomaticomaxillary complex fracture, showing discontinuities in the lateral wall of maxilla *(1)*, inferior orbital rim *(2)*, frontal process of zygoma *(3)*, and zygomatic arch *(4)*. **B,** Caldwell view more clearly shows the fracture at the zygomatico-frontal suture *(1)*, extending into the orbital process of the zygoma *(2)*.

FIG 2–36.
A, Waters view, showing a fracture passing from the buttress of the maxilla *(1)* to the inferior orbital rim *(2)* and separation at the zygomaticofrontal suture *(3)*. There appears to be a fracture in the mandible *(4)*. The patient also sustained a comminuted fracture of the frontal bone *(6)*. **B,** panoramic view confirms the fracture of the coronoid process *(4)* of the mandible and shows extension through the angle *(5)*.

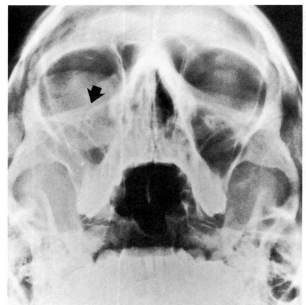

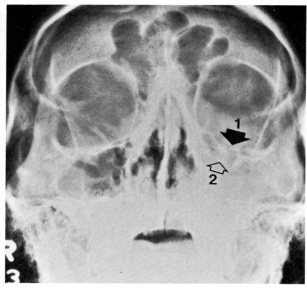

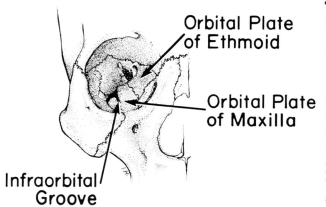

Orbital Plate of Ethmoid

Orbital Plate of Maxilla

Infraorbital Groove

FIG 2–37 (top left).
Waters view, showing an isolated fracture of the inferior orbital rim and anterior wall of the maxilla.

FIG 2–38 (top right).
Waters view of a comminuted fracture of the inferior orbital rim (1), with involvement of the posterior orbital floor (2).

FIG 2–39 (left).
Anatomy of the bony orbit.

FIG 2–40 (bottom left).
Waters view of a blow-out fracture of the left orbit. The inferior orbital rim (1) is intact, while the line representing the orbital floor is disrupted (2). A displaced fragment is seen on edge (3).

FIG 2–41 (bottom right).
Waters view of a blow-out fracture of the right orbit. The inferior orbital rim is intact (1). A soft tissue mass (2) occupies the roof of the antrum.

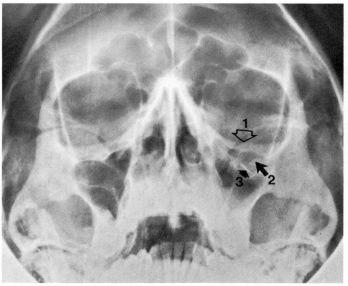

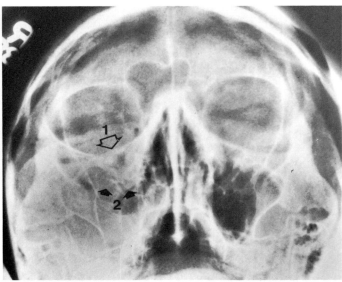

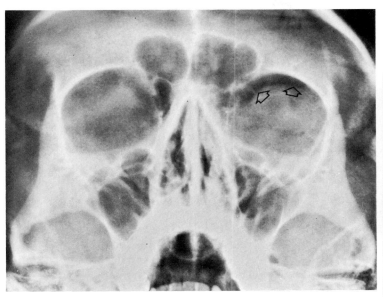

FIG 2–42.
Waters view, showing orbital emphysema.

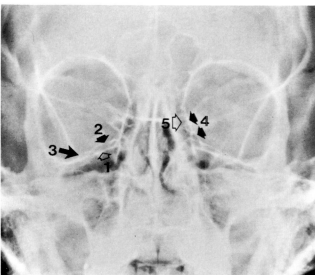

FIG 2–43.
Caldwell view. *1,* inferior orbital rim; *2,* orbital plate of the maxilla; *3,* posterior portion of the infraorbital groove; *4,* posterior portion of the ethmoid orbital plate; *5,* medial rim of orbit.

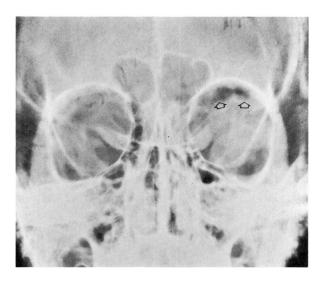

FIG 2–44.
Caldwell view, showing orbital emphysema.

jection obtained with the patient supine will not provide adequate detail. Re-examination will then be required following the initial presentation.

Le Fort Facial Fractures

The midfacial skeleton projects downward from the sloping base of the skull below the anterior and middle cranial fossae. Central support is supplied by the vomer and perpendicular plate of the ethmoid and the ethmoid lateral masses. Laterally, the processes of the zygoma connect the midface to the skull. Finally, the pterygoid processes of the sphenoid bone provide posterior support. This design allows the midfacial skeleton to resist the stress of mastication applied vertically. On the other hand, force applied from an anterior, superior, or lateral direction will tend to shear this complex from the skull base.

Understanding of the lines of fracture in the middle third of the face is attributable to experimental studies on cadaver heads performed by René Le Fort in 1901. He observed that the fracture lines could be divided into three categories (Fig 2–45).

A Le Fort I fracture begins at the lower lateral edge of the anterior nasal aperture. It passes laterally across the anterolateral wall of the maxillary antrum and dips below the buttress. It then inclines slightly upward through the posterolateral wall of the antrum and crosses through the lower portion of the lateral and medial pterygoid plates. The fracture line completes its circle by passing along the medial wall of the antrum to its starting point. A Le Fort I fracture usually develops bilaterally and is associated with a fracture through the vomer.

A Le Fort II fracture results from a violent force applied to the midfacial skeleton over an area extending from the glabella to the margin to the maxillary alveolus. The fracture starts transversely in the nasal bones, slightly below the frontonasal sutures, extends bilaterally across the frontal processes of the maxillae, and passes downward across the lacrimal bones. From this point the fracture line on each side passes forward and laterally to the inferior orbital rim, medial to the zygomaticomaxillary suture. Descending, the line traverses the anterolateral wall of the antrum, passing through or close to the infraorbital foramen. It then dips below the buttress of the maxilla, inclines upward abruptly, and passes across the posterolateral wall of the antrum. Fracture of the pterygoid plates occurs in their midportions. Within the nasal cavity, the medial walls of the maxillae are fractured, and a fracture extends through the nasal septum, involving both the perpendicular plate of the ethmoid and the vomer.

Le Fort III injuries usually result from a force inflicted over an even wider area from an anterior direction. Posterior displacement of the central facial structures splays apart the zygomatic bones. The fracture may also result from a lateral blow to the malar region that is too great to be entirely absorbed by fracturing of the zygoma. The midfacial skeleton will then hinge on the ethmoid bone, and the transmitted force will produce a laterally displaced fracture of the opposite zygoma. The fracture crosses the nasal bones and frontal processes of the maxillae adjacent to the frontonasal and frontomaxillary sutures. It then traverses the lacrimal bones and continues posteriorly across the orbital plate of the ethmoid bone. Comminution of the orbital plate usually occurs. The fracture line is deflected downward to the medial portion of the inferior orbital fissures. The fracture crosses the upper posterior surface of the maxillae in the sphenopalatine fossa to reach the posterior nasal cavity. The nasal surfaces of the lateral masses and the perpendicular plate of the ethmoid bone are fractured. The pterygoid plates are disrupted at their base from the sphenoid bone. Posterior displacement of the nasal bones may fracture the cribriform plate of the ethmoid bone, tearing the dura and resulting in CSF rhinorrhea. Additional fractures occur through the orbital and frontal processes of the zygomatic bones and through the zygomatic arches. Thus, the entire middle third of facial skeleton is detached from the skull base.

It is apparent that the Le Fort fractures characteristically involve the pterygoid plates. The lateral radiograph of the face (Fig 2–46) will show the interruption of the pterygoid plates and the posterolateral wall of the maxillae. The levels of the pterygoid plate fractures may suggest the severity of the injury. The lateral view of a Le Fort I injury will also show fractures involving the anterolateral walls of the maxillae (Fig 2–47). Le Fort II fractures will show disruption through the nasal bones and the frontal processes of the maxillae on the lateral view (Fig 2–48), while in Le Fort III fractures the separation occurs higher, at the frontonasal and frontomaxillary sutures (Fig 2–49).

The Waters view more precisely delineates the nature of injury. In Le Fort I, this view shows fractures of the lateral and medial maxillary walls and the vomer (Fig 2–50). The Le Fort II fracture is shown with disruption of the lateral maxillary walls and the inferior orbital rims (Fig 2–51). The nasal bones and the orbital processes of the maxillae may appear separated. Fracture of the nasal septum may also be visualized. In Le Fort III, the Waters view shows separation at the frontonasal and frontomaxillary sutures (Fig 2–52). The nasal bones, the frontal processes of

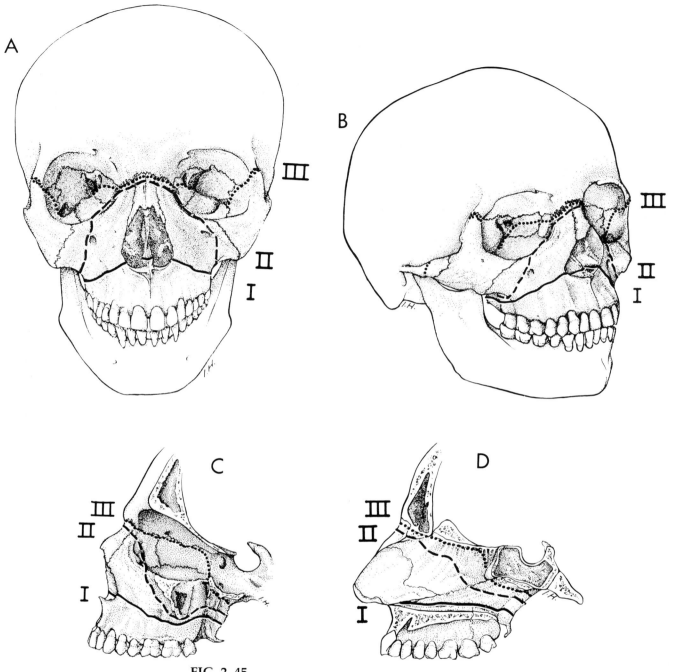

FIG 2–45.
A–D, schematic drawings of Le Fort fractures.

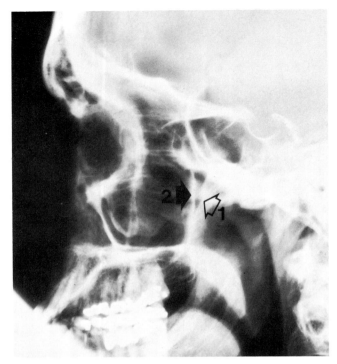

FIG 2–46.
Lateral view, showing anterior surface of pterygoid plate (1) and posterior wall of the maxilla (2).

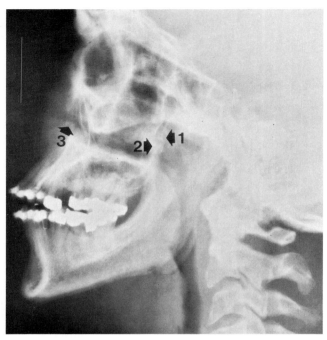

FIG 2–47.
Lateral view of Le Fort I fracture. There is a discontinuity in the pterygoid plate (1), the posterior wall of the maxilla (2), and the anterior maxillary surface (3).

FIG 2–48.
Lateral view of Le Fort II fracture. A lucency extends across the pterygoid plates (1), and there is a discontinuity in the posterior wall of the maxilla (2). A fracture line passes upward across the anterior wall of the maxilla (3) into the medial orbital wall (4). A fracture is present near the frontonasal suture (5).

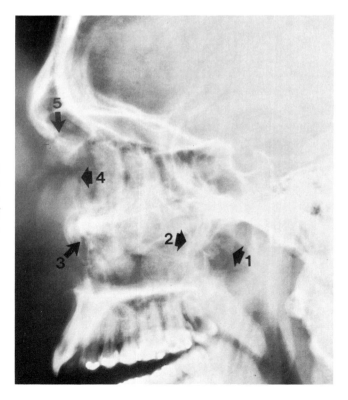

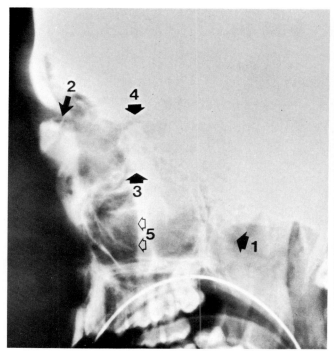

FIG 2–49.
Lateral view of Le Fort III fracture. The pterygoid plates are disrupted (1), and there is separation at the frontonasal suture (2). A fracture extends posteriorly in the medial wall of the orbit (3). Another lucent line (4) is due to fracture at the zygomaticofrontal suture. The fluid level (5) is due to blood in the maxillary sinuses.

FIG 2–51.
Waters view of Le Fort II fracture, showing disruption of the lateral walls of the maxillae (1) and inferior orbital rims (2).

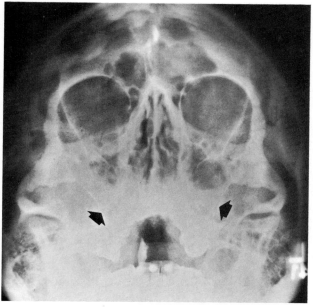

FIG 2–50.
Waters view of Le Fort I fracture, showing discontinuities in the lateral walls of the maxillae. A fluid level is seen in the left maxillary antrum, and extensive mucosal thickening is present in the right.

FIG 2–52.
Waters view of Le Fort III fracture, showing separation at the frontonasal suture (1) and disruption of the orbital plate of the ethmoid (2) made obvious by displacement of the midface toward the left. The frontal process of the zygoma is fractured on the left (3) and on the right (4). In addition, there are fractures involving the lesser (5 and 7) and greater (6 and 8) wings of the sphenoid.

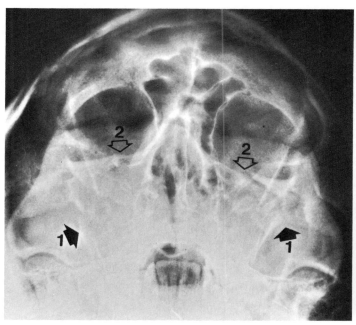

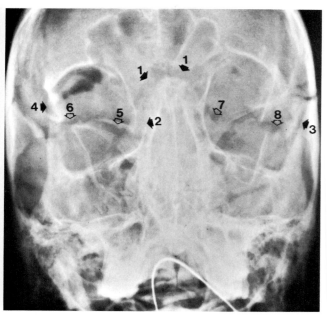

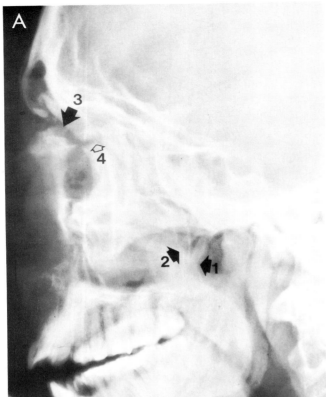

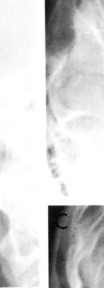

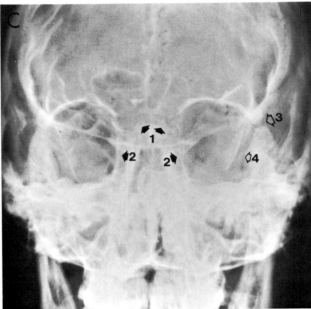

FIG 2–53.
A, lateral view showing disruption of the pterygoid plates *(1)* and posterior wall of maxilla *(2)*. There is a separation of the frontonasal suture *(3)* and one of the zygomaticofrontal sutures *(4)*. **B,** Waters view, showing fracture of the lateral walls of the maxillae *(1)*, inferior orbital rims *(2)*, nasofrontal suture *(3)*, and anterior orbital plate of ethmoid *(4)*, consistent with Le Fort II fracture. There is also fracture at the zygomaticofrontal suture *(5)* and zygomatic arch *(6)*. **C,** Caldwell view shows separation at nasofrontal suture *(1)* and orbital plates of the ethmoid *(2)*. The fracture at the zygomaticofrontal suture *(3)* extends into the orbital process of the zygoma *(4)*.

the maxillae, and the nasal septum may appear comminuted and displaced when there is an associated nasoethmoidal complex fracture. The separations of the zygomaticofrontal sutures are usually well demonstrated, and fractures of the zygomatic arches may even be evident. The lateral walls of the maxillae are shown to be intact in the pure Le Fort III injury.

Combinations of Le Fort fractures occur frequently, so that, once separation of a section of the midface has been confirmed on the lateral view, it may be more practical to identify the individual components evident on the Waters view rather than to classify by type (Fig 2–53).

Motor vehicle accidents are the major cause of Le Fort fractures. Peripheral skeletal and spine injuries are frequently present in these victims and may make positioning for optimum visualization of the midface hazardous. The lateral view of the face can be obtained with the patient supine in the "brow-up" position. A "reversed-Waters" view may also be obtained with the patient supine to roughly estimate the extent of injury. However, before definitive repair of the Le Fort II and III fractures is planned, more detailed information may be obtained with thin-section tomography.

Fractures of the Upper Third of the Face

Fractures of the upper third of the face include the superior orbital rim and the frontal sinus. Because of the contiguity of the central nervous system to these structures, assessment of neurologic function takes precedence over evaluation of the facial injury. Radiologic evaluation of intracranial structures by computed tomography may be more important than imaging of the suspected facial fractures.

The superior orbital rim may be fractured by localized trauma. The Waters view shows interruption of the dense cortical line representing the superior rim (Fig 2–54,A). On the Caldwell view, the palpable superior orbital rim does not produce a distinct cortical line but appears as a zone of slightly increased density in the upper orbit (Fig 2–54,B). The dense cortical line above this represents the roof of the orbit. The Caldwell view does show superior rim fractures, especially when the fragments are displaced downward.

Fractures of the medial portion of the superior orbital rim may also involve the frontal sinus (Fig 2–55,A). More commonly, the frontal sinus is fractured by itself. The fracture may be restricted to the anterior wall or involve both the anterior and posterior walls. Isolated linear fractures of the posterior wall of the frontal sinuses are rare. Fractures involving primarily the superior portions of the frontal bone may also extend into the frontal sinuses, involving one or both walls (Fig 2–56).

The fracture may be linear or comminuted; the fragments may be nondisplaced or depressed. While exposure of the fracture by a soft tissue laceration clearly represents a compound injury, a fracture that tears the mucosal lining is also compound, due to communication with the exterior via the frontonasal ducts.

The Caldwell view will show a linear fracture of the frontal sinus as a radiolucent cleft (see Fig 2–55,B). A decrease in the radiolucency of the sinus may be due to mucosal edema or hemorrhage. A fluid level is uncommon. When the fracture is comminuted and depressed, the decrease in radiolucency may be due more to overlap of fragments (Fig 2–57,A). The lateral view of the face shows the anterior and posterior surfaces of the frontal sinuses at the midline. Depression of fracture fragments and involvement of the posterior wall will be more evident (Fig 2–57,B). However, linear fractures, especially those which are not oriented transversely or which involve the lateral portions of the sinus, will not be clearly seen. Determination of damage to the dura mater by a linear fracture of the posterior wall may be difficult unless the lateral view shows intracranial air.

Computed Tomography in Facial Trauma

Computed tomography (CT) is an essential radiologic study for assessment of patients with head trauma. High resolution techniques can also be used to study facial fractures in great detail.

Most localized fractures can be adequately defined using routine radiographs. However, complex midface fractures, orbital blow-out fractures, and severe fractures of the frontal sinuses are often incompletely assessed with plain radiographs. CT also has the major advantage of being able to demonstrate soft-tissue complications associated with the bony injuries (Figs 2–58 and 2–61,D).

CT scans of the face are most easily obtained in the transverse plane. Standard scans are taken parallel to the infraorbital-meatal line using 2-mm to 5-mm thick collimation. These scans provide the best assessment of the anterior and posterior walls of the maxillary sinuses, the medial and lateral walls of the orbit, the zygomatic arch, and the anterior and posterior walls of the frontal sinuses.

Analysis of transverse scans is usually sufficient to classify a midface fracture. Le Fort I fractures show disruption of both maxillary sinuses while the medial and lateral orbital walls appear normal (Fig 2–59). Le

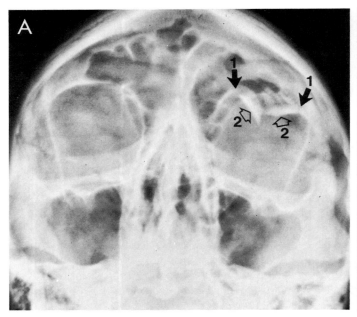

FIG 2–54.

A, Waters view, showing disruption of the superior orbital rim *(1)* and downward displacement of the fragments *(2)*. **B,** Caldwell view showing downward displacement of the fragmented left superior orbital rim *(1)*. The roof of the orbit *(2)* is intact. On the right, the normal roof of the orbit *(3)* and edge of the superior orbital rim *(4)* are indicated.

FIG 2–55.

A, Waters view, showing interruption of the superior orbital rim *(1)* and a linear fracture *(2)* extending across the frontal sinuses. The radiolucency of the sinus has been reduced by localized mucosal hemorrhage or edema. **B,** Caldwell view showing the frontal sinus fracture and loss of radiolucency more clearly.

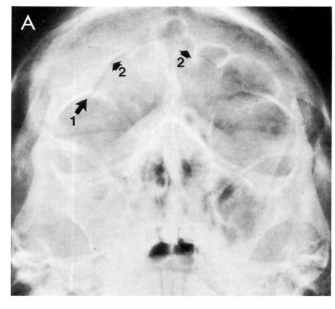
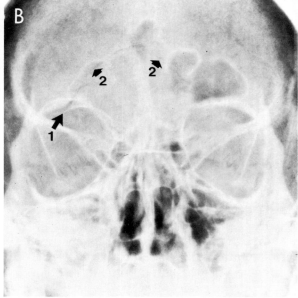

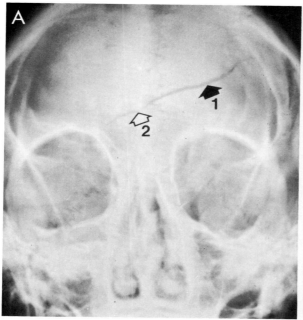

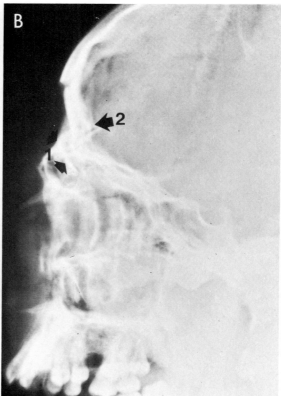

FIG 2–56.
A, Caldwell view, showing a frontal bone fracture *(1)* extending into the frontal sinuses *(2)*. The sinuses are opaque due to hemorrhage. **B,** lateral view, showing the linear frontal bone fracture *(1)* extending into the frontal sinus *(2)*.

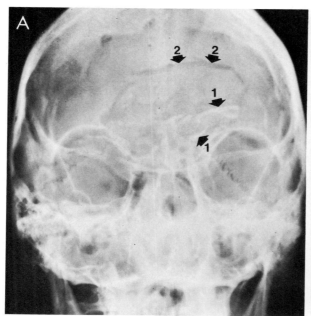

FIG 2–57.
A, Caldwell view of a comminuted, depressed frontal sinus fracture. Overlap of fragment causes increased density *(1)*, while separation produces irregular radiolucencies *(2)*. **B,** lateral view shows depression of fragments of the anterior *(1)* and posterior *(2)* walls.

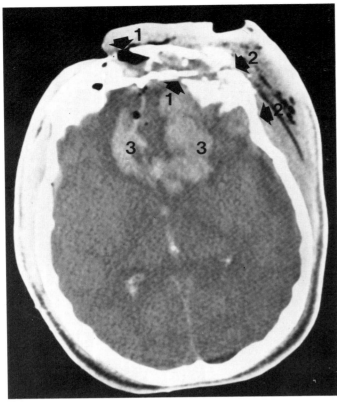

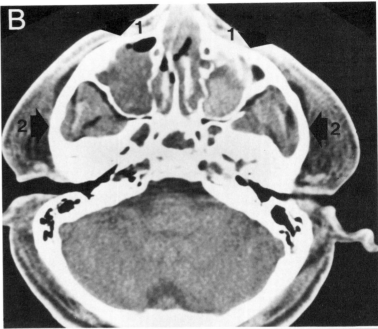

FIG 2–59.

A, transverse CT scan of a Le Fort I fracture showing disruption of the walls of the maxillae *(1)*, the nasal septum *(2)*, and the pterygoid plates *(3)*. **B,** transverse CT scan showing that the inferior orbital rims *(1)* and the zygomatic arches *(2)* are intact. **C,** transverse CT scan demonstrates that the lateral *(1)* and medial *(2)* orbital walls are also intact.

FIG 2–58.

Transverse CT scan showing fractures of the anterior and posterior walls of the frontal sinus *(1)* and the frontal bone *(2)*. There is extensive soft-tissue swelling and subcutaneous emphysema. Hemorrhage is present in both frontal lobes of the brain *(3)*.

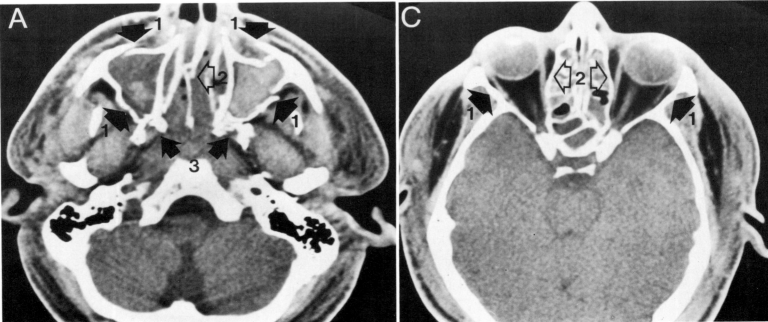

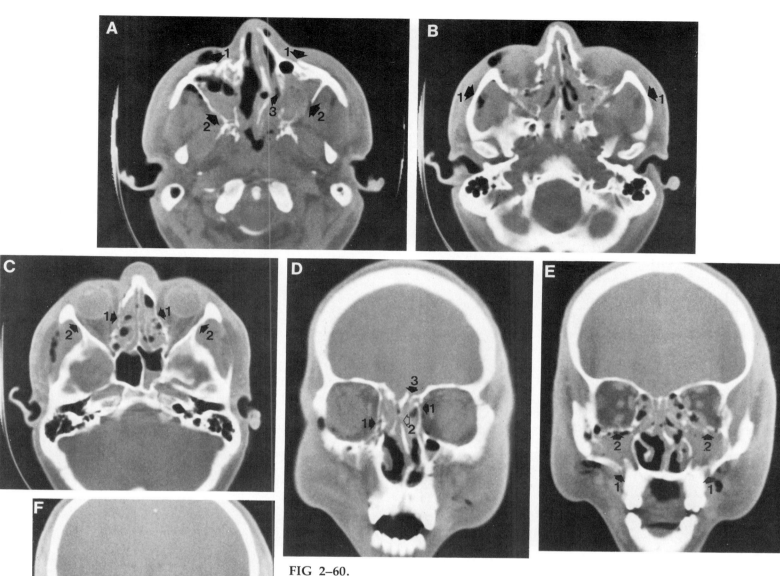

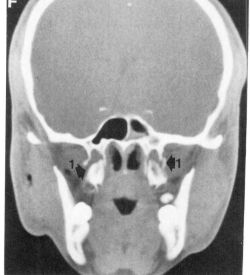

FIG 2–60.
A, transverse CT scan of Le Fort II fracture showing disruption of the anterior *(1)* and lateral *(2)* walls of the maxillae and of the nasal septum *(3).* **B,** transverse CT scan showing the zygomatic arches *(1)* are intact. **C,** transverse CT scan showing fractures of the medial orbital walls *(1).* The lateral orbital walls *(2)* are not damaged. **D,** coronal CT scan showing fractures of the medial orbital walls *(1),* nasal septum *(2),* and cribriform plate *(3).* **E,** coronal CT scan showing disruption of the lateral walls of the maxillae *(1)* as well as the orbital floors *(2).* **F,** coronal CT scan demonstrating pterygoid process fractures *(1).*

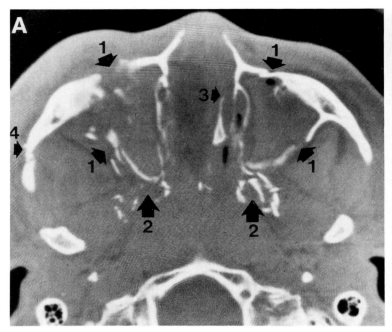

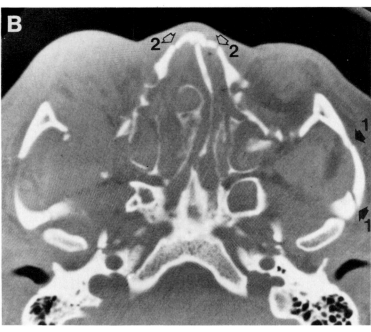

FIG 2–61.

A, transverse CT scan of Le Fort II and III fractures showing extensive bilateral maxillary fractures *(1)*. Fractures of the pterygoid processes *(2)*, nasal septum *(3)*, and right zygomatic arch *(4)* are also demonstrated. **B,** transverse CT scan showing fractures of the left zygomatic arch *(1)* and the nasal bones *(2)*. **C,** transverse CT scan demonstrating fractures of the lateral *(1)* and medial *(2)* orbital walls and the nasofrontal region *(3)*. **D,** transverse CT scan showing soft tissue swelling over the eye and a hematoma within the orbit *(1)*. The ethmoid and sphenoid sinuses are filled with blood.

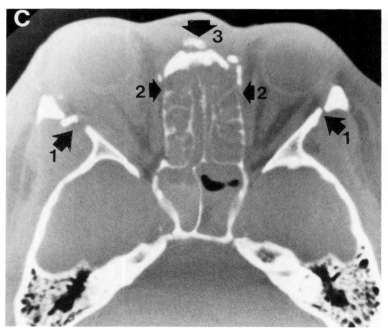

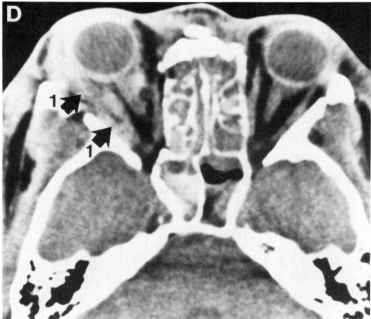

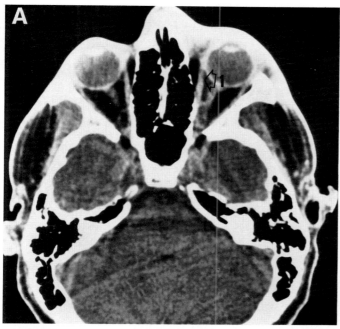

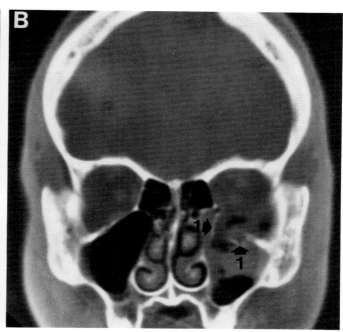

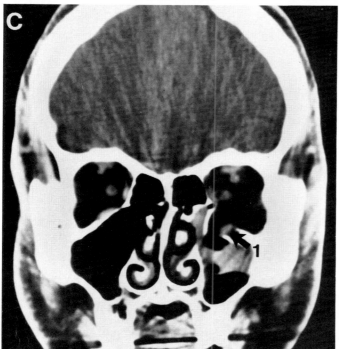

FIG 2–62.
A, transverse CT scan through the orbits demonstrates the relationship of the medial wall to the medial rectus muscle *(1).* **B,** coronal CT scan showing fracture of the orbital floor with displacement of fracture fragments *(1)* into the maxillary sinus. The sinus is partially opacified by hemorrhage. Air is present within the orbit. **C,** coronal CT scan showing displacement of the inferior rectus muscle *(1)* into the maxillary sinus.

Fort II fractures involve the medial orbital walls bilaterally as well as both maxillary sinuses. The lateral orbital walls, however, remain intact (Fig 2–60,A–C). Le Fort III fractures are recognized by bilateral damage to the maxillary sinuses and the medial and lateral orbital walls, as well as the zygomatic arches (Fig 2–61).

Complete assessment of a midface fracture requires additional scans in the coronal plane. The patient's neck must be hyperextended to allow scans to be obtained parallel to the ramus of the mandible. These scans give the best view of the orbital floor and roof, the cribriform plate, the medial wall of the maxillary sinus, and the pterygoid process (see Fig 2–60,D–F). Unfortunately, other injuries may preclude placing a trauma victim in position for coronal scans, and many other patients may find it just too uncomfortable to tolerate. Attempts to obtain coronal scans in patients with extensive dental fillings will also be unsuccessful because of image degradation by metal artifact.

Orbital blow-out fractures are also best assessed using both transverse and coronal scans. Transverse scans show the relationship between the fractured medial wall and the medial rectus muscle (Fig 2–62,A), while coronal scans better demonstrate displacement of the fragments. Coronal scans are critical for recognizing the orbital floor fractures and displacement of bone fragments into the maxillary sinus (Fig 2–62,B). Herniation of orbital fat and the inferior rectus muscle can usually be recognized on coronal scans (Fig 2–62,C). However, the precise relationship of the inferior rectus muscle to the floor fracture is best demonstrated by oblique sagittal images produced by computer reformation of transverse scans or by special patient positioning.

Suggested Reading

1. Towe NL, Killey HC: *Fractures of the Facial Skeleton,* ed 2. London, E & S Livingstone Ltd, 1968.
2. Harris LE, Harris MW: *The Radiology of Emergency Medicine,* ed 2. Baltimore, Williams & Wilkins, 1981.
3. Gerlock AJ, Sinn DP, McBride KL: *Clinical and Radiographic Interpretation of Facial Fractures.* Boston, Little, Brown & Co, 1981.
4. Hammeslag SB, Hughes S, O'Reilly GV, et al: Another look at blow-out fractures of the orbit. *AJNR* 1982; 3:331–336.
5. Hammerslag SB, Hughes S, O'Reilly GV, et al: Blow-out fractures of the orbit: A comparison of computed tomography and conventional radiography with anatomical correlation. *Radiology* 1982; 143:487–492.
6. Rowe LD, Miller E, Brandt-Zawadzki M: Computed tomography in maxillofacial trauma. *Laryngoscope* 1981; 91:745–757.
7. Jend HH, Rossman IJ: A systematic approach to the diagnosis of transethmoidal fractures in CT. *Europ J Radiol* 1985; 5:8–11.
8. Gentry LR, Manor WF, Turski PA, et al: High-resolution CT analysis of facial struts in trauma: 1. Normal anatomy. *AJR* 1983; 140:523–532.
9. Gentry LR, Manor WF, Turski PA, et al: High-resolution CT analysis of facial struts in trauma: 2. Osseous and soft-tissue complications. *AJR* 1983; 140:533–541.
10. Kreipke DL, Moss JJ, Franco JM, et al: Computed tomography and thin-section tomography in facial trauma. *AJR* 1984; 142:1041–1045.
11. Ball JB: Direct oblique sagittal CT of orbital wall fractures. *AJNR* 1987; 8:147.

Normal Variants

Theodore E. Keats, M.D.

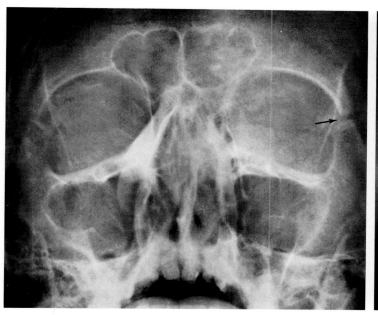

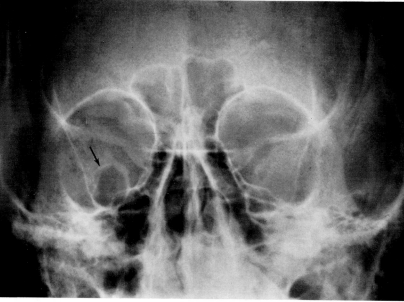

FIG 2–63 (top left).
Simulated fracture through zygomatic-frontal suture produced by a slight rotation of the head.

FIG 2–64 (top right).
Unusual appearance produced by extension of a sphenoidal air cell into the greater wing of the sphenoid.

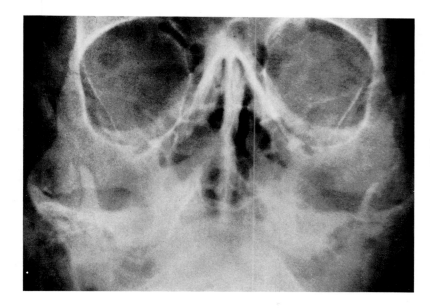

FIG 2–65.
Hypoplasia of both antra simulating sinus disease.

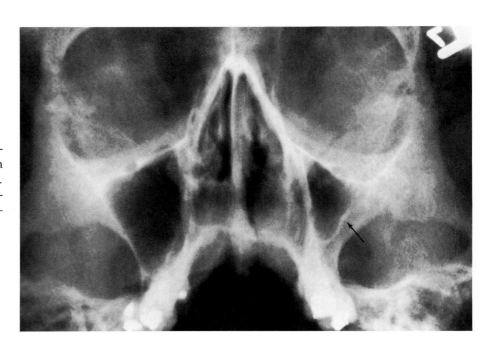

FIG 2–66.
Hypoplasia of the maxillary antrum. Note enlargement of the orbit on the same side, a finding which frequently accompanies hypoplasia of the antrum. (Ref: Bierny JP, Dryden R: Orbital enlargement secondary to paranasal sinus hypoplasia. *Am J Roentgenol* 1977; 128:850.)

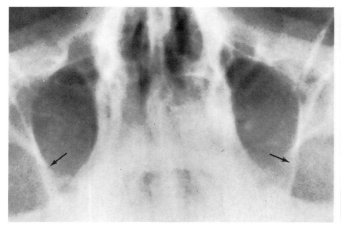

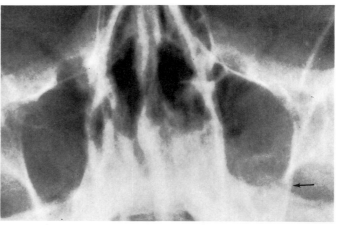

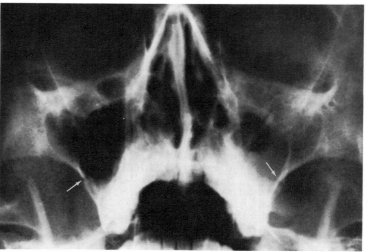

FIG 2–67.
Simulated fractures of the lateral wall of the maxillary antrum produced by the posterior superior alveolar canal. (Ref: Chuang VP, Vines FS: Roentgenology of the posterior superior alveolar foramina and canals. *Am J Roentgenol* 1973; 118:426.)

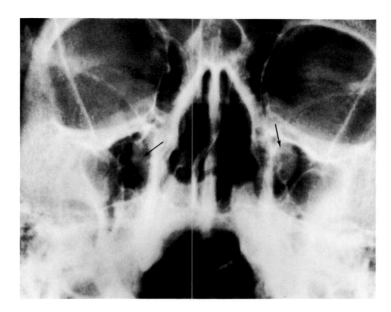

FIG 2–68.
The nares superimposed on the antra simulating polyps.

FIG 2–69.
Two examples of simulated tumor of the antrum produced by superimposition of the turbinates on the coronoid process of the mandible.

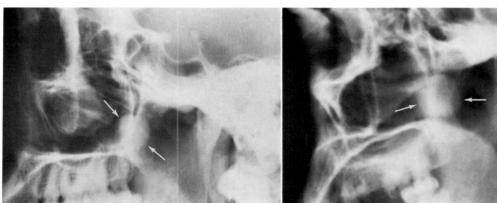

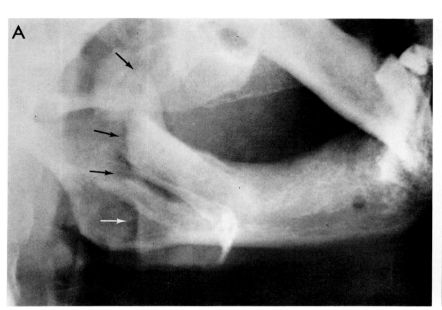

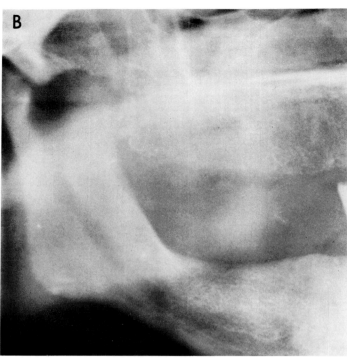

FIG 2–70.
A, pharyngeal air shadow over the base of the tongue superimposed on the mandible simulates a fracture. **B,** panorex film made at same session shows that no fracture is present.

FIG 2–71.
Superimposition of the airway producing an apparent fracture of the mandibular condyle.

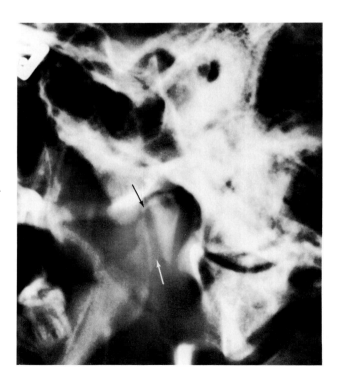

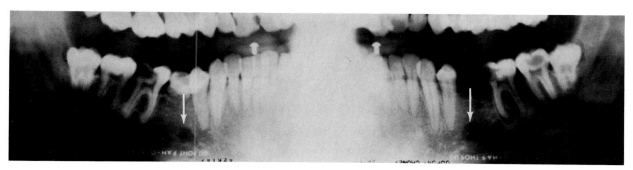

FIG 2–72.
The normal mental foramina.

FIG 2–73.

The normal nasal bone. Note the nasomaxillary suture (*arrow*) and the grooves for the nasociliary nerves (*notched arrows*). No grooves should cross the nasal bridge. (Ref: de Lacey GJ, et al: The radiology of nasal injuries: Problems of interpretation and clinical relevance. *Br J Radiol* 1977; 50:412.)

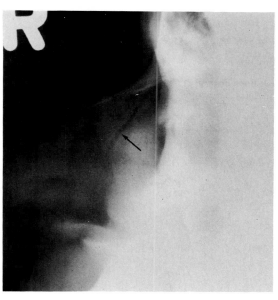 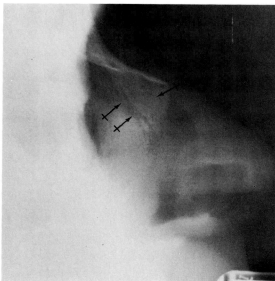

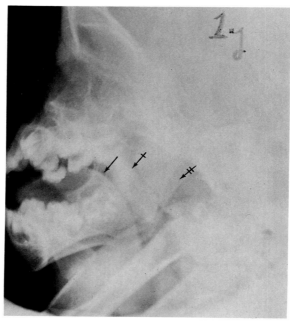

FIG 2–74.
Normal configuration of the soft tissues of the mouth and oropharynx in a 1-year-old infant during swallowing, showing tongue *(arrow)*, soft palate *(notched arrow)*, and adenoids *(double-notched arrow)*.

FIG 2–75.
The shadow of the ear lobe, simulating a mass in the nasopharynx.

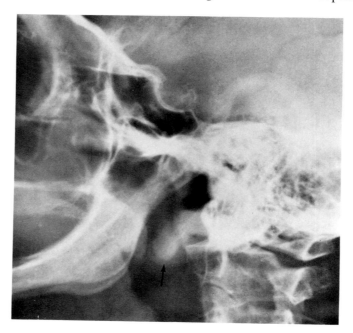

3
Spine

Thomas Lee Pope, Jr., M.D.
Hans O. Riddervold, M.D.

We will first describe cervical spine trauma and follow this with a discussion of combined thoracolumbar injuries. Commonly encountered nontraumatic causes of spine pain will then be presented.

The Cervical Spine

Traumatic injuries to the spine in general and to the cervical spine in particular are ever-increasing concerns for the emergency room physician. Radiographic evaluation of the cervical spine presents one of the most challenging situations in the trauma setting. The potentially serious nature of the injuries, together with the sometimes confusing anatomy in this region, make the cervical spine a difficult area to evaluate.

There are a number of treatises on the intricacies of cervical spine trauma.[1-3] Most of these are in-depth discussions designed specifically for radiologists or orthopedists. Awareness of few basic anatomical and pathologic patterns, some pitfalls and normal variations should, however, enable emergency room physicians to identify possible serious injuries and allow them to "get through the night."

Techniques

Most patients with suspected cervical spine injury will arrive at the hospital with the head and upper neck immobilized by a cervical collar or similar device. This obviously makes thorough physical examination difficult. Plain films of the cervical spine are essential in the acute trauma setting. Since in certain situations ER physicians may be called on to screen routine plain films, we will stress familiarity with this examination. It is unlikely that the ER physician will be asked to interpret spinal computed tomography (CT) or tomography. However, knowledge of the potential strengths and weaknesses of these and other

ancillary examinations in the trauma setting is important and will be discussed later.

The first and most important film to obtain of the cervical spine is a well-positioned, adequately penetrated, cross-table brow-up lateral projection in the neutral position. All seven cervical vertebrae and the upper thoracic vertebrae should be seen in all patients because the cervicothoracic junction is a common site of traumatic injury. Easily diagnosed fractures or dislocations in this region can be missed if this basic rule is not followed. Adequate demonstration of the C-7–T-1 region may require special maneuvers such as traction on the shoulders (Fig 3–1) or the so-called swimmer's projection. If none of these is successful, tomography (Fig 3–2) or computed tomography may be required for a thorough examination.

If the brow-up lateral film shows no abnormality, the rest of our routine series includes anteroposterior (AP), right and left oblique, and open-mouth odontoid views. We do not consider any examination complete until we have seen the odontoid in all patients. If our plain films are normal and the clinical suspicion remains high, we may obtain flexion-extension views. The patient must be able to move himself for these views. They should never be performed if someone else has to move the patient's head. Flexion-extension views may show unsuspected serious pathology even when the routine views are normal (Fig 3–3). Fluoroscopy may be useful during flexion extension to check for widening or subluxation, particularly at the C-1–C-2 interspace. However, we rarely use this maneuver. If the flexion-extension views are normal or inconclusive and clinical suspicion remains high, there are other plain films that may be helpful. The pillar view, a special projection, shows the lateral masses en face, has been advocated by some authors,[4] but its efficacy in the trauma setting has been questioned.[5] We have not found this view particulary helpful. Angulated 60° "trauma" oblique views are another alternative view and have the advantage of

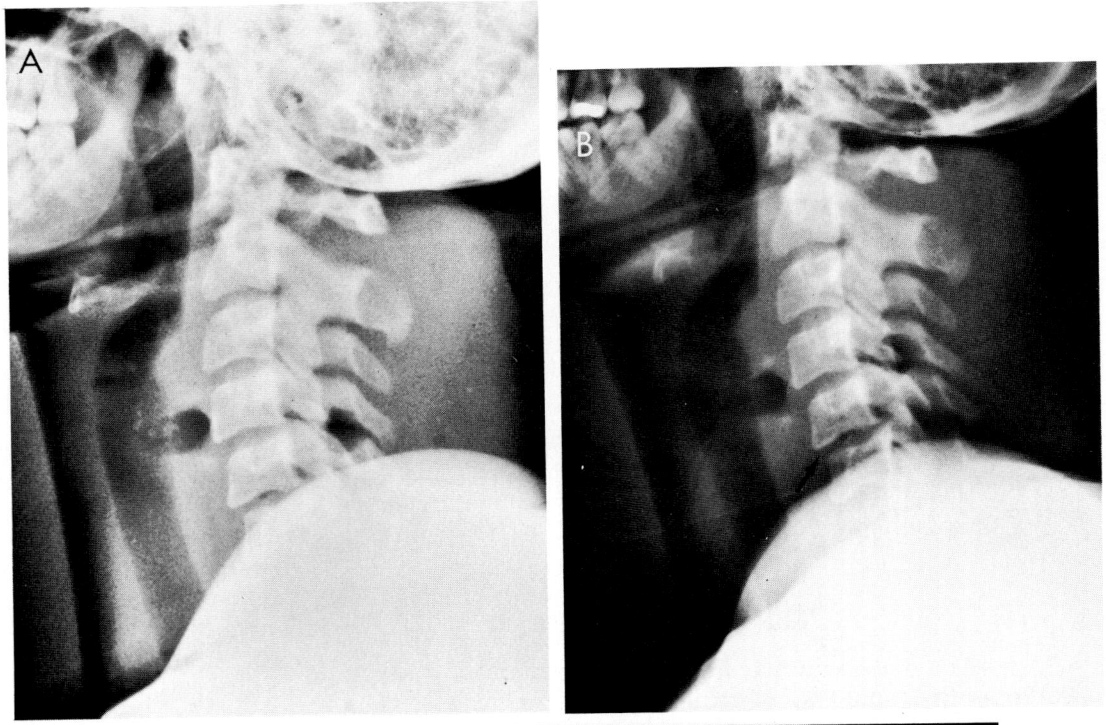

FIG 3–1.
A, lateral cervical spine showing only C-1 through upper border of C-6. **B,** repeat lateral film of cervical spine with traction on shoulders showing C-1 through upper border of C-7. Anterior subluxation of C-5 on C-6 (*arrow*) was missed on the initial film. In every situation possible, all cervical vertebrae should be seen.

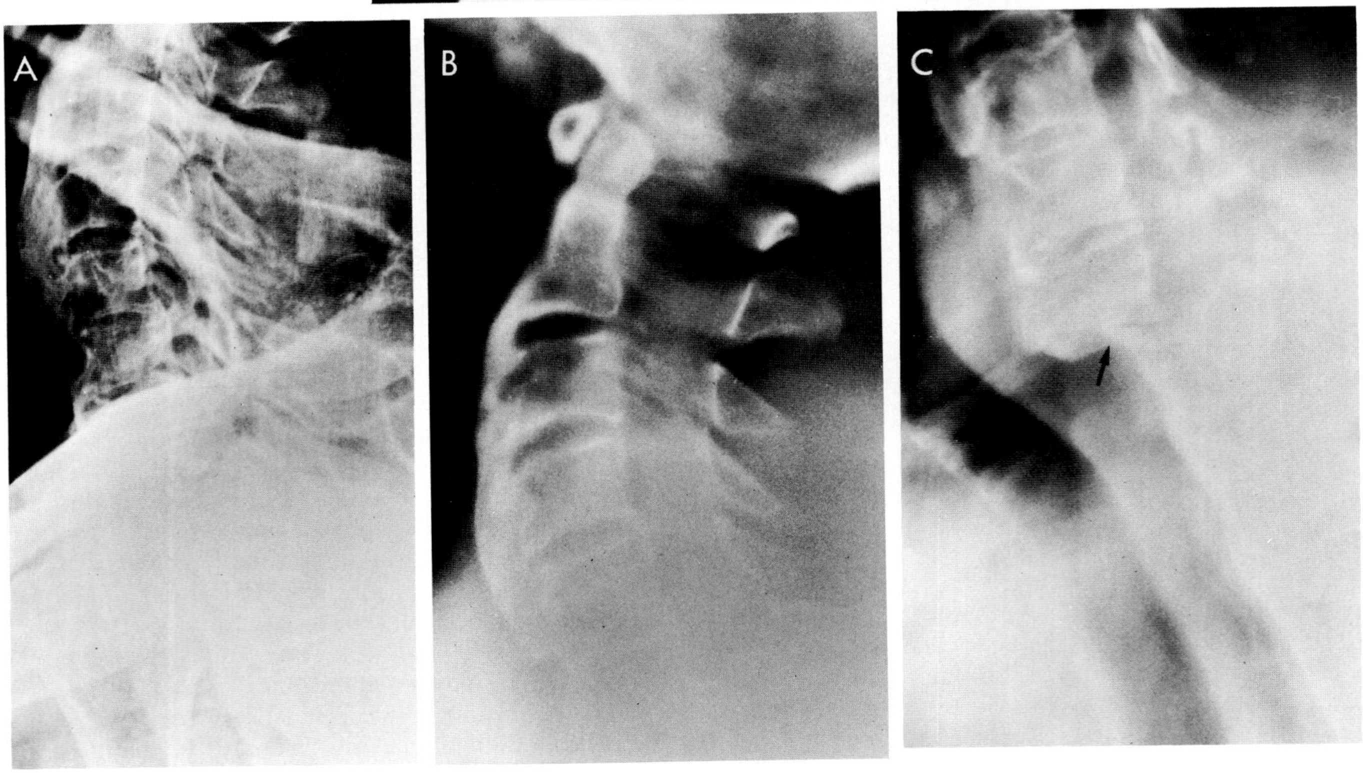

FIG 3–2.
A, lateral cervical spine of 65-year-old patient with ankylosing spondylitis who fell downstairs. Upper border of C-7 is seen; no fracture was identified. **B,** lateral tomogram the following day, showing no fracture. Only the lower border of C-6 is seen. **C,** re-peat lateral tomogram 3 weeks later because of continued pain shows 17 mm of anterior subluxation of C-7 on T-1 (*arrow*). Fortunately, the patient was still essentially neurologically intact. Lower cervical and upper thoracic vertebrae should be seen in all cases of suspected cervical spine trauma.

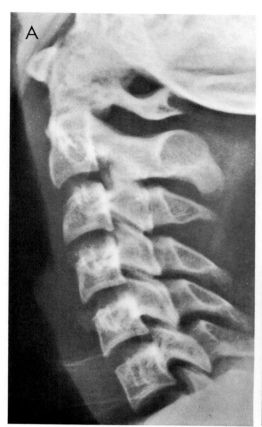

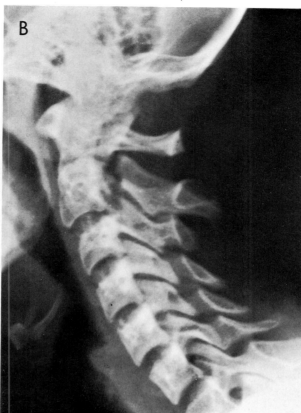

FIG 3–3.
A, lateral brow-up view of cervical spine of 40-year-old man in an automobile accident shows no abnormality. **B,** because of pain, flexion view was obtained. Unsuspected hangman's fracture of C-2 was demonstrated. Flexion-extension views can be invaluable in demonstrating subtle pathology or in the appropriate clinical setting. In this situation, the patient must move his head himself.

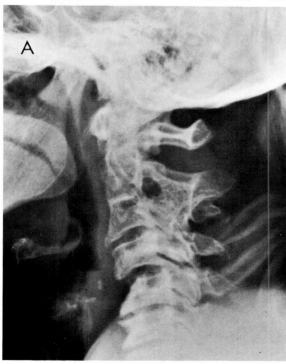

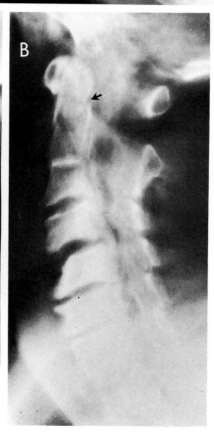

FIG 3–4.
A, brow-up lateral view of cervical spine in a 68-year-old man involved in an accident. Anterior subluxation of C-4 on C-5, no fracture, cervical spondylosis, and congenital fusion of C-2–3 were noted. Patient was neurologically intact. **B,** because of continued pain and subluxation, tomography was performed. Fracture of the odontoid was demonstrated (*arrow*). Tomography is important in cervical spine trauma.

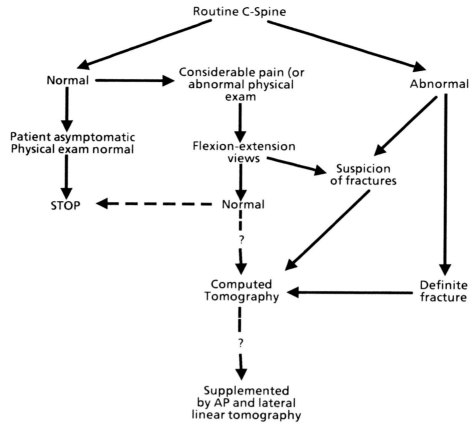

FIG 3–5.
Our approach to the potentially injured cervical spine. Computed tomography is not performed on every patient and has not yet found its true role at our institution. (Modified from Maravilla KR, Cooper PR, Sklar FH: The influence of thin section tomography on the treatment of spine injuries. *Radiology* 1978; 127:131. Used with permission.)

allowing the patient to remain immobilized. These views are particularly good for facet dislocations, but we have not found them particularly useful in identifying pathology not suspected from the brow-up lateral film.

If there is still a high clinical suspicion after these maneuvers or if a fracture or subluxation has been demonstrated, we then recommend high resolution computed tomography. This examination is advantageous because it is quickly performed and the patient may remain immobilized on the table. In addition, it shows soft tissue and potential spinal cord damage as well as bony pathology.[6-8] Although it is sensitive, CT still has certain limitations. It may not show pedicle, lateral mass, pars interarticularis, and mild compression fractures, and if these injuries are suspected clinically, CT may need to be supplemented with linear tomography.[9,10] We still commonly use linear tomography to supplement CT in this setting because subtle minimally displaced fractures can often best be seen by this technique (Fig 3–4).

Magnetic resonance imaging has been used in the acute setting of cervical spine trauma at some institutions.[11,12] Its immediate advantages are not significantly superior of those of CT, and it is more costly and time-consuming. Our experience with MRI in the acute setting is limited. Finally, computerized tomography of the cervical spine has been recommended by some authors in the trauma setting,[7,8] but we believe that all patients should have a routine cervical spine series performed before CT is done (Fig 3–5).

Anatomy

Basic anatomical landmarks (Figs 3–6 to 3–8) should be familiar to most emergency physicians. There are seven cervical vertebrae, all of which are enveloped in a supportive framework of muscles and ligaments. The cervical spine usually has a smooth lordotic curvature. Reversal of this curve may be normal in as many as two persons in ten, and hence is not always pathologic. The basic bony structures of all vertebrae are the body, the pedicles, the transverse processes, the laminae, and the posterior extension of the "posterior elements," the spinous processes. The vertebrae are connected by articular facets to their adjoining superior and inferior vertebral bodies.

In the upper cervical area, the relationship of the atlas (C-1) to the axis (C-2) is unique in that it allows flexion, extension, rotation, gliding, and tilting. The odontoid, a bony extension of the axis through the anterior aspect of the ring of C-1, is frequently and easily injured and should be visualized in all cases of trauma.

The soft tissues anterior to the cervical spine should be evaluated in each case. Normally the soft tissue distance between the anteroinferior aspect of C1–3 and the pharynx should not exceed 7 mm in adults or children. The retrotracheal space (from the anteroinferior aspect of the body of C-6 to the posterior tracheal wall) should not exceed 14 mm in children or 22 mm in adults. Any increase in this distance may indicate unsuspected pathology.[13] Calcifications in this region include the cricoid and thyroid cartilages. Of course, other anatomical areas visualized in the "corners" of the film should always be scrutinized for pathology.

Pathology

A variety of simple and complex injuries occurs in the cervical region. The C1–2 articulation and the C4–T1 region are the two areas most commonly involved, probably because of the unique forces applied to the cervical spine by its support of the calvarium.

Soft tissue changes in the prevertebral region should be evaluated on every series of radiographs. The distance between the anteroinferior aspect of C-3 and the pharynx should not normally exceed 7 mm in the adult or child. However, radiographic technique may affect this relationship as films done at end expiration or with Valsalva maneuver may produce an appearance of prevertebral soft tissue swelling (Fig 3–9). If the technique is acceptable, the prevertebral soft tissues may be secondary to hemorrhage or edema from underlying bony injury (Fig 3–10). However, in our experience, this swelling is not apparent immediately after injury in many cases, but usually occurs later. In the absence of obvious fractures, later development of soft tissue swelling may herald an unsuspected odontoid or other fracture, which may require further diagnostic evaluation and therapy (Fig 3–11).[14]

Reversal of the normal lordotic curve on the lateral cervical spine x-ray has been reported to indicate muscle spasm and possible significant ligament damage. However, one author has reported that this reversal occurs normally in 20% of patients and that, if the chin is merely lowered one inch in the lateral projection, the number of reversed lordotic curves approaches 40% of normal patients.[4] Therefore, be wary of diagnosing muscle spasm with this reversal, and make sure the patient is in a true neutral position when the film is obtained.

Cervical spine fractures can be classified in many different ways. The simplest and most straightforward method, which covers the most common injuries, is to describe the pathology in relation to the

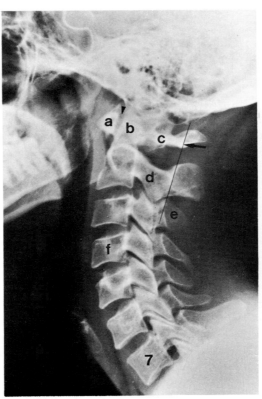

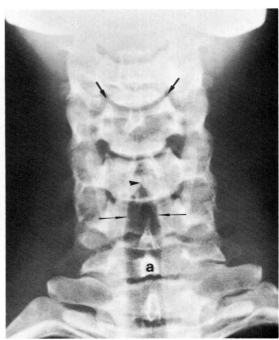

FIG 3–6 (near right).
Normal lateral cervical spine showing C1–7. *a* = anterior arch of C-1, *b* = odontoid, *c* = posterior arch of C-1, *d* = lamina, *e* = spinous process, *f* = vertebral body, *7* = body of C-7. *Arrow* designates posterior cervical line (see text); *arrowhead* indicates distance between anterior arch of C-1 and odontoid.

FIG 3–7 (far right).
Normal AP view of cervical spine. *a* = spinous process of C-7; *long arrows* indicate tracheal air shadow; *arrowhead* indicates glottis; *short arrows* indicate uncinate processes of C-4.

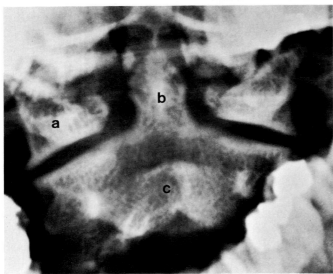

FIG 3–8 (left).
Normal open-mouth odontoid view. *a* = lateral mass of C-1; *b* = odontoid; *c* = body of C-2.

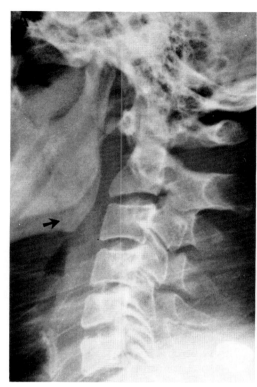

FIG 3–9.
A, lateral C-spine on a 32-year-old hit by car shows apparent prevertebral soft tissue swelling (*arrow*).

B, repeat study with good inspiration shows normal prevertebral tissues (*arrow*). No fractures were identified.

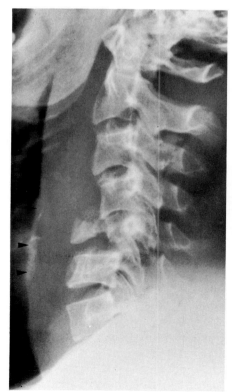

FIG 3–10.
Extensive soft tissue swelling (*arrowheads*) anterior to bursting flexion teardrop in 30-year-old patient who fell with a sudden onset of quadriparesis.

forces required to produce it. Simply, this means two broad categories, flexion and extension injuries. In applying such a classification, the history of the mechanism of trauma is obviously important in predicting likely injuries. If the patient is unconscious and a history is not available, associated clinically obvious fractures may help predict whether the major force was one of flexion or extension. More important, whether a cervical spine injury is *stable* or *unstable* is of the utmost concern. Injuries can be classified as follows (modified from Harris):[15]

> *Stable*
> Anterior subluxation
> Unilateral interfacetal dislocation
> Simple wedge fracture
> Burst fracture, lower cervical spine
> Posterior neural arch fracture, atlas
> Pillar fracture
> Clay shoveler's fracture (if lamina is not involved)
> *Unstable*
> Bilateral interfacetal dislocation
> Flexion teardrop fracture
> Extension teardrop fracture (stable in flexion, unstable in extension)
> Hangman's fracture
> Jefferson fracture of atlas
> Hyperextension of fracture-dislocation
> Clay shoveler's fracture (if lamina is involved)

Regardless of the classification of cervical spine injuries, one point should be stressed. Fractures of the cervical spine are usually not isolated. As many as 67% of obvious injuries will have associated abnormalities. Therefore, if a fracture or subluxation is noted on the plain films, tomography or CT should be performed to demonstrate other possible pathology and the full extent of the visualized plain film finding. Never stop looking after you find one fracture on the routine series (Figs 3–12 to 3–14). Furthermore, if you have an old fracture on the routine series, don't overlook possible new ones in the appropriate clinical setting (Fig 3–15).

Flexion injuries have been classified by Braakman and Penning into distractive and compressive hyperflexion:[16]

> *Distractive hyperflexion injuries*
> Hyperflexion "sprain"
> Unilateral facet dislocation
> Bilateral facet dislocation
> Compressive hyperflexion injuries
> Anterior wedge compression fracture
> Comminuted "teardrop" body fracture

In distractive hyperflexion injuries, the primary source is deceleration, with pulling on the cervical spine and possible distraction or separation of the vertebral elements. Forces are expended first along the posterior ligaments, then along the interspinous ligaments, next along the facet joint capsules themselves.

The hyperflexion "sprain" occurs when moderate force is applied to the posterior ligaments with incomplete interspinous ligament tearing. The neutral lateral cervical spine film is normal in most of these cases, and flexion-extension views may be required to make the diagnosis. On flexion, the spinous processes separate or "fan," indicating interspinous ligament disruption (Fig 3–16). These injuries should be followed closely.

Unilateral or bilateral facet dislocation is usually obvious radiographically. Unilateral dislocation can be diagnosed by malalignment of the spinous processes above the site of injury on the AP view and by displacement of less than 50% of one vertebral body on another on the lateral view (Fig 3–17). Bilateral dislocation occurs with significant flexion forces and usually results in "locked facets," which are manifested by greater than 50% displacement of one cervical body on another.[17]

With compressive hyperflexion injuries, axial compressive forces combine with flexion to damage the vertebral bodies. If the predominant force acts at the anterior aspect of the body, it produces a wedge compression fracture (Fig 3–18). If the posterior elements are intact, this fracture is stable. If the posterior elements are injured, this fracture is unstable. Teardrop fractures typically involve a comminuted fracture of the body and are usually obvious radiographically. However, the more important second component of this injury may involve a portion of the body being driven posteriorly into the spinal canal, with resulting cord damage. This complication should be looked for in all teardrop injuries (see Fig 3–10).

Extension injuries are less common, yet potentially just as severe, as flexion injuries. Severe hyperextension trauma may produce rupture of the anterior longitudinal ligament, inward bulging of the ligamentum flavum, or extrusion of the intervertebral disk, all of which have severe neurologic consequences.

Extension injuries may be categorized according to disruptive or compressive sequelae, as described by Burke.[18]

> *Disruptive hyperextension*
> Normal x-ray
> Anteroinferior marginal fracture (often C-2)
> *Compressive hyperextension injuries*
> Hangman's fracture
> Forward displacement with compression of posterior elements

Disruptive hyperextension apparently produces

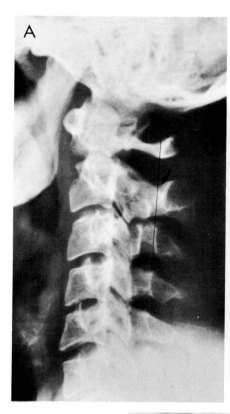

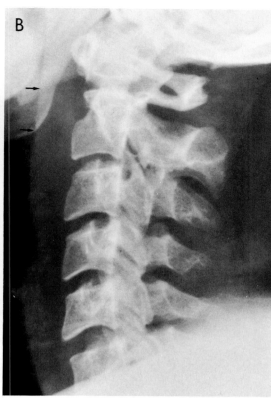

FIG 3–11.
A, lateral cervical spine of 26-year-old man in auto accident was originally read as normal, but posterior cervical line is abnormal (*arrow*). **B,** lateral cervical spine radiograph done 4 days later shows marked soft tissue swelling in prevertebral region (*arrows*).

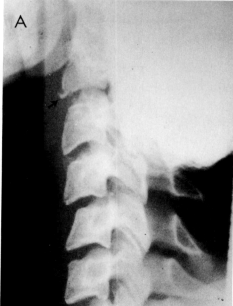

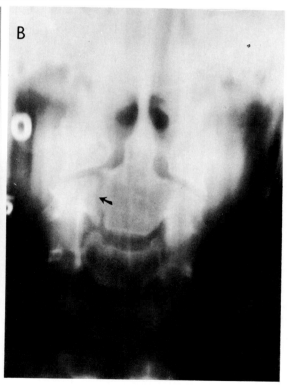

FIG 3–12.
A, neutral lateral cervical spine of 17-year-old in auto accident shows small chip fracture off anterior inferior surface of C-2 (*arrow*) and 4 mm of anterior subluxation of C-4 on C-5. **B,** tomography revealed four other fractures, including this linear fracture through the body of C-2. Tomography can show more extensive fractures than those suspected from the plain films.

FIG 3–13.
A, lateral C-spine on a 23-year-old in automobile accident shows C6–7 decreased disc space and 2 mm of anterior subluxation of C-6 on C-7 (*arrow*). **B,** CT shows multiple laminar fractures of C-5 and C-6 (*arrows*).

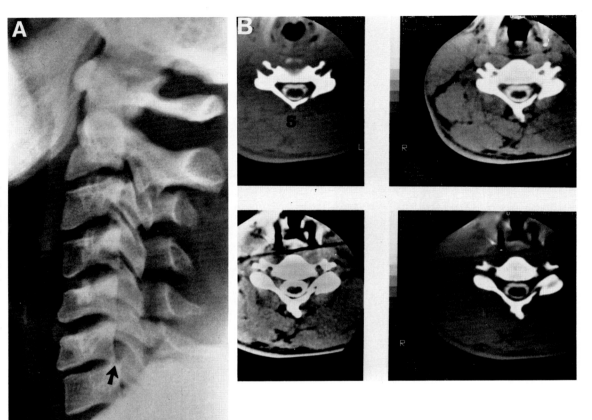

FIG 3–14.
A, lateral C-spine view of a 38-year-old involved in motor accident shows C-5 spinous process fracture (*arrow*) with minimal anterior subluxation and joint space narrowing of C4–5. **B,** single slice from CT shows multiple fractures of C-4 not recognized on the plain film (*arrows*). CT is the definitive study at present in the evaluation of spine trauma.

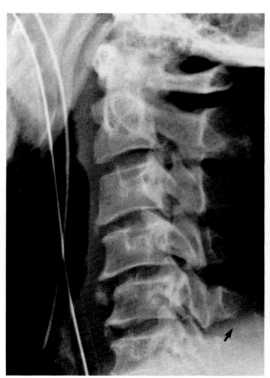

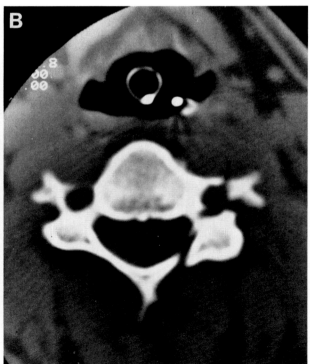

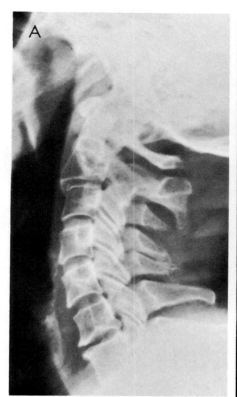

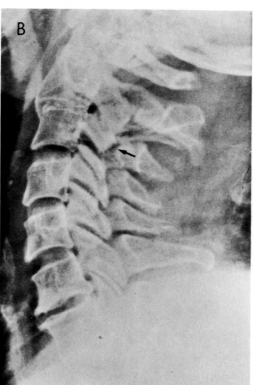

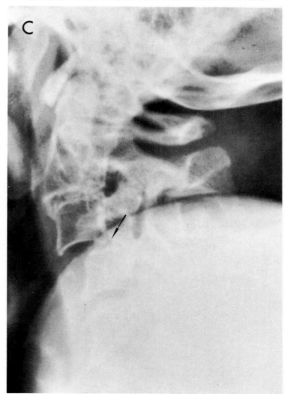

FIG 3-15.
A, lateral cervical spine in 54-year-old patient shows old healed fracture of C-2. **B,** lateral cervical spine of same patient 4 years later, after he sustained a fall with central cord syndrome. No fractures were seen on this view. *Arrow* denotes fractures through the lamina previously overlooked. **C,** coned-down view of lateral cervical spine done 3 days later shows marked anterior subluxation of C-3 on C-4 (*arrow*). Old trauma should not keep one from recognizing new injuries.

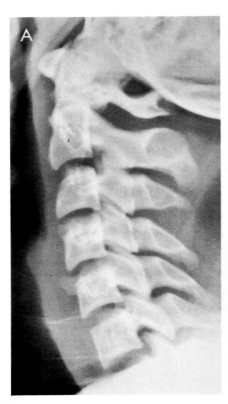 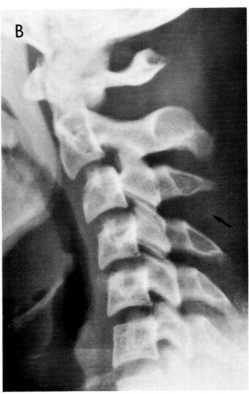

FIG 3–16 (top left and right).
A, lateral cervical spine of 25-year-old man in auto accident with loss of consciousness appears normal. **B,** flexion view with the patient moving himself shows "fanning" of the spinous processes between C-3 and C-4 and minimal subluxation at this level (*arrow*). Flexion-extension views may be important in delineating pathology not seen on the plain films. Furthermore, with this injury, if the patient is not treated, permanent subluxation and deformity of the neck may occur later.

FIG 3–17 (right).
Lateral cervical spine of 15-year-old injured in auto accident shows anterior subluxation of C-4 on C-5 of less than 50% of the vertebral width. Further examination revealed a unilateral locked facet at this level (*arrow*).

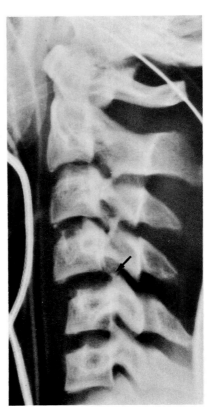

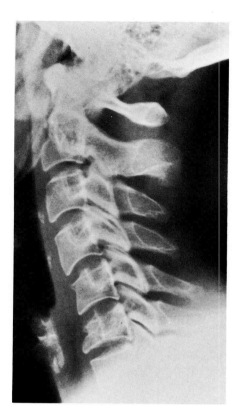

FIG 3–18 (left).
Lateral cervical spine of 40-year-old patient shows mild compression of C-5 and marked wedge compression of C-6. Tomography did not reveal any involvement of the posterior elements.

FIG 3–19 (right).
Lateral cervical spine of 30-year-old man injured in motorcycle accident with loss of consciousness shows a typical hangman's fracture *(arrow)*. Also note that the posterior cervical line is abnormal *(arrowhead)*.

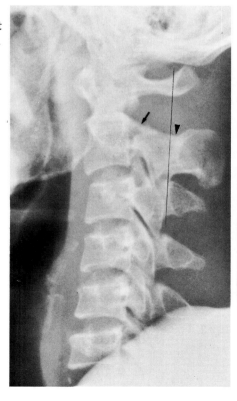

FIG 3–20.
A, lateral C-spine shows marked prevertebral soft tissue swelling and widening of the distance between the anterior arch of C-1 and the odontoid. Congenital fusion of C-2 and C-3 is also noted. **B,** AP view shows offset of left lateral mass C-1 in relation to C-2 (*arrow*). **C,** CT shows multiple fractures of the ring of C-1.

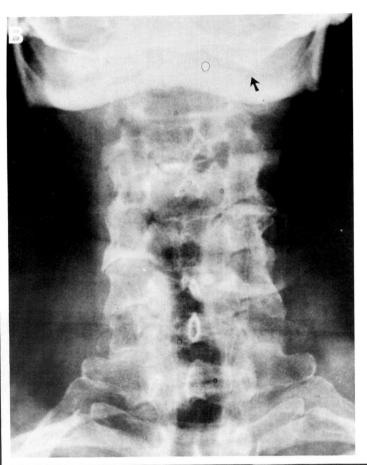

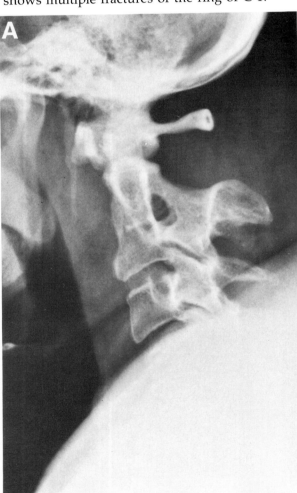

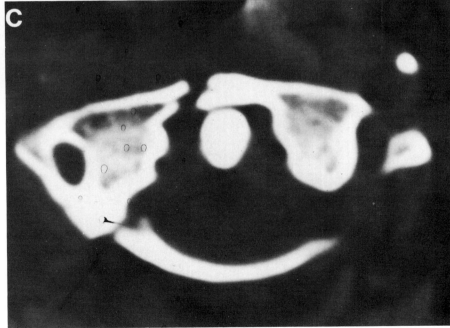

FIG 3–21.
A, open-mouth odontoid view of 20-year-old injured in motor-cycle accident with loss of consciousness shows posterior displacement of both lateral masses of C-1 on C-2 (*arrows*). **B,** lateral film shows fracture of the posterior arch of C-1. **C,** computerized tomographic scan shows multiple fractures of the "ring" of C-1. (Courtesy of Dr Anne Brower, Uniformed Services University, Bethesda, Md.)

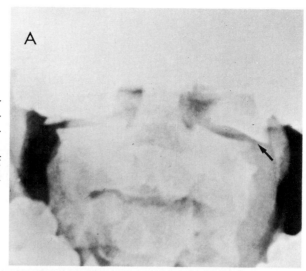

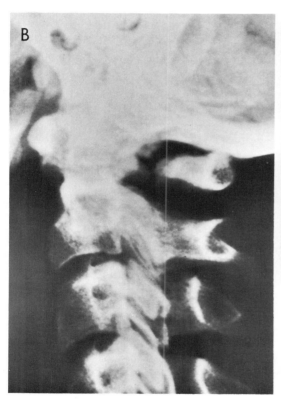

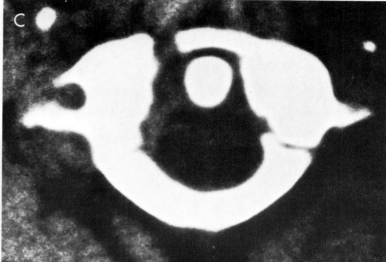

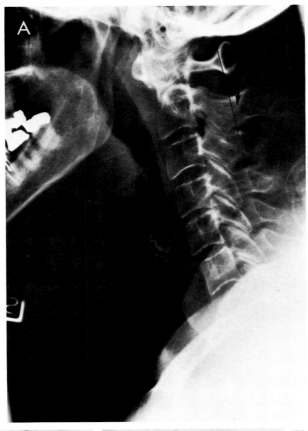

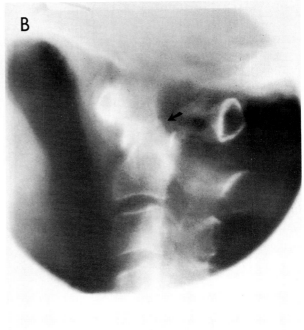

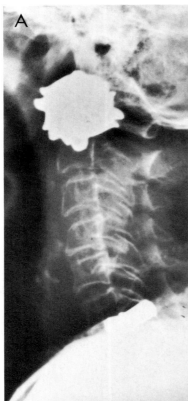

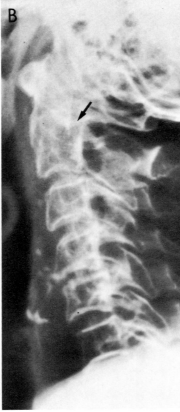

FIG 3–22 (top).
A, neutral lateral cervical spine of 40-year-old involved in automobile accident with loss of consciousness. The anterior cortical margin of the spinous process of C-2 is displaced behind the posterior cervical line more than 2 mm *(arrow).* **B,** tomography of upper cervical spine shows displaced fracture of the odontoid *(arrow).* The posterior cervical line can be helpful in odontoid fractures.

FIG 3–23 (left).
A, lateral cervical spine in the neutral position with earring overlying the odontoid. The posterior cervical line is abnormal. **B,** repeat film with the earring removed shows the fractured odontoid *(arrow).*

FIG 3–24.
A, lateral cervical spine in flexion on 12-year-old child shows pseudosubluxation of C-2 on C-3 *(arrow).* Note that the posterior cervical line is normal. Incidentally, note the unfused posterior arch of C-1. **B,** extension view, same patient, shows normal vertebral alignment. Pseudosubluxation of C-2 on C-3 should not be confused with acute traumatic injuries in the pediatric age group.

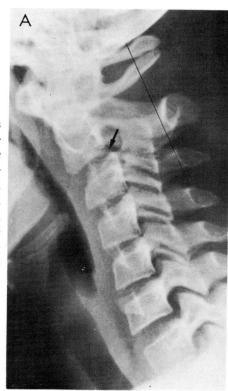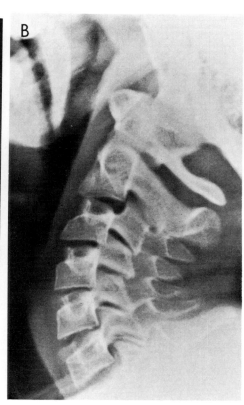

FIG 3–25.
A, neutral lateral cervical spine of 27-year-old involved in automobile accident. An os odontoideum is noted superior to the anterior arch of C-1. **B,** tomography confirms the presence of the os odontoideum. This is developmental in origin or related to old trauma. It should not be confused with an acute fracture.

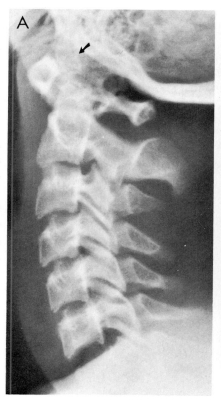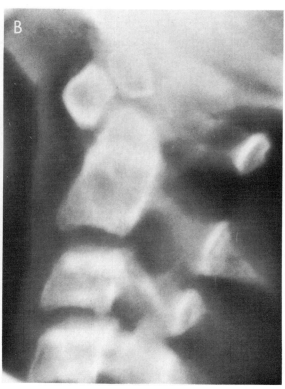

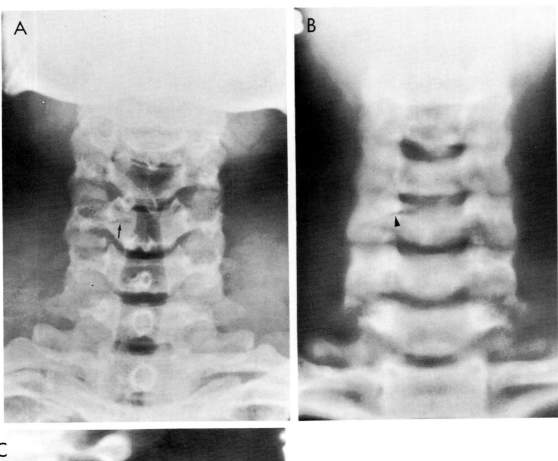

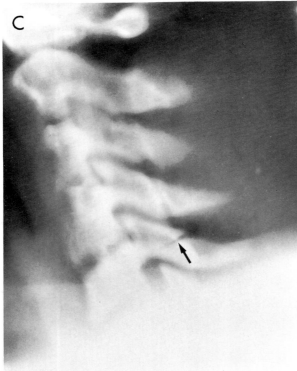

FIG 3–26.
A, AP view of cervical spine of 40-year-old involved in motorcycle accident. Lucent line superimposed on the body of C-5 *(arrow)* prompted further diagnostic study. **B,** tomography confirms fracture through the lamina of C-5 *(arrowhead).* **C,** lateral tomogram shows the lamina fracture to better advantage *(arrow).*

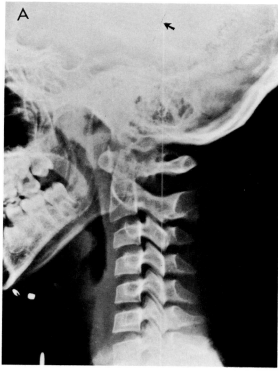

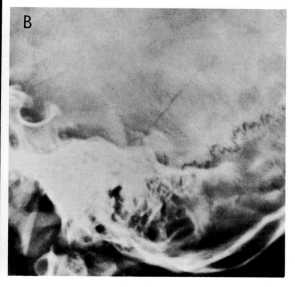

FIG 3–27.
A, lateral view of cervical spine of a 12-year-old child hit by a truck. The spine is normal. Note, however, the unsuspected parietal skull fracture lurking in corner *(arrow)* (retouched for detail). **B,** lateral view of skull confirms presence of fracture. Always look for "corner clues."

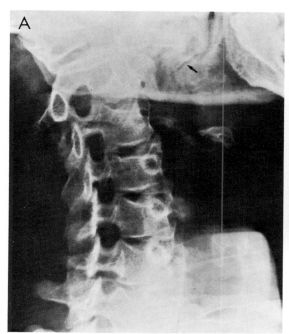

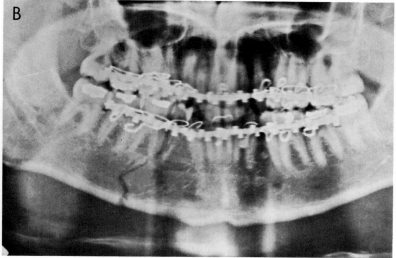

FIG 3–28.
A, oblique view of cervical spine in 28-year-old patient with closed head injury. Cervical spine is normal, but clinically unsuspected fracture of the mandible was initially missed *(arrow).* **B,** Panorex confirms "corner" fracture.

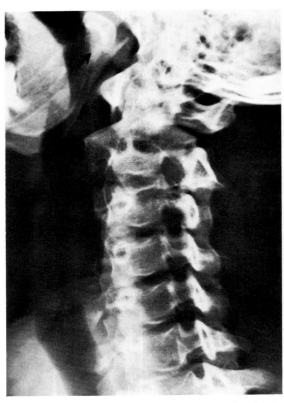

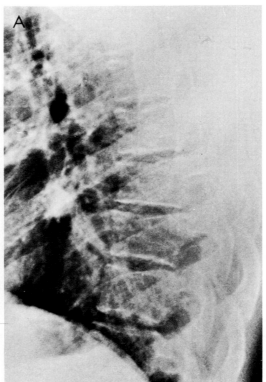

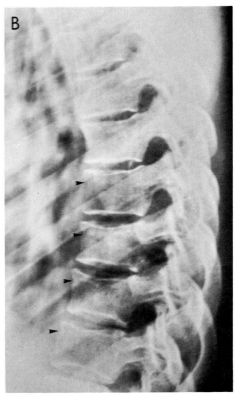

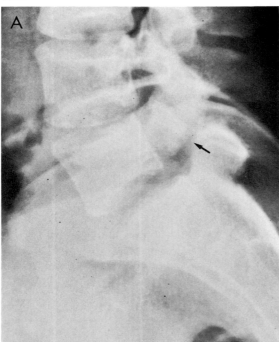

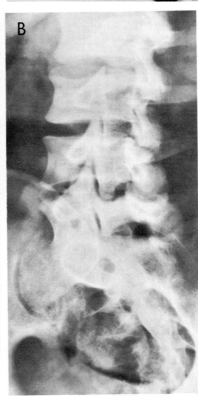

FIG 3–29 (top left).
Oblique view of cervical spine in patient injured in automobile accident shows a fracture of the mandibular condyle (*arrow*) unsuspected before this film was obtained.

FIG 3–30 (top middle and right).
A, lateral thoracic spine of middle-aged female who fell. Much of the bony detail is obliterated by overlying shadows. **B,** long exposure made during quiet breathing shows compression fractures not seen on the initial lateral film. Quiet breathing gives a tomographic effect and enhances bony detail.

FIG 3–31 (bottom left).
A, lower lumbar spine of an 18-year-old with back pain shows spondylolysis (*arrow*) and grade I spondylolisthesis of L-5 on S-1. **B,** oblique film, same patient, shows no apparent spondylolysis. Most instances of spondylolysis may be diagnosed from the lateral view of the lumbar spine.

damage by compressing the spinal cord between the ligamentum flavum and the intervertebral disk; plain films show an apparently "normal" cervical spine. In certain cases, marked soft tissue swelling will be present, and extension views will confirm the diagnosis. This injury is stable in flexion and unstable in extension.

The hangman's fracture is a bilateral pedicle break limited to the axis and resembling the injuries formerly inflicted by judicial hanging (Figs 3–3 and 3–19).

Injuries in the area of the C1–2 articulation deserve special attention. The Jefferson bursting fracture, an unusual injury resulting from a downward axial loading on the spine, is by definition a bilateral fracture of the anterior and posterior arches of the atlas. Its radiographic appearance consists of lateral displacement of both the articular masses of C-1 in the open-mouth odontoid view (Figs 3–20 and 3–21). Fractures of the odontoid may be notoriously difficult to demonstrate. In such injuries, attention should be paid to the posterior cervical line drawn between the anterior cortical margins of the spinous processes of C-1 to C-3. Normally, the anterior cortical margin of C-2 is within 1 mm to 1.5 mm of this line.[19] Displacement greater than 2 mm may indicate odontoid injuries, hangman's fracture, or posterior element pathology (Figs 3–22 and 3–23). It should be remembered that, in children and young adults, there may normally be anterior subluxation of C-2 on C-3.[19,20] This has been termed "physiologic pseudosubluxation of C-2" and should not be mistaken for traumatic injury (Fig 3–24). In these cases, the posterior cervical line will also be normal. Of course, the os odontoideum, a separate ossification center of the odontoid, or an old traumatic odontoid injury should not be confused with a recent fracture (Fig 3–25).

Finally, all the information available on the film should be used. Small fractures without dislocation are frequently difficult to identify. Any suspicious areas should be examined with linear tomography (Fig 3–26) and supplemented by CT as necessary. Clinically unsuspected injuries on the periphery of the film may be diagnosed if a determined effort is made to look for what we call "corner clues" (Figs 3–27 to 3–29).

The Thoracolumbar Spine

Radiographs of the thoracic and lumbar spine are commonly obtained in the emergency setting. The most common symptom that prompts the clinician to order a radiograph is low back pain. It has been reported that clinicians overuse lumbar spine films since, in one study, 46% of these films were absolutely normal.[21] It is possible that, with good physical examination, this figure could be lowered. Of course, other considerations are radiation dose and costs to patients. Lumbar spine films deliver large radiation exposures and cost about $500 million annually. Hence, all emergency room physicians should weigh the possible yield of the examination against the potential risks and costs. Only in this way can the diagnostic yield be increased and unnecessary patient radiation and costs reduced.

Techniques

As with suspected cervical spine injuries, patients with presumed thoracolumbar traumatic pathology are usually immobilized upon arrival at the emergency room. The most informative radiograph in both areas is the cross-table lateral view obtained without moving the patient.

For the thoracic film, a long exposure is used and the patient should breathe quietly. This gives a tomographic effect and helps eradicate some of the overlying rib and soft tissue shadows that may make interpretation difficult (Fig 3–30). We then obtain a standard well-collimated AP view to complete the study. The upper and lower extents of the thoracic vertebrae region should be included, especially if the clinical findings point to one of these areas. As mentioned in the cervical spine section, the swimmer's view can be helpful in demonstrating the upper thoracic and lower cervical spine.

The cross-table lateral lumbar film is taken with a long (11 in. by 17 in.) film and includes the lower thoracic vertebrae. Pain from a lower thoracic injury may be referred to the lumbar or sacral area and mimic lumbar spine pathology. Therefore, we try to see at least up to T-10 on every lumbar spine series done for trauma. If this view shows no obvious abnormality, an AP film is taken. This is our standard series and is usually sufficient.

If ligament injury is suspected, flexion-extension views may be indicated. However, their yield is low. Some authorities recommend oblique views to check for spondylolysis. In our experience, however, the spondylolysis and resulting spondylolisthesis are usually seen on the standard lateral view. We have seen a few cases where spondylolysis was seen on the lateral view, but was not confirmed by the obliques (Fig 3–31).

As in all traumatic injuries, one obvious fracture may have associated pathology, and tomography is often needed to delineate the true extent of such le-

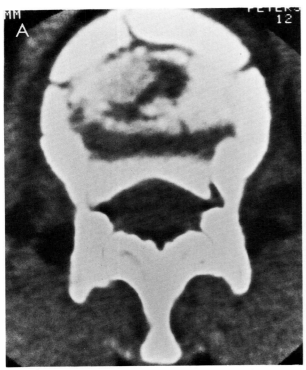

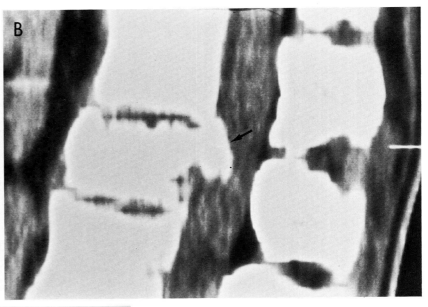

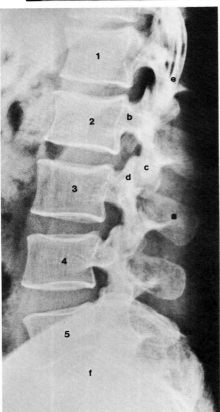

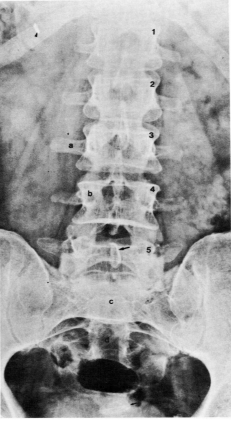

FIG 3–32 (top).
A, computerized tomographic cut from middle-aged patient with multiple trauma shows multiple fractures through the body and neural arch. **B,** sagittal reconstruction of this image shows a large bony extrusion into the spinal canal *(arrow)*. CT may be very helpful in determining bony extension. (Courtesy of Dr Victor Haughton, Medical College of Wisconsin, Milwaukee, Wisc.)

FIG 3–33 (bottom left).
Normal lateral lumbar spine. *a* = spinous process of L-3; *b* = pedicle of L-2; *c* = inferior articular facet of L-2; *d* = superior articular facet of L-3, *e* = T-12 rib; *f* = sacrum. Lumbar vertebrae 1 through 5 are numbered.

FIG 3–34 (bottom right).
Normal AP view of lumbar spine. *a* = spinous process of L-3, *b* = pedicle of L-4, *c* = sacrum, *d* = remainder of sacral complex. *Small arrow* indicates coccyx; *larger arrow* indicates spinous process of L-5. *Arrowhead* shows metallic density in right upper quadrant of abdomen. The lumbar vertebrae are numbered.

FIG 3–35.
A, supine chest x-ray of 25-year-old male injured in automobile accident shows marked bilateral paravertebral swelling in mid-thoracic region *(arrowheads).* **B,** lateral view of thoracic spine shows marked compression of a mid-dorsal vertebra *(arrow).* Paravertebral soft tissue swelling may be the only indication of a thoracic fracture.

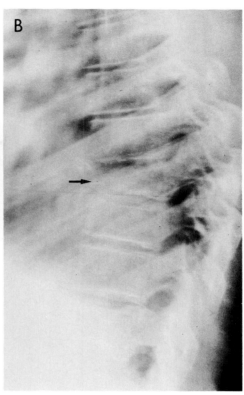

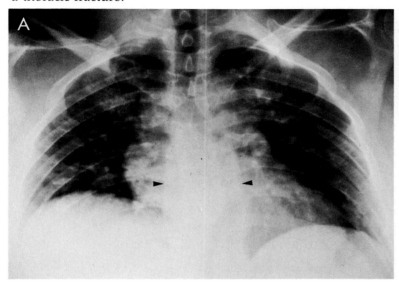

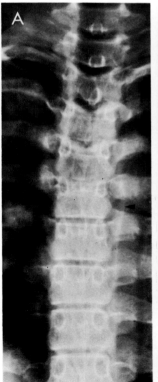
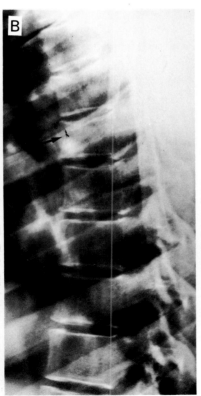
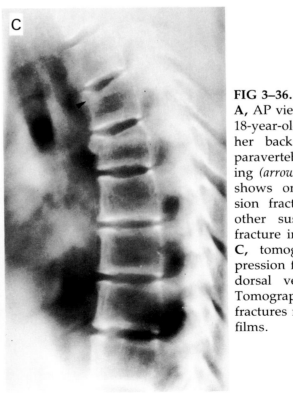

FIG 3–36.
A, AP view of thoracic spine of 18-year-old female who fell on her back. There is minimal paravertebral soft tissue swelling *(arrowhead).* **B,** lateral view shows one definite compression fracture *(arrow)* and another suspected compression fracture in the vertebra above. **C,** tomogram confirms compression fractures of both mid-dorsal vertebrae *(arrowheads).* Tomography may delineate fractures not apparent on plain films.

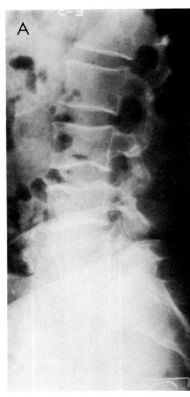
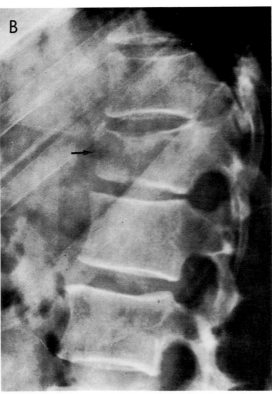

FIG 3–37.
A, lateral lumbar spine of 48-year-old man with acute flexion injury. Highest level seen is the upper aspect of L-1. **B,** close-up lateral view of thoracolumbar spine shows compression fracture of T-12. Thoracic spine injury may present as pain referred to lumbar area. Using longer film (11 in. × 17 in.) and making sure the lower dorsal vertebrae are seen can help eliminate such mistakes.

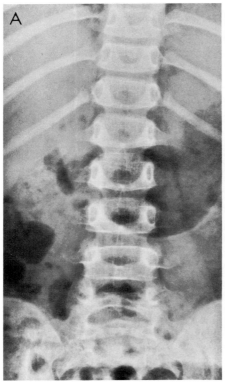
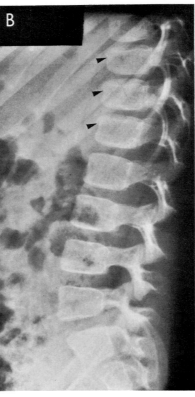

FIG 3–38.
Young child with injury and pain in lower lumbar region. **A,** AP view of thoracolumbar spine shows no fracture or paraspinal soft tissue swelling. **B,** lateral thoracolumbar spine shows at least three compression fractures of T-11, T-12, and L-1 *(arrowheads).* These were originally missed.

FIG 3–39.
A, lateral thoracic spine of young patient injured in automobile accident was read as normal. **B,** lateral lumbar spine shows compression fracture of L-1 *(arrow).* Patients with apparent thoracic pain may have lumbar spine injuries.

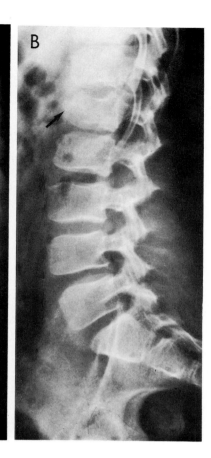

FIG 3–40.
A, lateral lumbar spine of 17-year-old patient injured in motorcycle accident shows a comminuted compression fracture of L-2. **B,** tomogram shows a large bony fragment in the spinal canal *(arrows).* Tomography may be helpful in delineating the full extent of such injuries.

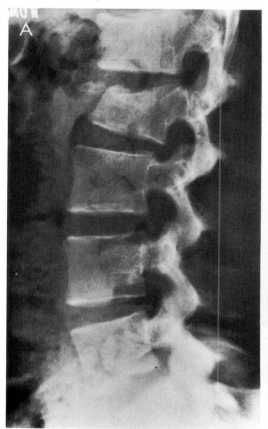

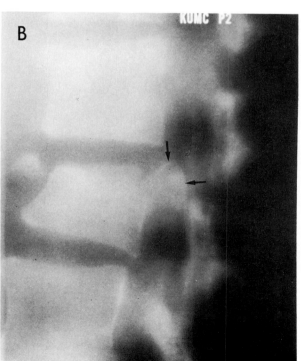

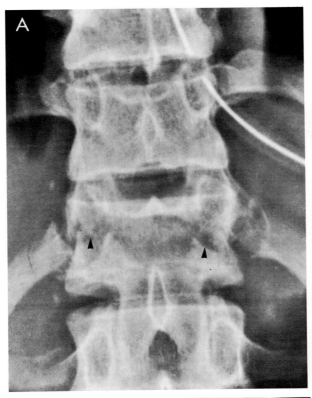

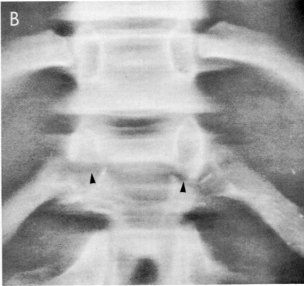

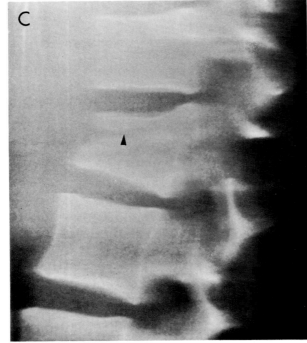

FIG 3–41.
A, coned-down AP view of lower thoracic spine of 28-year-old injured in automobile accident shows a fracture line through the body of T-12 *(arrowheads).* **B,** tomographic cut in the AP projection shows the previously described fracture line extending through both pedicles *(arrowheads).* **C,** lateral tomogram shows to better advantage the fracture line extending throughout the body of T-12 *(arrowhead)* and through the spinous process. The Chance fracture is unstable and should be treated accordingly.

FIG 3–42.

A, AP view, of lower lumbar spine of 48-year-old female after a motor vehicle accident shows marked separation of the spinous processes of L-3 and L-4 *(arrows* lie beside spinous processes). **B,** lateral lumbar spine, same patient, shows compression of L-4 *(long arrow),* separation of the articular facets at L-3 and L-4 *(short arrow),* and widening of the spinous processes *(arrowheads).* Widened spinous processes on the AP film can suggest serious pathology.

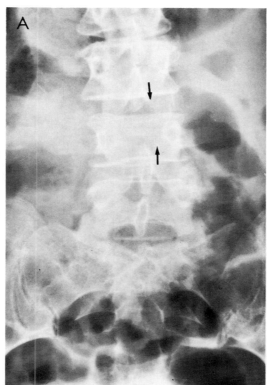

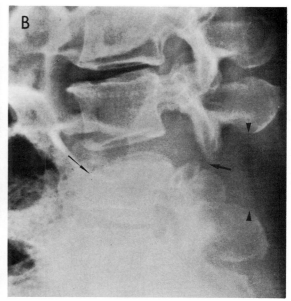

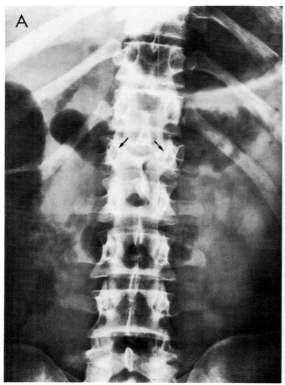

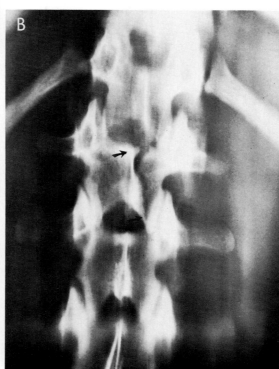

FIG 3–43.

AP view of lower thoracic and lumbar spine of a 19-year-old who fell from a bridge shows widening of the interpedicular distance at L-1 *(arrows).* **B,** AP tomogram shows fracture through the posterior elements of this vertebra *(arrows).* Widening of the interpedicular distance should always be looked for on the AP film.

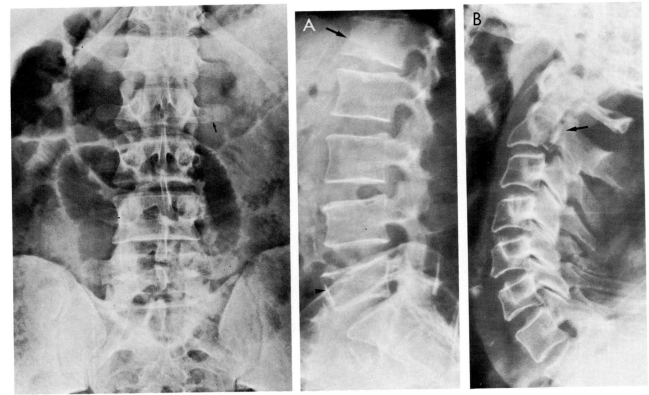

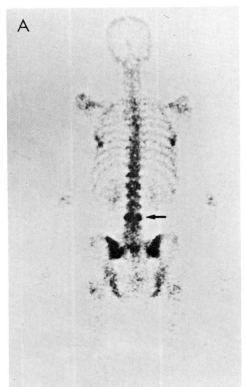

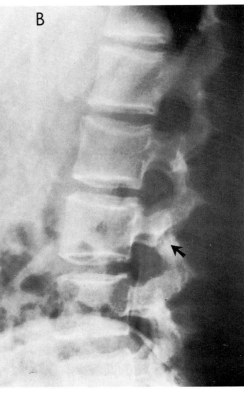

FIG 3–44 (top left).
AP view of lumbar spine of 34-year-old patient thrown from a car shows localized small bowel ileus. Fracture of transverse process of L-2 *(arrow)* was initially missed. Localized ileus can be a secondary sign of bony trauma.

FIG 3–45 (top middle and right).
A, lateral lumbar spine of 65-year-old patient in automobile accident shows compression fracture of L-1 *(arrow)* and compression of L-5 *(arrowhead)*. **B,** cervical spine, same patient, shows hangman's fracture. A thoracic spine fracture (not shown) was also present. When one fracture is found, others should be looked for assiduously.

FIG 3–46 (bottom left).
A, posterior view of nuclear bone scan of 16-year-old patient who fell on ice 10 months earlier shows "hot" spot at L-3. **B,** lateral view of lumbar spine, taken 1 week before nuclear scan, was initially read as normal. Review of the radiograph after nuclear scan revealed spondylolysis *(arrow)*. In certain patients, special studies may be required to delineate subtle pathology.

FIG 3–47 (top near right).
AP view of thoracic spine of 18-year-old patient involved in automobile accident. Fractures of posterior aspects of 8th, 9th, and 10th ribs were best seen on this film *(arrows)*. In trauma cases always look at all of the information provided on films.

FIG 3–48 (top far right).
Lateral thoracic spine of young patient involved in automobile accident. The thoracic spine is normal, but a clinically unsuspected sternal fracture was seen on this view *(arrow)*.

FIG 3–49 (bottom left).
Lateral lumbar spine of 26-year-old patient injured in automobile accident. The fracture of T-11 *(arrowhead)* was initially missed because it was hidden under the top of the viewbox. Always use all of the information provided on the films.

FIG 3–50 (bottom middle and right).
A, lateral cervical spine of elderly man with diffuse idiopathic skeletal hyperostosis and marked osteophytic changes, particularly at the C-6–7 region. The patient presented with dysphagia. **B,** barium swallow shows compression of the esophagus from the marked osteophyte formation at this level.

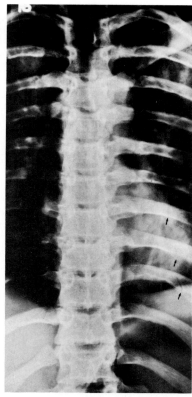
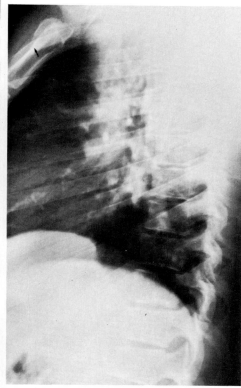
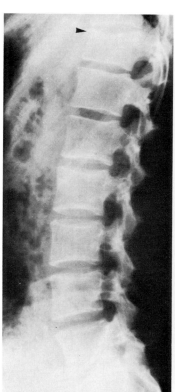
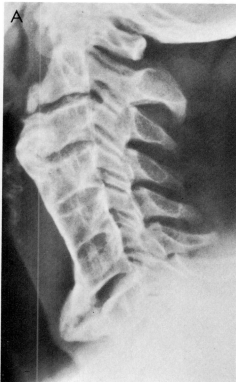
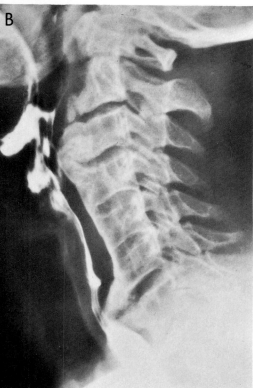

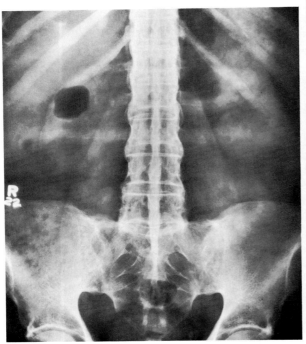

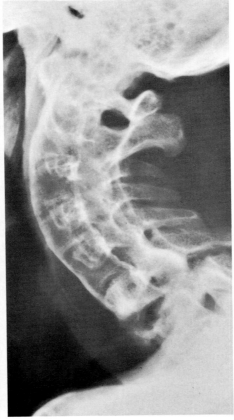

FIG 3–51 (top far left).
AP view of lumbar spine of man with 6-month history of back pain shows "bamboo" spine and ankylosis of both sacroiliac joints, characteristic of ankylosing spondylitis.

FIG 3–52 (top near left).
Lateral cervical spine of patient with known ankylosing spondylitis injured in automobile accident. Fracture through C-6–7 is demonstrated. Patients with ankylosing spondylitis have very brittle bones with characteristic fractures.

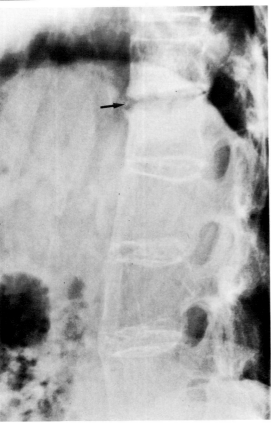

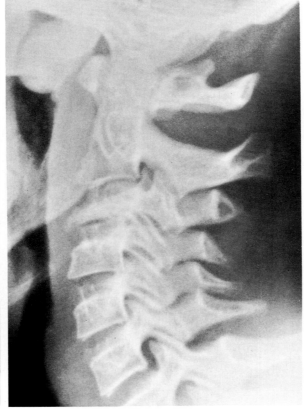

FIG 3–53 (bottom far left).
Lower thoracic spine of patient with known ankylosing spondylitis shows pseudarthrosis of T-11–12 *(arrow)* following a traumatic episode months earlier.

FIG 3–54 (bottom near left).
Lateral cervical spine of 11-year-old patient shows vertebra plana at C-3. The patient had known eosinophilic granuloma.

FIG 3–55.

A, lateral cervical spine of 50-year-old patient shows a small bony chip at the anterior aspect of C-5. This was read by the radiology department as degenerative change and by the orthopedic resident as an acute fracture. The patient was placed in tongs. **B,** lateral cervical spine tomography in same patient shows that the previously described bony chip was a degenerative osteophyte. Degenerative disease should not be mistaken for acute trauma.

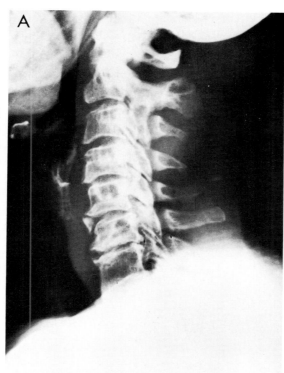
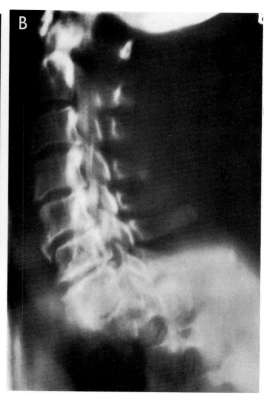

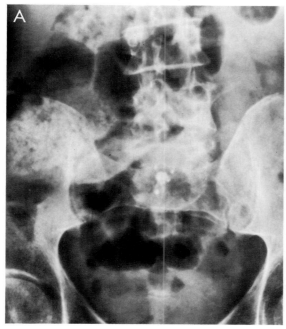
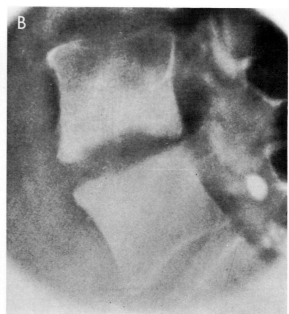

FIG 3–56.

A, AP view of lumbar spine of 60-year-old man after laminectomy at L4–5. Myelographic contrast is noted in the lower caudal sac. There is also loss of vertebral height of L-4. **B,** lateral lumbar spine, same patient, shows marked sclerosis at the end plates of L-4 and L-5 with bone destruction. This is characteristic of disk space infections.

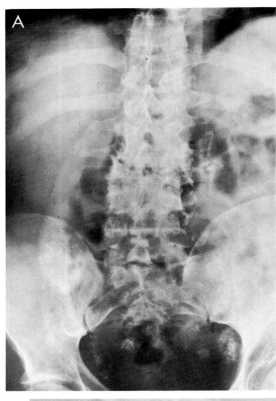

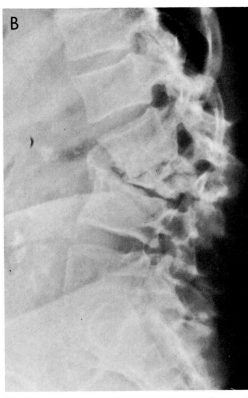

FIG 3–57 (top left).
A, AP view of lumbar spine of 37-year-old with a history of tuberculosis and back pain shows extensive bony destruction of L-2 and L-3, with marked adjacent soft tissue calcifications. **B,** lateral lumbar spine, same patient, shows characteristic ''gibbous'' deformity associated with tuberculosis.

FIG 3–58 (bottom left and middle).
A, coned-down AP view of thoracolumbar spine in 40-year-old with back pain shows some loss of joint space and paravertebral calcification at the L-1–2 interspace *(arrow).* **B,** lateral lumbar spine, same patient, shows bony destruction *(arrow).* This area showed tuberculosis on culture.

FIG 3–59 (bottom right).
Lateral lumbar spine of 29-year-old with known sickle cell disease (SC trait) shows the characteristic H-shaped vertebrae.

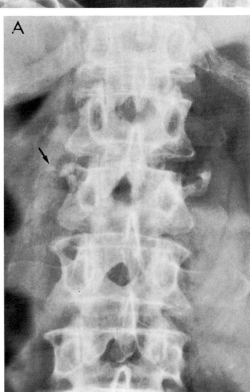

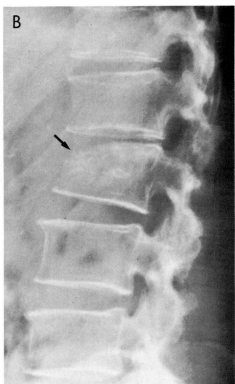

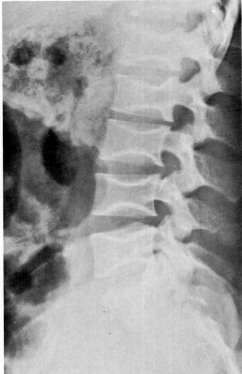

FIG 3–60 (top right).
AP pelvis and lower lumbar spine view of 75-year-old man with known prostatic carcinoma shows diffuse metastases, including marked sclerosis of L-2 *(arrowheads)*. This bony sclerosis is characteristic of metastatic prostatic carcinoma.

FIG 3–61 (bottom left and middle).
A, AP view of thoracolumbar spine in 54-year-old woman with known breast cancer shows marked paravertebral soft tissue swelling *(arrow)*, as well as loss of a pedicle at this mid-dorsal vertebra *(arrowhead)*. **B,** myelogram performed on this patient shows marked extradural compression on the subarachnoid space at this level *(arrowheads)*. At surgery, this proved to be extradural metastases from a breast carcinoma.

FIG 3–62 (bottom right).
Lateral lumbar spine of patient with known Paget's disease shows some compression of L-1. There was no history of recent trauma and this appearance should not be mistaken for acute pathology.

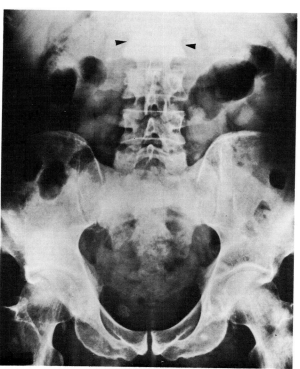

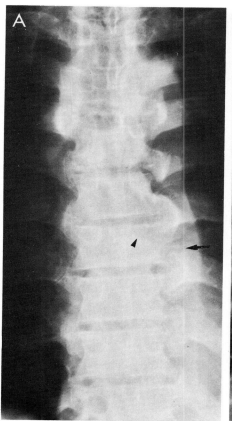

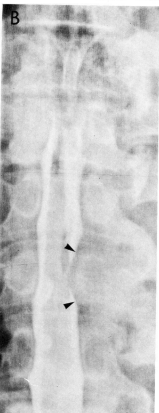

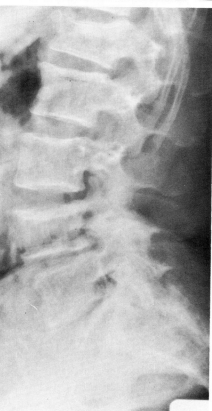

sions. Computed tomography may also prove helpful in such cases, especially if there is a question of bony extension into the spinal canal (Fig 3–32).[6–8] Finally, in some cases, nuclear bone scanning may show a cause for clinical symptoms when plain films are unrevealing.

Anatomy

The anatomy of both the thoracic and the lumbar spine is straightforward, and the basic framework of the vertebrae is very similar to that of C3–7. The anatomy of the lumbar spine is shown in Figures 3–33 and 3–34.

Pathology

Injuries to the thoracic region may first be noticed on a supine chest x-ray. Paravertebral soft tissue swelling is a reliable secondary sign of hemorrhage, edema, or infection adjacent to the thoracic spine (Fig 3–35). However, it should not be relied upon totally, as there can be multiple fractures with minimal soft tissue changes. Of course, if a fracture is identified, other associated injuries should be suspected. Tomography may also help delineate subtle abnormalities not suspected on the routine AP and lateral films (Fig 3–36).

Use of the long film for the lateral view on many occasions has proved helpful in diagnosing thoracic compression fracture causing referred lower back pain in adults and children (Figs 3–37 and 3–38). Likewise, in patients with pain in the thoracic region, always include the upper lumbar spine (Fig 3–39). In patients with severe injuries, the possibility of bony fragments extending into the canal should always be kept in mind. Computed tomography is the best second diagnostic exam to perform, but linear tomography, as with the cervical spine, can be supplemental (Fig 3–40).

The Chance fracture, or seatbelt injury, deserves special attention.[22] This injury involves horizontal fractures through the vertebral body and the posterior elements, including the spinous process (Fig 3–41). This is an unstable injury and should be treated immediately. Another unstable injury is the fracture-dislocation. Ligamentous disruption should be sought carefully and is manifest on the AP radiograph by a gap in the spinous processes (Fig 3–42). Widening of the interpedicular distance on the AP view also indicates a disruption of the neural arch making up the posterior elements. This fracture is unstable and is therefore important to recognize (Fig 3–43). Transverse process fractures, commonly overlooked, can

also be diagnosed on this view. They are usually associated with a localized ileus and may cause retroperitoneal hemorrhage (Fig 3–44).

In the spine, multiple injuries may present a diagnostic challenge. Therefore, whenever a fracture is seen, others should be diligently sought (Fig 3–45).

Of course, there may be situations where plain films and tomograms are negative and high clinical suspicion of pathology remains. In such circumstances, nuclear bone scanning may prove beneficial (Fig 3–46).

The corners of the film may also hide unsuspected pathology. Rib fractures can be seen on the AP view of the thoracolumbar spine (Fig 3–47). Fractures of the sternum can be detected on lateral thoracic spine views (Fig 3–48). Finally, the pathology may be hidden by the radiology view box (Fig 3–49). Always be on the lookout for these "corner clues."

Remember that all spine pain in the emergency setting is not secondary to fractures or dislocations. Always look for evidence of other disease. For example, extensive degenerative disease in the cervical region is one cause of such pain or dysphagia (Fig 3–50). Ankylosing spondylitis, a cause of spine pain, has a characteristic radiographic appearance (Fig 3–51). These patients may present in the trauma setting with unusual fractures (Fig 3–52), and these injuries may also develop into pseudoarthrosis (Fig 3–53).

Although most commonly involving the thoracic region, eosinophilic granuloma with its "vertebra plana" can affect any region and cause pain (Fig 3–54). Degenerative disease in any region may mimic pathology. Its presence should not be misinterpreted as acute disease (Fig 3–55).

Infections involving the spine are not uncommon in the emergency setting. Bacterial infection involving the vertebrae is usually manifest by destruction of bone and cartilage (Fig 3–56). Tuberculosis of the spine, an indolent chronic disease, can be quite blatent producing the so-called gibbous deformity (Fig 3–57), or it may be subtle and more difficult to diagnose (Fig 3–58).

Hematologic diseases such as sickle cell trait or sickle cell disease may also cause back pain. The characteristic infolding of the vertebral endplates, or H-shaped vertebrae, should not be overlooked (Fig 3–59).

And finally, the spine is a favorite site for metastatic spread, particularly from prostate (Fig 3–60) and breast (Fig 3–61) carcinomas. Of course, as in the pelvis, Paget's disease of the spine can mimic metastatic disease (Fig 3–62).

References

1. Kattan KR: *"Trauma" and "No-Trauma" of the Cervical Spine.* Springfield, Ill, Charles C Thomas, Publisher, 1975.
2. Gehweiler JA, Osbourne RL, Becher RF: *The Radiology of Vertebral Trauma.* Philadelphia, WB Saunders Co, 1980.
3. Harris JH, Edeiken-Monroe B: *The Radiology of Acute Cervical Spine Trauma,* ed 2. Baltimore, Williams & Wilkins Co, 1987.
4. Weir DC: Roentgenographic signs of cervical injury. *Clin Orthopaed* 1975; 109:9–17.
5. Vines FS: The significance of "occult" fractures of the cervical spine. *Radiology* 1969; 107:493–504.
6. Handel SF, Lee Y: Computed tomography of spinal fractures. *Radiol Clin North Am* 1981; 19:69.
7. Brown BM, Brant-Zawadski M, Cann C: Dynamic CT scanning of spinal column trauma. *AJR* 1982; 139:1177.
8. Post MJD, Green BA, Quencer RM, et al: The value of computed tomography in spinal trauma. *Spine* 1982; 7:417.
9. Keene JS, Goletz TY, Lilleas F, et al: Diagnosis of vertebral fractures. *J Bone J Surg* 1981; 64A:586.
10. Pech P, Kilgore DP, Pojunas KW, et al: Cervical spine fractures: CT detection. *Radiology* 1985; 157:117.
11. McAedle CB, Crofford MJ, Mirfakhrale M, et al: Surface coil MR of spinal trauma: Preliminary experience. *AJNR* 1986; 7:885.
12. Tarr RW, Drolshagen LF, Kerner TC, et al: MR imaging of recent spinal trauma. *JCAT* 1987; 11:412.
13. Clark MW, Gehweiler JA, Laib R: Twelve significant signs of cervical spine trauma. *Skeletal Radiol* 1979; 3:201–205.
14. Andrew WK, Willinson AE: Prevertebral soft tissue swelling as a sign of undisplaced fracture of the odontoid process. *South Afr Med J* 1978; 53:672.
15. Miller MD, Gehweiler JA, Martinez S, et al: Significant new observations on cervical spine trauma. *AJR* 1978; 130:659–663.
16. Braakman R, Penning L: *Injuries of the Cervical Spine.* Amsterdam, Excerpta Medica, 1971, pp 53–62.
17. Beatson TR: Fractures and dislocations of the cervical spine. *J Bone Joint Surg* 1963; 45B:21–35.
18. Burke DC: Hyperextension injuries of the spine. *J Bone Joint Surg* 1971; 53B:3–12.
19. Swischuk LE: Anterior displacement of C2: Physiologic or pathologic. *Radiology* 1977; 122:759–763.
20. Harrison RB, Keats TE, Winn HR, et al: Pseudosubluxation of the axis in young adults. *J Can Assoc Radiol* 1980; 31:176–177.
21. Scavone JG, Latshaw RF, Rohner V: Use of lumbar spine films. *JAMA* 1981; 246:1105–1108.
22. Chance CQ: Note on a type of flexion fracture of the spine. *Br J Radiol* 1948; 21:249.

Suggested Reading

Harris JG, Harris WH: *The Radiology of Emergency Medicine,* ed 2. Baltimore, Williams & Wilkins Co, 1981.

Harris JH, Edeiken-Monroe B: *The Radiology of Acute Cervical Spine Trauma,* ed 2. Baltimore, Williams & Wilkins Co, 1987.

Rogers LF: *Radiology of Skeletal Trauma,* vols. 1 and 2. New York, Churchill Livingstone, 1982.

Normal Variants

Theodore E. Keats, M.D.

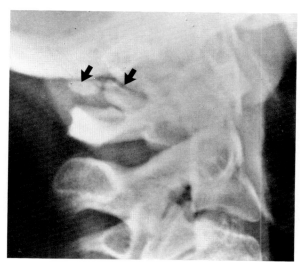

FIG 3–63.
Accessory osseous elements between the base of the skull and the spinous process of C-1.

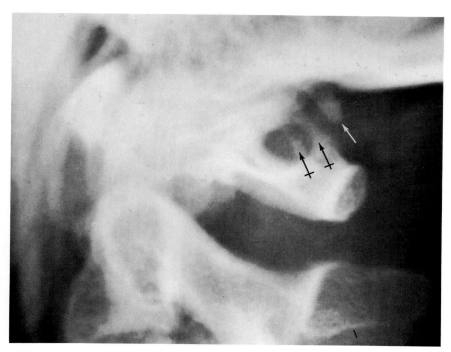

FIG 3–64.
Bony spur arising from the base of the skull, simulating a neural arch (*arrow*). The complete bony rings are the arcuate foramina (*notched arrows*).

FIG 3–65.
A, normal cleft in the neural arch of the atlas in a 1-year-old child. **B,** normal cleft in the neural arches of all the cervical vertebrae in an 11-month-old child.

These neurocentral synchondroses may persist until the 3rd to 6th years and may persist unilaterally for several months after the other side has closed.

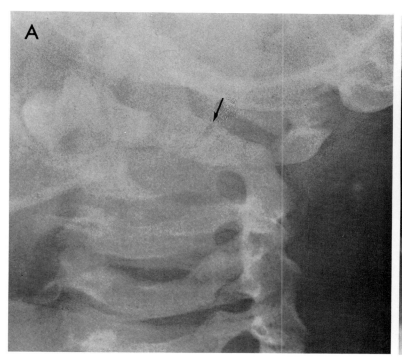

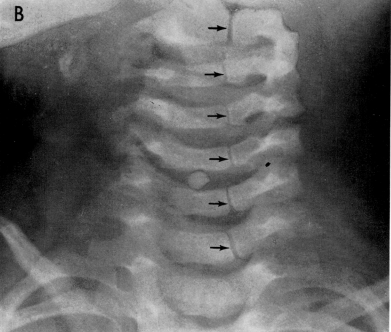

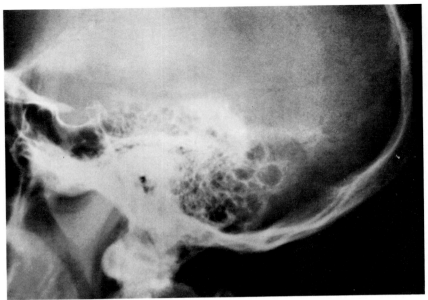

FIG 3–66.
Complete absence of the posterior neural arch of C-1. (Ref:
Dalinka MK, et al: Congenital absence of the posterior arch
of the atlas. *Radiology* 1972; 103:581.)

FIG 3–67.
Two examples of incomplete formation of the posterior neural arch of C-1.

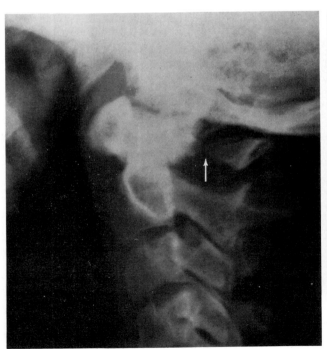

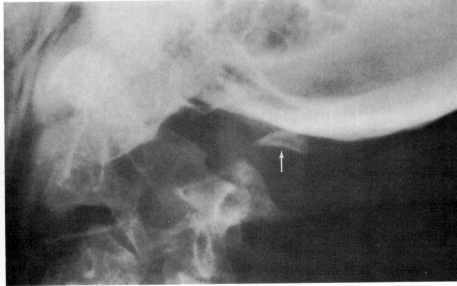

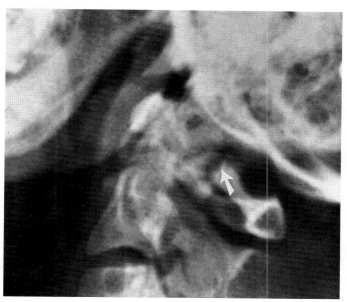

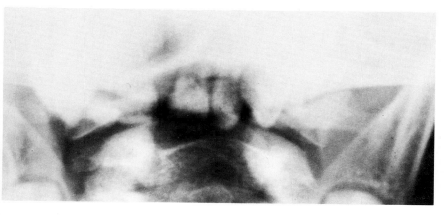

FIG 3–68 (left).
Unilateral spondylolysis of the neural arch of C-1.

FIG 3–69 (right).
Bilateral offsets of the lateral masses of C-1 and C-2 in children. This appearance in an adult would be presumptive evidence of fracture of the neural arch of C-1. This entity is believed to be secondary to a disparity of growth of the atlas and axis vertebrae in children and is seen in children most commonly about the age of 4 years. (Ref: Suss RA et al: Pseudospread of the atlas. False sign of Jefferson fracture in children. *Am J Roentgenol* 1983; 140:1079.)

FIG 3–70.
Two examples of anomalous development of the base of the odontoid. Note the corresponding deformity of the lateral masses of C-1.

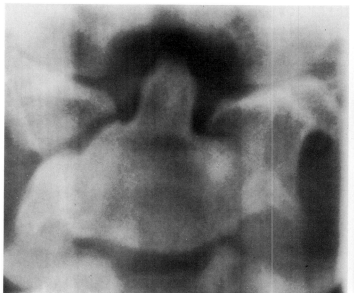

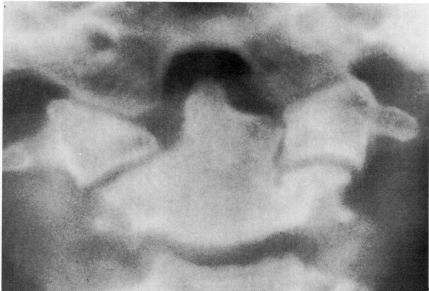

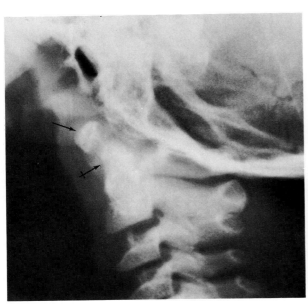
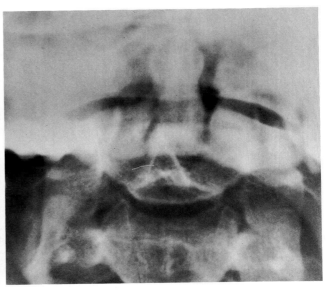

FIG 3–71 (left).
Normal position of the anterior process of C-1 (*arrow*) with relationship to the odontoid (*notched arrow*) when head is in extension. This may be mistaken for a post-traumatic event.

FIG 3–72 (right).
Pseudofracture of the body of C-2 produced by overlapping shadows of the teeth.

FIG 3–73.
A, normal asymmetry of the intervals between the odontoid and the lateral masses of C-1 produced by rotation of the head. **B,** same patient with head in neutral position.

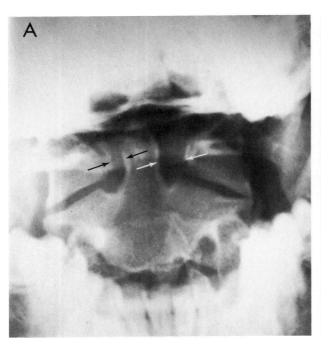
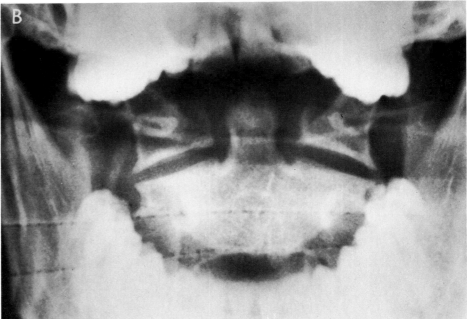

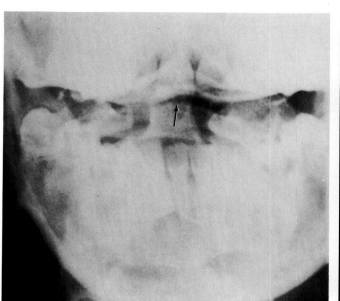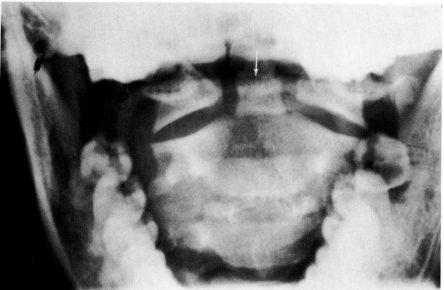

FIG 3–74.
Pseudofractures of the odontoid produced by overlapping shadows of the central maxillary incisors.

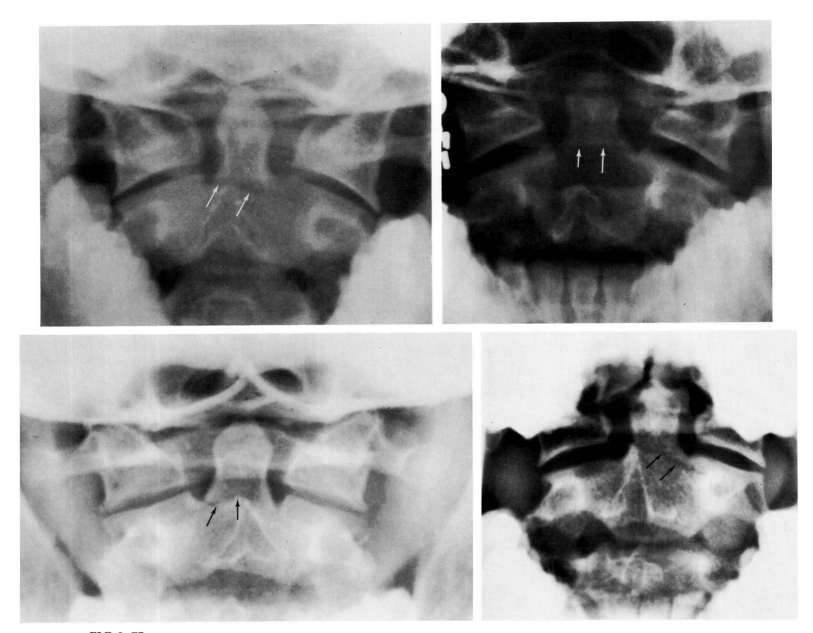

FIG 3–75.
Pseudofractures of the base of the odontoid produced by the Mach effect from overlapping of the posterior arch of C-1, the tongue, or the occiput. Each was proved a pseudofracture by laminography. (Ref: Daffner RH: Pseudofracture of the dens: Mach bands. *Am J Roentgenol* 1977; 128:607.)

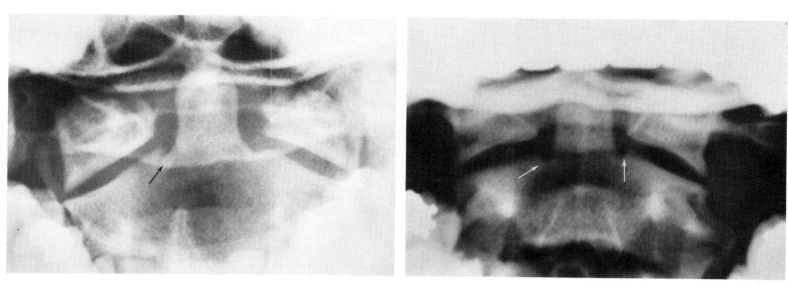

FIG 3–76.
Normal developmental clefts at the base of the odontoid.

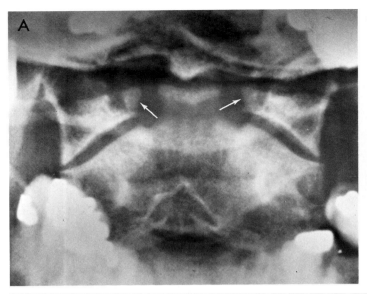

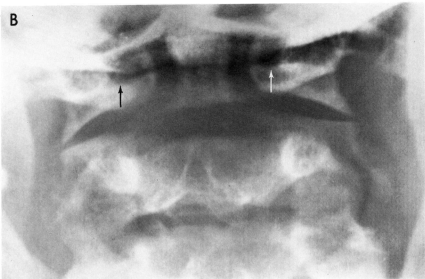

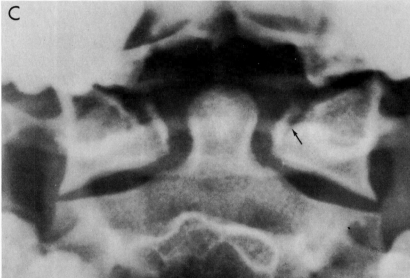

FIG 3–77.
Normal variations in the appearance of the lateral masses of C-1. **A,** spur-like configurations of the medial borders; **B,** foramen-like configuration of the medial borders; **C,** pseudofracture. These variants should not be mistaken for manifestations of trauma. (Ref: Meghrouni V, Jacobson G: The pseudonotch of the atlas. *Radiology* 1959; 72:260.)

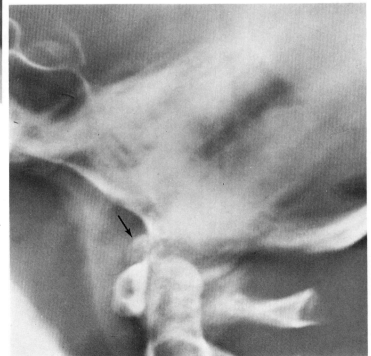

FIG 3–78.
An accessory ossicle above the anterior process of C-1. (Ref: Lombardi G: The occipital vertebra. *Am J Roentgenol* 1961; 86:260.)

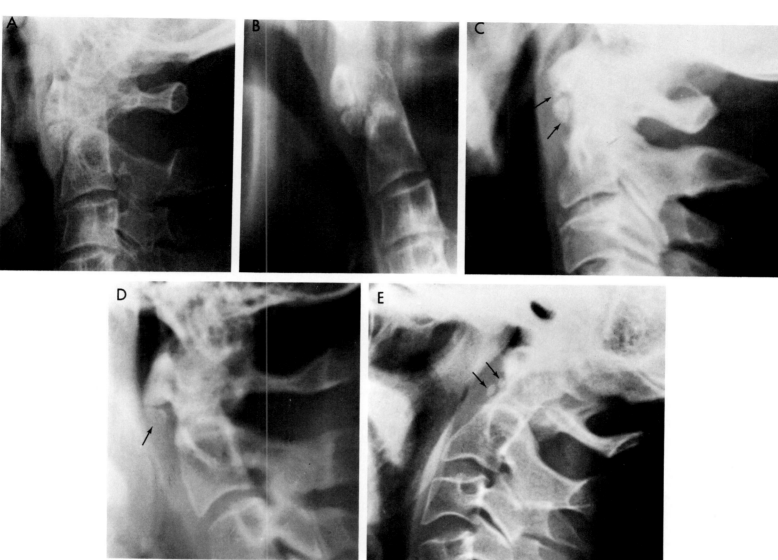

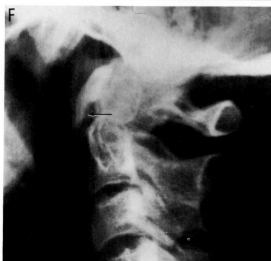

FIG 3–79.
Six examples of the variable appearance of the accessory ossicle of the anterior arch of the atlas. The laminagram in **A** indicates an articulation with the inferior aspect of the anterior arch of C-1. This articulation may be confused with a fracture. In **F**, the ossicle is fused to the anterior process of C-1. (Courtesy of Dr. Armand Fortin, Montreal, Canada.) (Ref: Keats TE: The inferior accessory ossicle of the anterior arch of the atlas. *Am J Roentgenol* 1967; 101:834. Used by permission.)

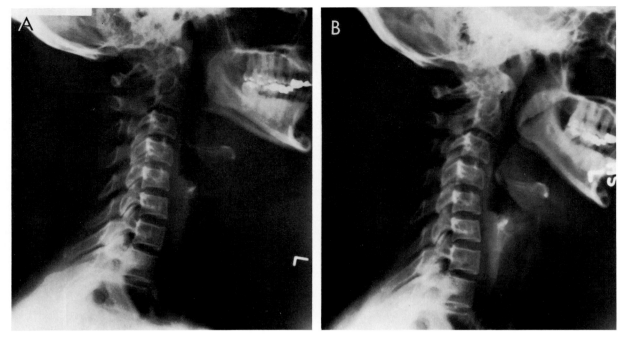

FIG 3–80.
Normal cervical spine. **A,** neutral position; **B,** flexion. Note the striking alteration in curvature which can be produced with only slight alteration in head position.

FIG 3–81.
The superimposed lobe of the ear may produce shadows that simulate fracture (*arrow*). Note in **B** the cleft in the anterior aspect of the vertebral body, which is probably a remnant of the synchondrosis for the odontoid process (*notched arrow*).

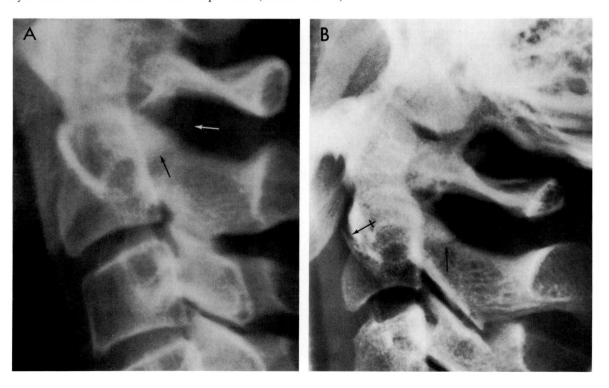

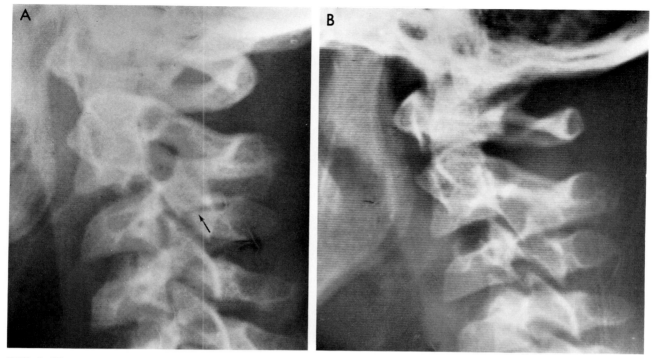

FIG 3–82.
A, simulated fracture of the posterior neural arch of C-3 produced by rotation; **B,** corrected rotation. No fracture is seen.

FIG 3–83.
A, simulated fracture of the neural arch of C-3 produced by rotation; **B,** repeat examination with correction of rotation shows restitution to normal appearance. Note also the absence of lordotic curve in **A.**

This is a common variation, especially between the ages of 8 and 16 years. (Ref: Cattell HS, Filtzer DL: Pseudosubluxation and other normal variations in the cervical spine in children. *J Bone Joint Surg* 1965; 47A:1295.)

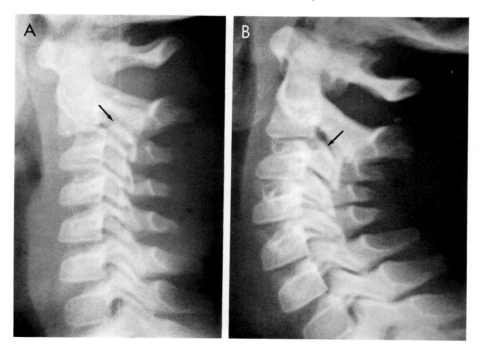

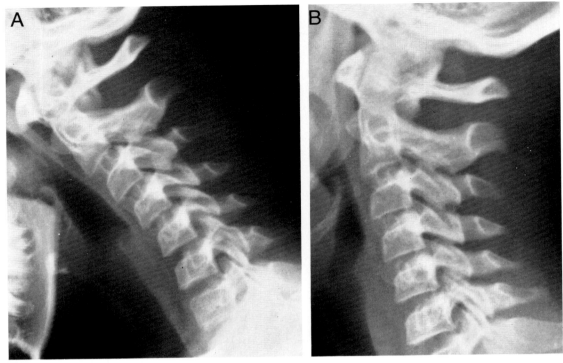

FIG 3–84.
A, pseudosubluxation of C-2 and C-3 in a 9-year-old boy. This is the normal area of maximum movement in the child and is seen regularly in flexion. **B,** with the head in neutral position, normal relationships are restored. This phenomenon may also be seen in young adults. (Ref: Jacobson G, Beeckler HH: Pseudosubluxation of the axis in children. *Am J Roentgenol* 1959; 82:472.)

FIG 3–85.
A, simulated fracture of C-3 (*arrow*) produced by uncovertebral joint degeneration. **B,** the frontal projection demonstrates the degenerated joint (*arrows*) responsible for the simulated fracture.

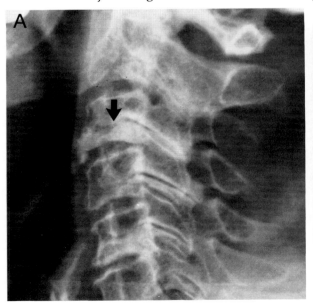

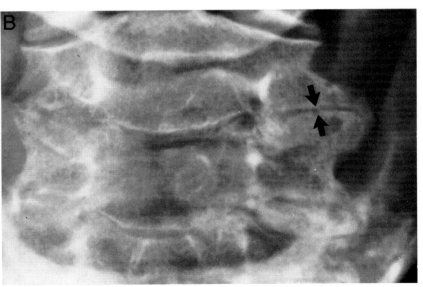

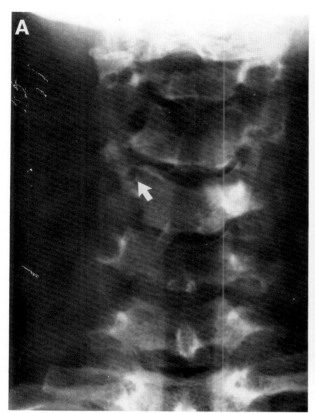

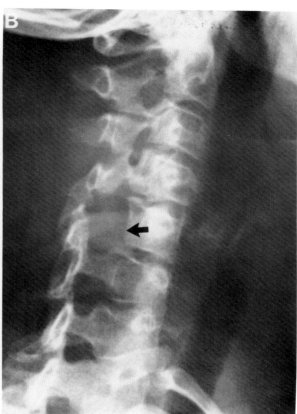

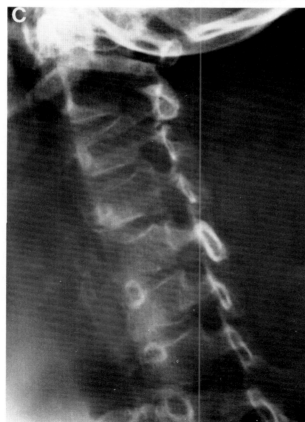

FIG 3–86.
A, congenital absence of the pedicle (*arrow*) on the right side of C-5. Compare oblique projection **(B)** with the opposite side **(C)**. This congenital lesion may be mistaken for a destructive process. (Ref: Chapman M: Congenital absence of cervical pedicle. *Skel Radiol* 1976; 1:65.)

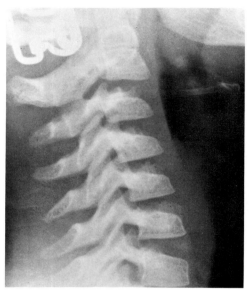

FIG 3–87.
Normal wedge shape of juvenile cervical vertebral bodies, which should not be confused with compression fracture.

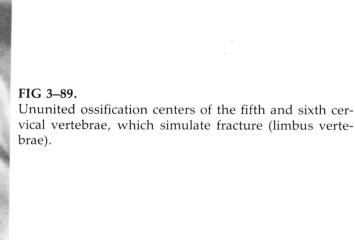

FIG 3–88.
Wedge-shaped vertebral bodies in a 13-year-old boy. Note particularly the marked wedging of C-3, mistaken for a compression fracture.

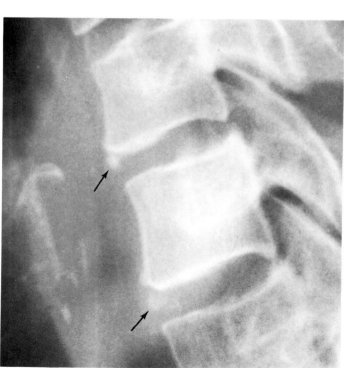

FIG 3–89.
Ununited ossification centers of the fifth and sixth cervical vertebrae, which simulate fracture (limbus vertebrae).

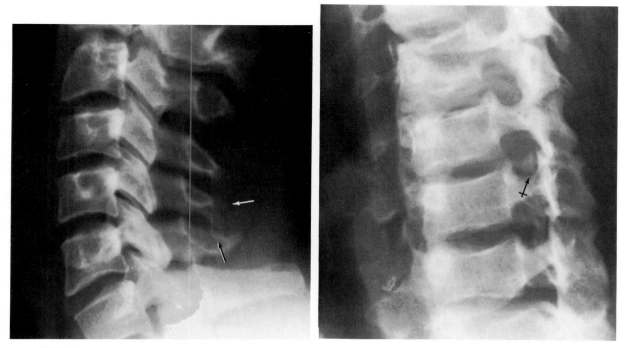

FIG 3–90.
A bifid spinous process (*arrows*) may project into the neural foramen and simulate a fracture (*notched arrow*).

FIG 3–91 (left).
Calcification of the ligamentum nuchae.

FIG 3–92 (right).
Failure of union of the apophysis of the spinous process of C-7 simulating a fracture.

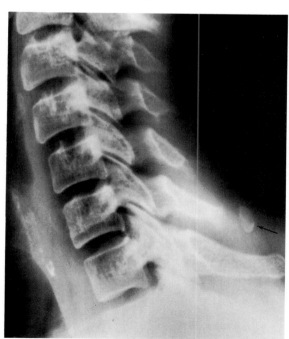

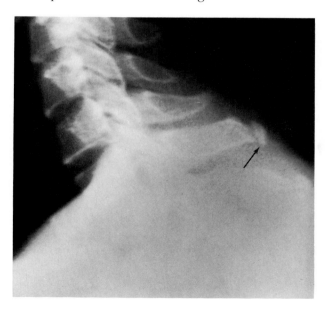

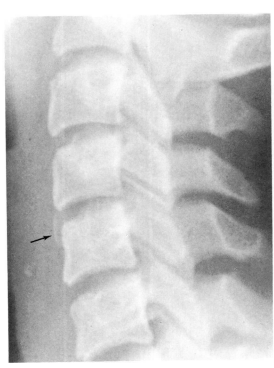
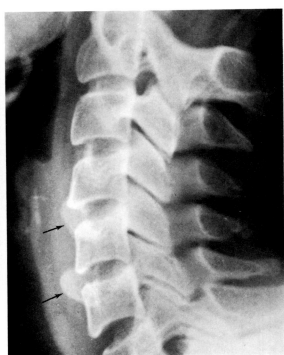
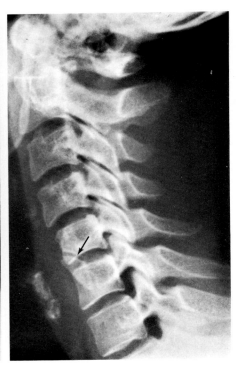

FIG 3–93.
Three examples of normal elongation of the transverse processes of C-5 and C-6, producing an unusual appearance anterior to the vertebral bodies. (Ref: Laypayowker MS: An unusual variant of the cervical spine. *Am J Roentgenol* 1960; 83:656.)

FIG 3–94.
Oblique projection of the cervical spine showing the anterior tubercle of the transverse process, the structure responsible for the shadows in Figure 3–98.

FIG 3–95.
Ossification centers at the distal ends of the transverse processes of T-1 in an adolescent.

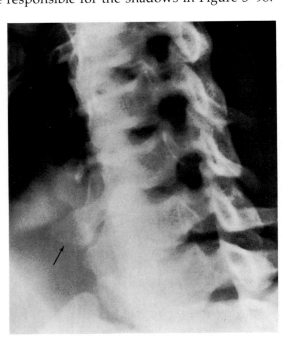
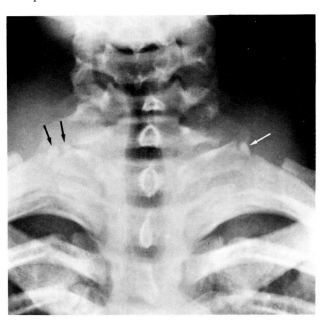

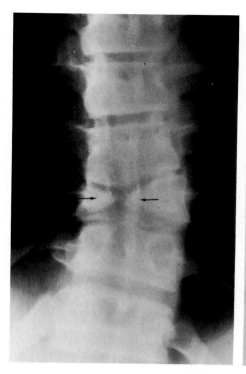
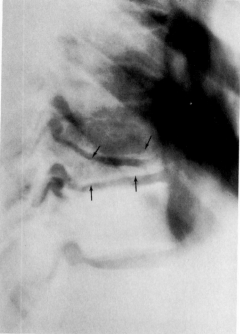
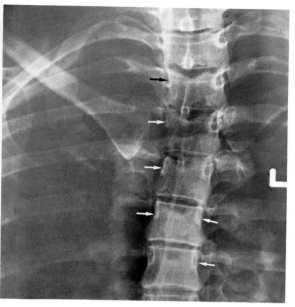

FIG 3–96 (left and middle).
Congenital butterfly vertebra. Note overgrowth of adjacent vertebrae.

FIG 3–97 (right).
Minor scoliosis producing simulated pedicle erosion.

FIG 3–98.
Pseudofractures of the dorsal spine. **A,** superimposition of the glenoid process of the scapula on the dorsal spine, simulating a vertebral compression fracture.

B, pseudofracture of the second dorsal vertebra, produced by superimposition of the superior margin of the manubrium.

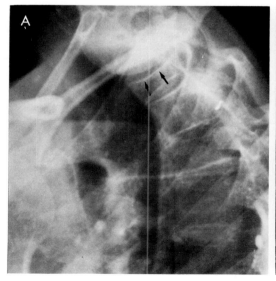
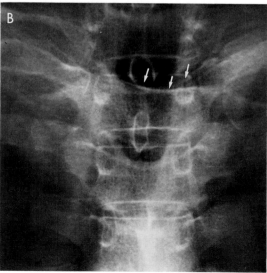

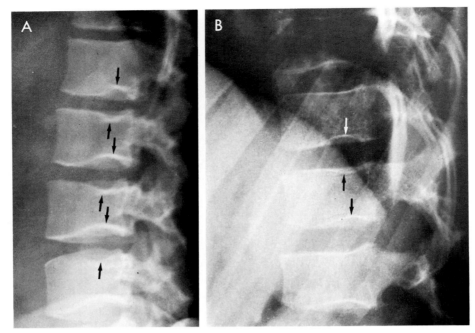

FIG 3–99.
Two examples of end-plate depressions secondary to notochordal remnants. Indentations of this type in the end-plates of normal vertebrae of young people indicate the site of the notochordal recession into the intervertebral disk. They should be differentiated from Schmorl's nodes. **A,** a 27-year-old man; **B,** a 12-year-old girl. (Ref: Dietz GW, Christensen EE: Normal "Cupid's bow" contour of the lower lumbar vertebrae. *Radiology* 1976; 121:577.)

FIG 3–100.
Ununited secondary ossification center (limbus vertebra) simulating a fracture of L-5. **A,** plain film; **B,** laminagram.

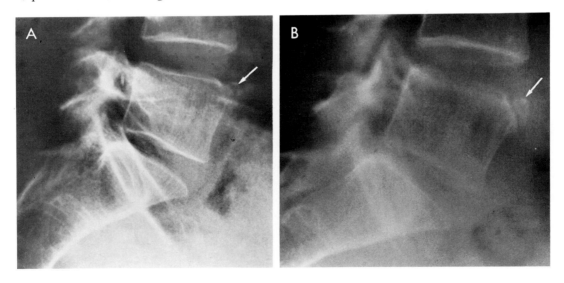

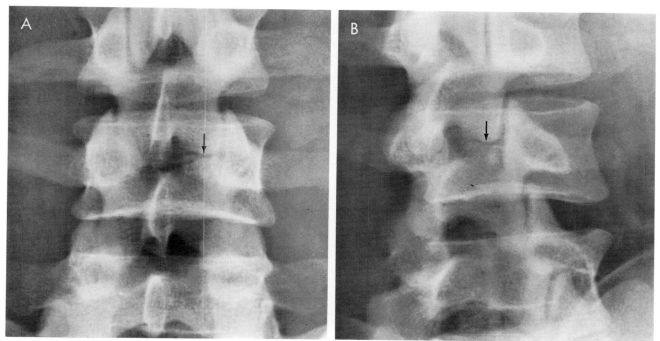

FIG 3–101.
Ununited ossification center of the end of the inferior articulating process of L-4, which may be mistaken for fracture. **A,** frontal projection; **B,** oblique projection.

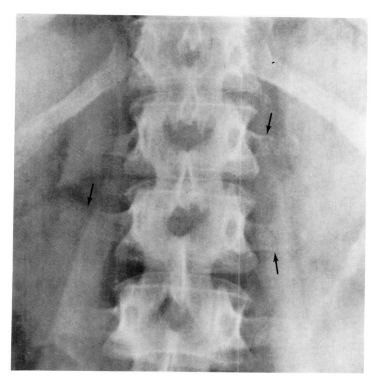

FIG 3–102.
Simulated fractures of the transverse processes produced by the crossing shadow of the psoas muscle.

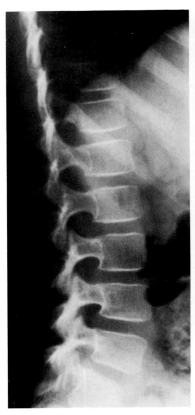

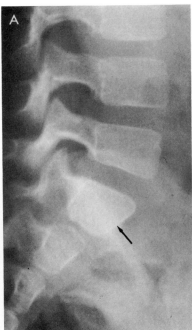

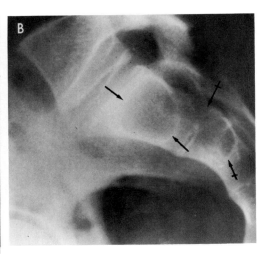

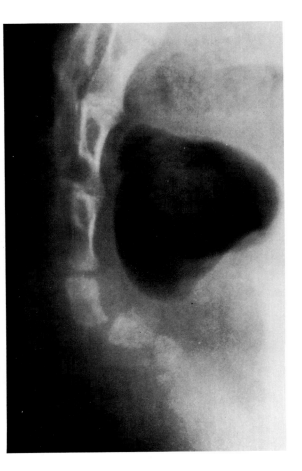

FIG 3–103 (top left).
Posterior scalloping of the posterior aspects of the vertebral bodies may be seen as a normal variant, particularly in adolescence.

FIG 3–104 (top middle and right).
Normal variations in the appearance of the first sacral segment. **A,** normal relative increase in density in a 2-year-old boy. This is, at times, mistaken for osteosclerosis. **B,** pseudocyst of the sacrum (*arrows*) in a young adult due to the large amount of cancellous bone with suggestion of a similar appearance in the second sacral segment. Note also the posterior widening of the S-1–2 interspace (*notched arrows*). This represents a normal variant in sacral development in youth. (Ref: Cacciarelli AA: Posterior widening of the S-1–2 interspace in children: A normal variant of sacral development. *Am J Roentgenol* 1977; 129:305.)

FIG 3–105 (bottom right).
Normal anterior angulation of the coccyx. The position of the coccyx is not useful, in itself, in the identification of trauma.

4
Chest

Peter Armstrong, M.D.

A wide range of intrathoracic diseases can be diagnosed with the imaging techniques available in the modern radiology department. The first test is invariably a plain chest radiograph and, depending on the findings at chest radiography, more complex tests may follow. Computed tomography (CT) of the chest is an increasingly used modality. Techniques such as ultrasound, magnetic resonance imaging, radionuclide examinations, and angiography all have specific indications, which are discussed in the appropriate sections of this chapter.

The first step in categorizing any abnormality detected by plain chest radiography is to decide its location, particularly whether it lies in the lung, the pleura, the mediastinum, the diaphragm, or the chest wall. The next step is to determine the shape of the lesion, and finally to analyze the density of each portion. CT provides more information than the chest radiograph in every aspect of this analysis. The multiple sections provide the equivalent of a three-dimensional display and therefore provide superb localization and delineation of the shape of any abnormality. CT is also far superior to plain films in showing cavitation, calcification, and air within a lesion. Most fluid collections can be distinguished from adjacent soft tissues, including consolidated lung. Also, the excellent contrast resolution of CT allows one to see the fat planes which outline the mediastinal structures, thus providing details of mediastinal pathology. Despite all of these advantages, however, it should be emphasized that CT is only cost effective in a limited number of circumstances. Usually, the chest film provides the information necessary for management decisions. In this chapter, therefore, the emphasis will be on plain film findings.

Plain Chest Radiographs

The routine views of the chest are the posteroanterior (PA) and the lateral views (Fig 4–1). Ideally, both should be exposed at full inspiration with the patient in the erect position. If the patient cannot stand, an acceptable alternative is to obtain a film with the patient sitting, utilizing an anteroposterior (AP) or PA projection. For patients who can neither sit nor stand,

a supine AP film may be the only practical solution, but supine films are often difficult to interpret due to poor inspiration and magnification of the heart and anterior mediastinum. Also, such films are frequently made with mobile x-ray machines, which require longer exposure times and produce a blurred image in patients who are unable to hold their breath.

There are many ways of looking at chest films. The trained radiologist often uses a problem-oriented approach: he or she varies the search pattern according to features present on the films, constantly integrating clinical information. Those with less radiologic experience need a routine to avoid overlooking important information. One approach is presented here.

The upper surface of the diaphragm should be clearly outlined by air in the lung from one costophrenic angle to the other, except where the heart and the pericardial fat are in contact with the diaphragm. The costophrenic angles are usually sharp, but if the hemidiaphragms are flattened, the angles may become meniscus-shaped, simulating pleural fluid. Failure to clearly see the diaphragm outline indicates either pleural or pulmonary disease.

The right hemidiaphragm is usually 1 to 3 cm higher than the left, but may be level with, or even slightly below it, and still be normal; on average, the midpoint of the right hemidiaphragm is level with the anterior end of the sixth rib.

The lateral borders of the heart and superior mediastinum should be clearly defined from the clavicles to the diaphragm. Any lack of clarity of these borders indicates pulmonary or, less often, pleural disease. Above the clavicles the mediastinal border may be indistinct.

On the PA view the center of the trachea lies midway or slightly to the right of the midpoint, between the medial ends of the clavicles, even if the patient is rotated. The trachea courses vertically or slightly to the right as it descends into the chest. The position of the heart is variable, making it difficult to diagnose all but the most severe degrees of cardiac displacement. On average, one third of the heart lies to the right of the midline, but the normal range varies from one fifth to one half of the cardiac diameter lying to the right of the midline.

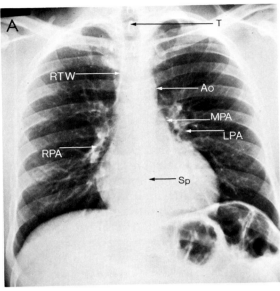
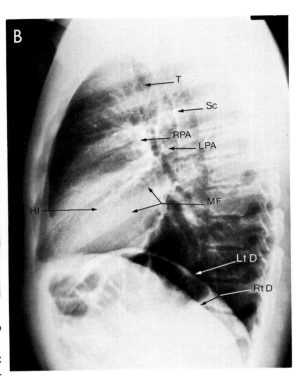

FIG 4–1.
A and **B**, normal PA and lateral chest radiographs. *Ao* = aorta; *Ht* = heart; *MF* = major fissure; *MPA* = main pulmonary artery; *LPA* = left pulmonary artery; *RPA* = right pulmonary artery; *Lt D* = left hemidiaphragm; *Rt D* = right hemidiaphragm; *T* = trachea; *RTW* = right tracheal wall; *Sc* = scapula; *Sp* = spine.

FIG 4–2.
Normal thymic shadow in a 4-month-old child. The characteristic "sail shape" is seen projecting to the right of the superior mediastinum. This appearance should not be confused with right upper-lobe consolidation or collapse.

FIG 4–3.
Azygos lobe fissure. During intrauterine development the azygos vein migrates through the lung. In some individuals, the pleural invagination, together with the azygos vein deep within it *(arrow)*, persist as a fissure.

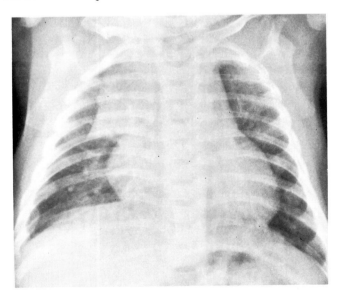

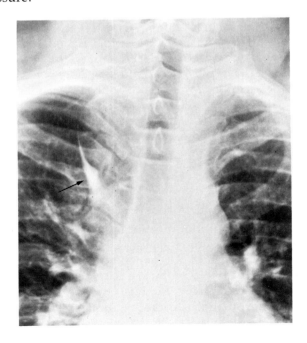

The right superior mediastinal border, formed by the right innominate vein and superior vena cava, is usually straight or slightly curved as it passes downward to merge with the right heart border. The left superior mediastinal border above the aortic knob is formed by the left subclavian artery and is often ill defined. The knob should be well defined and have a transverse diameter of 2 to 3 cm. Aortic unfolding often modifies the appearance of the superior mediastinum, sometimes hiding pathology and often simulating significant disease.

Air in the major bronchi can be recognized, but the bronchial walls are usually not visible except when seen end-on. It is occasionally possible to diagnose narrowing of the major bronchi, but this is difficult because of the variable visualization of air within the bronchi.

In children the thymus is often visible as an anterior mediastinal mass. It is rarely identifiable on plain films of patients above the age of seven. Its shape is variable, a "sail" configuration being characteristic (Fig 4–2), but rounded outlines are frequent and may be mistaken for true mediastinal masses or pulmonary infiltrates. An important feature of the thymus is that it is soft and does not deform adjacent structures, such as the trachea.

The hilar shadows are produced by the pulmonary arteries and veins. The hilar lymph nodes cannot be identified as separate shadows, and the walls of the bronchi are thin and contribute little to the image seen on the radiograph. The left hilum is usually slightly higher than the right.

The lower lobe arteries are 9 to 16 mm in diameter, with parallel walls except where they branch. Any lobulation of the hilar shadow, any local expansion, or increase in density compared with the opposite side indicates a mass. Enlargement of the pulmonary arteries can usually be recognized by noting the branching nature of the shadows and realizing that vascular enlargement is usually bilateral and accompanied by enlargement of the heart and main pulmonary artery.

The only structures that can be identified within the normal lungs are the blood vessels, the walls of certain bronchi seen end-on, and the interlobar fissures. The blood vessels show an orderly decrease in diameter from the hila outward. In the upright patient the vessels equidistant from the hila are smaller in the upper zones than they are in the lower zones. This difference is not seen if the patient is examined supine. The fissures can be seen only if they lie tangential to the x-ray beam. Usually, only the minor fissure is visible in the frontal projection, running from the right hilum to the sixth rib in the axilla; it can be identified

in over half the population. In about 1% of the population an extra fissure, the so-called azygos fissure (Fig 4–3), is visible in the frontal view. Each major fissure on the lateral view runs obliquely across the chest from the T-4–5 vertebral bodies to a point on the hemidiaphragm close to where the hemidiaphragm meets the anterior chest wall. Intrathoracic shadows or lucencies arising in, or projected over, the lungs are signs of disease. Care should be taken not to confuse chest wall structures such as pectoral muscles, breasts, or costal cartilages with intrathoracic disease. In particular, the nipples or skin lumps may mimic pulmonary nodules, and hair braids or clothing can cause shadows that mimic pulmonary densities. The nipples are usually in the fifth anterior rib space and, in general, if one nipple is visible, the other will also be seen.

Finding abnormal shadows in the frontal film is usually fairly easy, since it is possible to compare one lung with the other. This is best done zone by zone (Fig 4–4). Detecting shadows in the lateral view may be difficult. It is helpful to bear in mind that as the eye travels down the vertebrae to the diaphragm each vertebral body should appear more lucent than the one above (Fig 4–5). Also, but less reliably, the density of the retrocardiac space in most patients is similar to that of the retrosternal space, and the density over the heart is uniform with no abrupt change.

The *ribs*, *sternum*, *clavicles*, *scapulae*, and *spine* need to be examined for fractures and areas of lysis and sclerosis. The upper cortical line of the ribs is continuous and easy to assess. The inferior cortical line is indistinct in the posterior portions of the ribs in normal persons and should be not misdiagnosed as a lytic lesion. Each scapula casts two linear shadows on the lateral view that could be mistaken for disease or misplaced fissures.

Rib disease may be accompanied by soft tissue swelling and, not infrequently, the swelling is more obvious than the bone abnormality. Therefore, when the ribs are examined, the outer lung edge should be scanned for extrapleural soft tissue swelling, and the frontal film should be reviewed for ill-defined densities that may lead to the discovery of a rib lesion (Fig 4–6). Soft tissue swelling may be the only sign of a rib disorder in the standard views. Recognizing this swelling calls for detailed rib views, which may then lead to identification of the responsible rib lesion. There are two basic methods of reviewing the ribs on a plain chest radiograph. One can trace each rib in turn, or one can view the posterior portions, anterior portions, and midportions separately. The latter method is much quicker and, somewhat surprisingly, is an equally accurate if not a better technique.

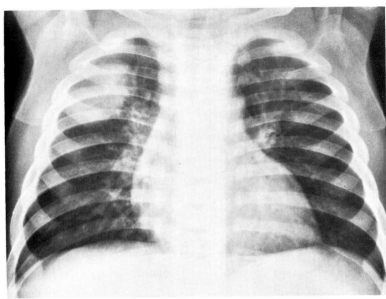

FIG 4–4.
Right upper-lobe pneumonia. The infiltrate could be overlooked if the two lungs are not consciously compared.

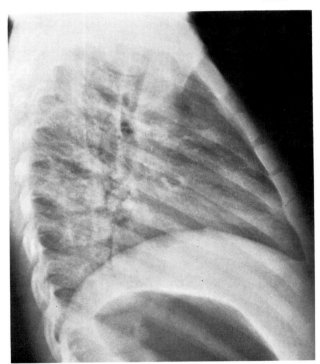

FIG 4–5.
Lateral chest radiograph showing collapse and consolidation due to pneumonia in the left lower lobe. The vertebral bodies should appear more lucent as one travels down the thoracic spine (see Fig 4–1). In this case, the lower thoracic vertebrae appear denser due to the pulmonary disease projected over them. Another feature to note is the increased retrocardiac density. The retrocardiac area should be the same density as the upper retrosternal area. (The frontal view of this patient is illustrated in Fig 4–24.)

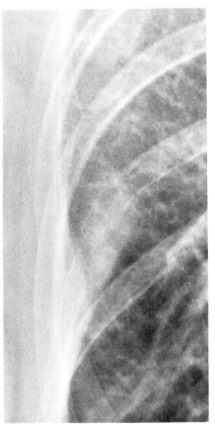

FIG 4–6.
Soft tissue swelling in association with a rib metastasis. The density of the soft tissue swelling may be a useful sign guiding the eye to the ill-defined lytic lesion in the rib.

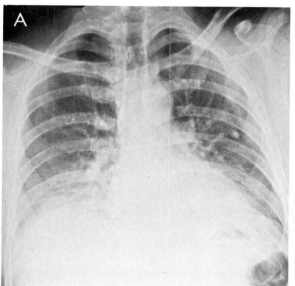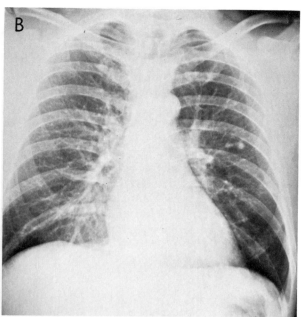

FIG 4–7.
Effects of expiration on a chest radiograph. **A,** expiration; **B,** inspiration. On expiration, the heart appears larger and the lung bases are hazy. It would be easy to falsely diagnose heart failure or bilateral pneumonia.

Technical evaluation of a film is necessary, since incorrect exposure, poor centering, or faulty projection may either hide or mimic disease. The correctly exposed routine PA chest film is one in which the ribs and spine behind the heart can be identified. Unless one can see through the heart, lower-lobe lesions may be completely overlooked. A straight film is one where the medial ends of the clavicles are equidistant from the edges of the thoracic vertebrae. Unless the film is exposed on full inspiration, the heart may appear enlarged and the lung bases may be hazy or show ill-defined densities (Fig 4–7). Such an appearance may mimic pulmonary edema, pneumonia, or pulmonary infarction, and it is, therefore, wise to check the degree of inspiration, which is adequate if the right hemidiaphragm lies in the sixth anterior interspace.

Additional Plain Films of the Chest

There are a number of extra views of the chest that may provide details of a lesion seen on routine films or may even enable a previously invisible abnormality to be detected.

LORDOTIC VIEWS.—Lordotic views are usually taken to show the upper zones of the lungs. The apical lordotic view projects the clavicles above the lung apices. This improves visualization of apical lung lesions and allows one to distinguish a pulmonary from a bony density.

EXPIRATION VIEWS.—Expiration views are used to diagnose small pneumothoraces that are either not visualized or are doubtful on standard inspiratory films. Despite its popularity, the expiration view is rarely of help since most pneumothoraces are readily diagnosed on conventional views. It should never be used as a substitute for the inspiratory film since it is inferior in every way except for detecting a small pneumothorax.

DECUBITUS VIEWS.—Lateral decubitus views are not, as the name implies, lateral views; they are frontal projections taken with the patient lying on one side or the other. Their principal use is to demonstrate mobile fluid in the pleural cavities (see Fig 4–4). Lateral decubitus views can be used to decide the size of the effusion and to determine how much of the fluid is mobile. On occasion, they are also used to establish the presence of pleural fluid where this is in doubt on the standard views. The lateral decubitus view also can help occasionally in diagnosing pneumothorax or pulmonary disease that is hidden by pleural fluid in both PA and lateral projections, but revealed when the fluid moves away when the patient changes position.

RIB VIEWS.—Since the ribs are curved, multiple projections may be needed to show each part of the rib. Consequently, oblique views are often taken to find a fracture or to improve the demonstration of known or suspected abnormality. The degree and direction of obliquity depends on which portion of the rib is suspect. The standard oblique view is taken AP at 45 degrees with the patient turned toward the appropriate side.

Computed Tomography

Nowadays, computed tomography has effectively replaced conventional tomography in the evaluation of the chest. The chief indications for urgent chest CT in emergency room patients are to diagnose:

1. Aortic dissection (see page 199).
2. Esophageal rupture (see page 211).
3. Empyema when the plain film findings are ambiguous (see page 174).

A standard CT examination of the chest consists of contiguous 1-cm thick sections from the lung apices to the posterior costophrenic angles. The examination may require 30 to 40 sections. The precise technique is often tailored to the clinical problem. For example, intravenous contrast medium is essential for the evaluation of aortic dissection, whereas it may not be necessary to detect suspected empyema. Also, for patients with suspected aortic dissection, the examination need not cover the whole chest.

Normal Chest CT

Just as with the plain chest radiograph, the only structures that are seen within the normal lungs are the blood vessels, the pleural fissures, and the walls of the larger bronchi. Vessels within the lung are recognized by their shape rather than by contrast opacification. When seen in cross section, the vessels appear round and may be indistinguishable from small lung nodules. Fortunately, most metastases and granulomas are located peripherally where the vessels are smallest, and true diagnostic confusion is, therefore, unusual. The fissures are seen infrequently as a line; their position is recognizable by a relatively avascular zone within the lung.

The mediastinal anatomy is complex and beyond the scope of this chapter. The normal appearances at selected levels are shown in Figure 4–8.

Basic Technical Factors in CT

The basic principle of CT is that each picture element—known in computer jargon either as a pixel

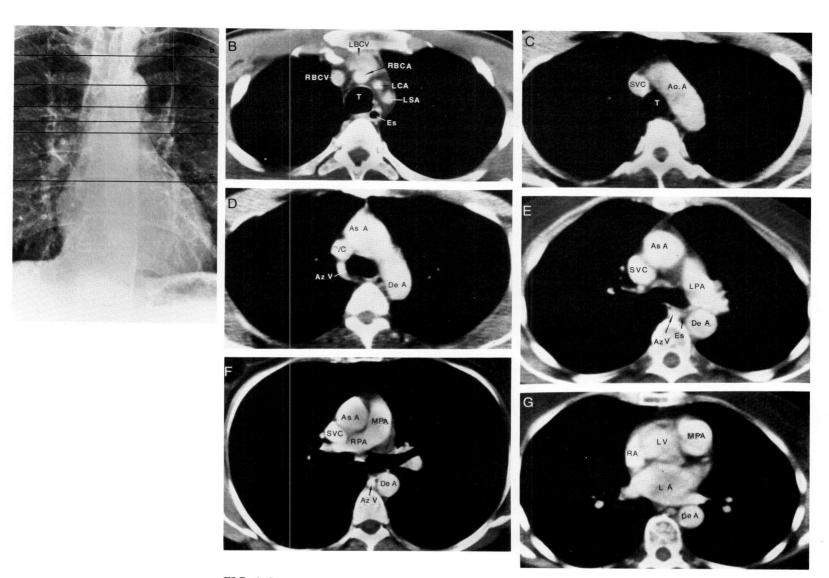

FIG 4–8.
CT of normal mediastinum. The levels of the individual sections are shown in **(A)**. *Ao A* = aortic arch; *As A* = ascending aorta; *Az V* = azygos vein; *De A* = descending aorta; *Es* = esophagus; *LA* = left atrium; *LBCV* = left brachiocephalic vein; *LCA* = left carotid artery; *LPA* = left pulmonary artery; *LSA* = left subclavian artery; *LV* = left ventricle; *MPA* = main pulmonary artery; *RA* = right atrium; *RBCA* = right brachiocephalic artery; *RBCV* = right brachiocephalic vein; *RPA* = right pulmonary artery; *SVC* = superior vena cava; *T* = trachea.

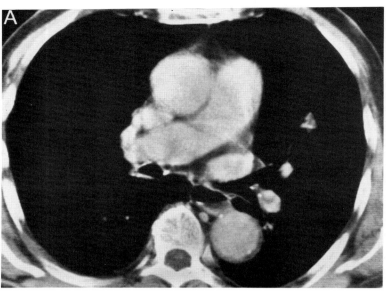
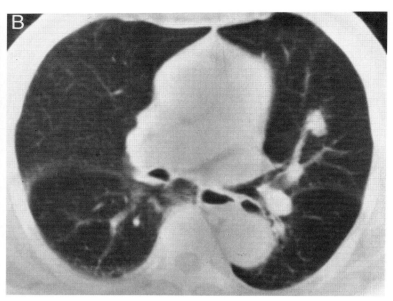

FIG 4–9.
Window widths and centers in CT. **A,** a narrow window width of 300 H units and a center corresponding to soft tissue (30 to 50 H units) are used for displaying mediastinal structures. **B,** a wide window (more than 1200 H units) with a center close to air (−400 H units) is used to display lung detail. Note that mediastinal details are not visible in **(B)** and corresponding lung details are not visible in **(A)**.

FIG 4–10.
Partial volume artifact. **A,** the apparent mass adjacent to the ascending aorta (*x*) is in fact the left pulmonary artery which has been partially included in the section. The correct interpretation becomes self-evident once the section below **(B)** is examined. The exact correspondence of the shadow to the left pulmonary artery can then be seen.

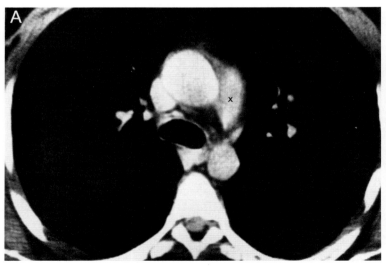
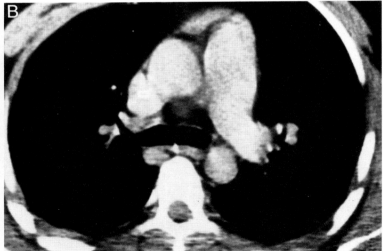

(picture element) or a voxel (volume element)—represents the absorption of x-rays by tissue. The attenuation values are expressed on an arbitrary scale with the density of water set at zero; air is minus 1,000 units and dense bone is plus 1,000 units. These density units are known as Hounsfield units to commemorate the man who played such an important part in developing CT scanning. The human eye can only appreciate approximately 22 shades of gray and, therefore, the information obtainable from CT cannot all be presented at one time. The range and levels of density displayed on the TV monitor (or on the film photographed from the monitor) can be selected by the operator. The range of densities displayed is known as the "window width" and the average level is known as the "window level" or "center." With a wide window all the structures are visible, but fine details of density differences cannot be appreciated. With a narrow window, differences in density of just a few units can be recognized, but much of the image is either totally black or totally white and, in these areas, no useful information is provided. In chest work, two distinct window and level settings are used: one for mediastinal structures and one to show details of pulmonary or pleural disease (Fig 4–9). When information about the bones is needed, a specialized wide window image is usually obtained.

The technical aspects of reconstructing images need not concern us, but there are two artifacts that need to be kept constantly in mind:

1. *Partial volume effect.* Since each voxel has a definite thickness, often 10 mm, a structure may be partly in and partly out of the section. The image displayed is the mean attenuation for the entire voxel, so the density of any object "partially in the volume" may not be truly representative of that structure, nor may its size be correctly represented (Fig 4–10).

2. *Streak artifacts.* Streak artifacts may be seen radiating from high-density objects, particularly if they move during the exposure of the image. They are commonly encountered radiating from intravascular catheters, metallic implants, and surgical clips, as well as from dense calcifications in the walls of the aorta or other vessels. They are also seen radiating from densely-calcified lymph nodes which move with the beating of the heart and large arteries. These streaks may degrade the images of surrounding structures. They pose a particular problem in patients with suspected aortic dissection because one of the low-density streaks may resemble an intimal flap when projected over the aortic lumen and may, therefore, lead to a false positive diagnosis of aortic dissection.

The Abnormal Plain Chest Radiograph

The first steps when viewing an abnormal density on a plain chest film are to determine whether the abnormality is situated in the lung, pleura, mediastinum, or chest wall, and to decide its shape and extent. Only then does one move on to answer the question, "What is it?" Clearly, the differential diagnosis will differ substantially, depending on the site of origin of the lesion. Accurate localization frequently requires two views; this is one of the major reasons why lateral views are useful in so many cases.

The location of an abnormality is usually obvious, but when a lesion is at the boundary between the lung and the chest wall, mediastinum, or diaphragm, it may be difficult to decide its site of origin. If the shadow has a broad base with smooth, well-defined, convex borders projecting into the lung, it is likely to be pleural, extrapleural, or mediastinal in origin (Fig 4–11).

Changes of shape with change in position of the patient can be helpful in localizing disease. It may be impossible to distinguish pleural effusion from a lower-lobe infiltrate but, if the effusion is free, it will move to the dependent portion of the chest on a lateral decubitus film, allowing a confident diagnosis of pleural effusion (see Fig 4–32).

Shadows in the hilar region on the frontal view should be accurately localized to the hilum or overlying lung since the causes of hilar shadows differ from those of pulmonary shadows. Another pitfall in localization is falsely diagnosing a pulmonary shadow in cases of pleural fluid in one of the fissures (Fig 4–12).

The information on a chest film is largely dependent on the transradiancy of air in the lung compared with the density of the heart, blood vessels, mediastinum, and diaphragm. An intrathoracic lesion in contact with the heart, mediastinum, or diaphragm will make their normal borders ill-defined or invisible. This sign, known as the silhouette sign, may be very helpful both in recognizing and localizing chest disease (Figs 4–13 and 4–14; see also Fig 4–23). The silhouette sign makes it possible to localize a shadow by observing which borders are lost (e.g., loss of the heart border must mean that the shadow lies in the anterior half of the chest). Alternatively, loss of part of the diaphragm outline indicates disease of the pleura or lower lobes.

The silhouette sign also makes it possible, on occasion, to diagnose disorders such as pulmonary consolidation, even when one is uncertain whether an

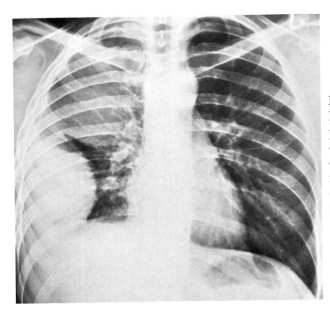

FIG 4–11.
Loculated pleural fluid, in this instance an empyema. The pleural location of the right lower-zone density is revealed by the broad base against the chest wall and the well-defined convex edge pushing into the lung. There is another loculation of the empyema based against the posterior chest wall in the upper zone.

FIG 4–12.
Frontal **(A)** and lateral **(B)** views of pleural fluid loculated in the left major fissure *(arrows)*. Note that, from the frontal view alone, it would not be possible to distinguish between loculated pleural fluid and a pulmonary lesion such as pneumonia or carcinoma.

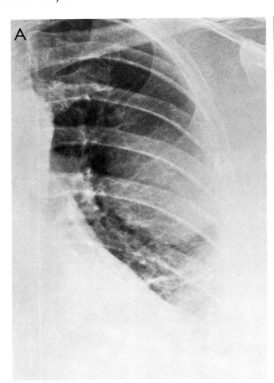

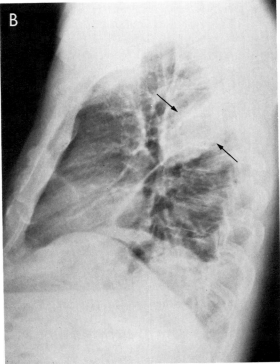

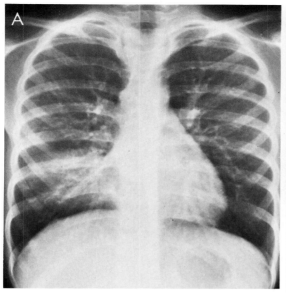

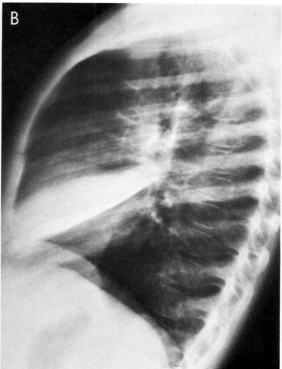

FIG 4–13.
A and **B,** the silhouette sign. This child with middle-lobe collapse and consolidation shows an indistinct right heart border on the frontal projection because the pulmonary density "silhouettes out" the adjacent heart border (compare to Fig 4–14).

FIG 4–14.
A and **B,** a pulmonary infiltrate, in this case due to pneumonia. Note the ill-defined edge of the pulmonary density, except where it abuts the major fissure. The lack of clarity of the diaphragm adjacent to the infiltrate is well demonstrated. Note that the right heart border is visible in this case because the adjacent middle lobe is normal (compare Fig 4–13).

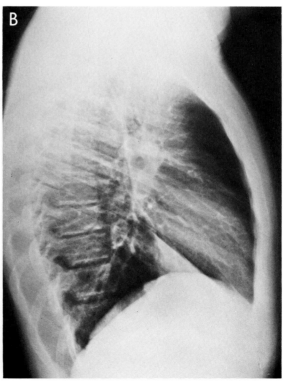

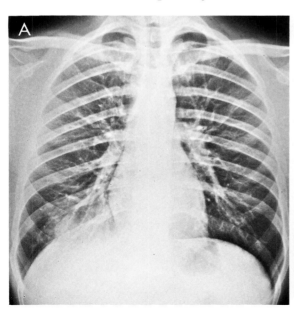

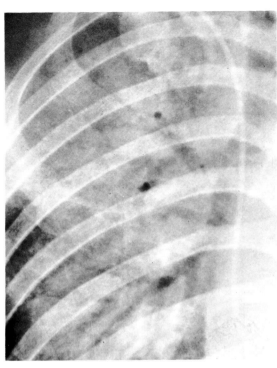

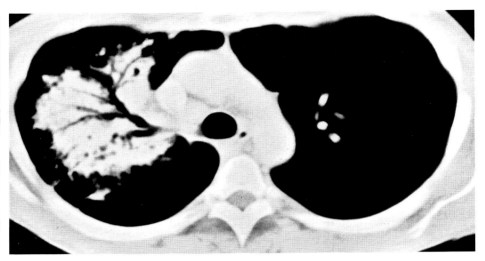

FIG 4–15 (left).
Air bronchogram within a pulmonary infiltrate. In this case, the pulmonary density is due to pulmonary edema.

FIG 4–16 (right).
Air bronchogram shown by CT in a case of pneumonia.

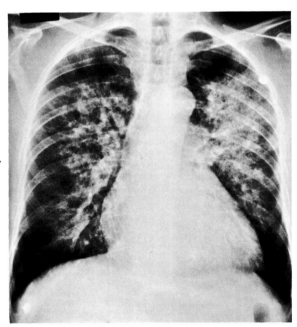

FIG 4–17.
Pulmonary edema, showing the typical "bat's wing" or "butterfly" pattern.

opacity is present. It is a surprising fact that a wedge- or lens-shaped opacity may be very difficult to see because of the way the shadow fades out at its margin, but if such a lesion is in contact with the mediastinum or diaphragm, it causes loss of their normally sharp boundaries. It must be stressed, however, that, as a completely isolated sign, lack of clarity of one of these borders is of limited value in diagnosing intrathoracic disease. To be meaningful, this loss of clarity must be accompanied by a density in at least one projection.

Interpretation of Radiological Findings

Occasionally it is possible to base a specific diagnosis on radiological examination alone. More often, there are several possible diagnoses for any particular finding. It is, therefore, helpful to try to categorize abnormalities in order to limit the differential diagnostic possibilities. One method is to try to place each abnormality into one or more of the following broad categories.

A. Pulmonary shadows
   1. Air-space filling
      a. Pulmonary edema
      b. Pulmonary consolidation (alveolar infiltrates with or without atelectasis)
   2. Spherical shadows
   3. Line shadows
   4. Widespread small shadows
B. Pleural processes
   1. Free pleural fluid
   2. Loculated pleural fluid
   3. Pleural thickening (fibrosis, tumor)
   4. Pneumothorax
C. Mediastinal/hilar disease
D. Diaphragm disease
E. Chest wall disease

The presence of cavitation or calcification should be noted. On CT it is also possible to distinguish fluid and fat from other soft tissue densities and, with intravenous contrast enhancement, it is possible to separately identify blood circulating in the vessels.

The classification listed above depends primarily on accurately localizing any abnormality. The more projections one has, the more accurate the localization becomes. The localization may be self-evident from the frontal chest radiograph alone, but two views at least are usually required, the lateral being the common accompaniment to the frontal projection.

Air-space Filling

"Air-space filling" (pulmonary infiltrates) represents the replacement of air in the alveoli by fluid or, rarely, by tumor or other substances. The fluid can be either a pulmonary edema or an exudate. The causes of an alveolar exudate include infection, infarction, pulmonary contusion, hemorrhage, collagen vascular disease/vasculitis, and eosinophilic pneumonia.

The radiographic sign associated with air-space filling is a shadow with ill-defined borders, except where the disease process is in contact with a fissure, in which case the shadow has a well-defined edge corresponding to the fissure (see Fig 4–14). In order to diagnose a pulmonary infiltrate, a shadow that cannot be accounted for by normal anatomical structures must be seen. Conversely, it is important not to misdiagnose shadows from structures projected over the lung (e.g., chest wall, breast, spine, scapula).

An air bronchogram may be visible within the density (Fig 4–15). Air bronchograms are often easy to see on CT scans (Fig 4–16). Normally it is impossible to identify air in the bronchi deep within the lung on either plain films or CT because the walls of the bronchi are too thin and are surrounded by air in the alveoli. If the alveoli are filled with fluid, however, the air in the bronchi contrasts with fluid within the lung. The air bronchogram is a very useful sign, because it signifies that the shadow must be intrapulmonary. An infiltrate containing an air bronchogram is almost always due to either pneumonia or pulmonary edema.

The heart, mediastinal, or diaphragmatic border adjacent to an infiltrate may be lost because of the silhouette sign (see page 159).

Pulmonary Edema

Radiographically, there are two forms of pulmonary edema—interstitial and alveolar. Since the edema fluid initially collects in the interstitial tissues of the lungs, all patients with alveolar edema also have interstitial edema. Alveolar edema is always acute. The causes can be divided into (1) those due to circulatory problems, e.g., acute left ventricular failure and fluid overload from renal failure or overtransfusion; and (2) noncardiogenic pulmonary edema—the so-called adult respiratory distress syndrome.

Alveolar edema (Fig 4–17) is almost always bilateral, involving all the lobes. The shadowing is greatest close to the hila and fades out peripherally, leaving a relatively clear zone around the edges of the lobes. This pattern of edema is sometimes called the "butterfly" pattern or the "bat's wing" pattern. Although the classic description is a bilaterally symmetric appearance, symmetry is in fact unusual, and the edema often predominates on one side or the other and varies in severity from lobe to lobe. An appear-

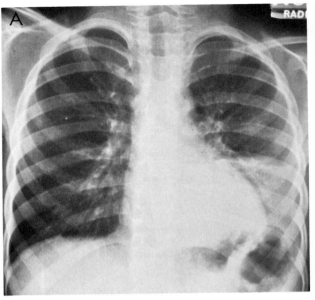

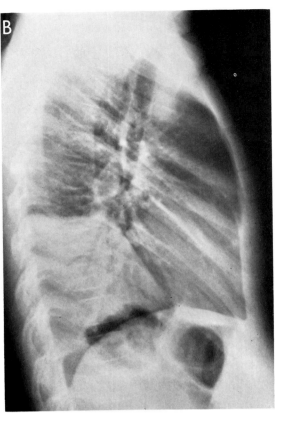

FIG 4–18.
A and **B**, consolidation of the left lower lobe due to bacterial pneumonia. Part of the superior segment is spared in this particular example.

FIG 4–19.
Widespread patchy consolidation in a case of bronchopneumonia.

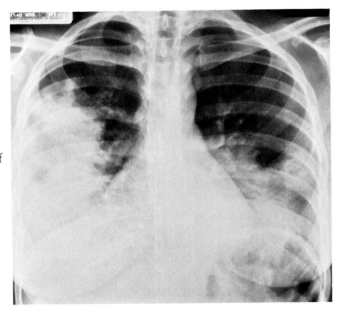

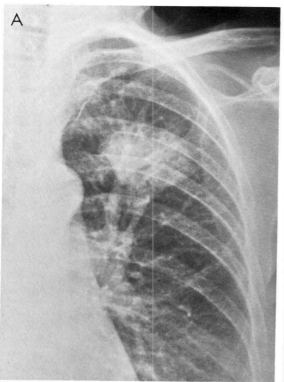

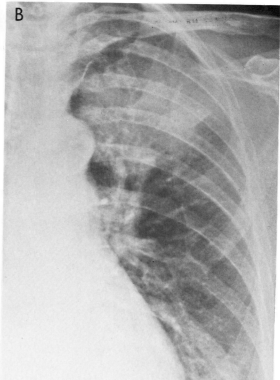

FIG 4–20.
Round pneumonia. **A,** the round shadow could be confused with a lung tumor, but one day later **(B)** the rapidly expanding shadow clearly indicates its inflammatory nature. Diagnosis of pneumonia was obvious clinically. The organism was the pneumococcus.

FIG 4–21 (left).
Cavitation within consolidation due to pneumonia. The air-fluid level within the right upper lobe is obvious. There is also some solid debris floating in the fluid. The pneumonia prior to cavitation is illustrated in Figure 4–53.

FIG 4–22 (right).
Pneumatoceles in a child with staphylococcal pneumonia.

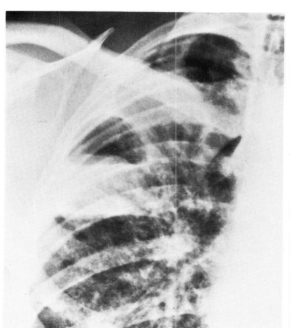

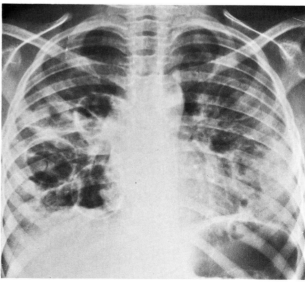

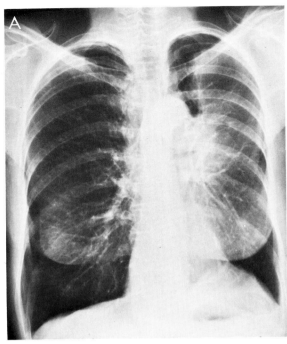

FIG 4–23.
Collapse of the left upper lobe. Note the ill-defined edge of the shadow of the collapsed lobe in the frontal view **(A).** The lack of clarity of the left heart border due to the silhouette sign is well demonstrated. In the

lateral view **(B)** the major fissure, which forms the posterior boundary, is clearly displaced anteriorly *(arrows).*

FIG 4–24.
Collapse of the left lower lobe. There is a large retrocardiac density with a well-defined lateral edge *(arrows).* Notice that the structures of the left lower hilum are invisible because they are surrounded by the atelectatic lung. (See Fig 4–5 for the lateral view of this patient.)

FIG 4–25.
Collapse of the right lower lobe. The obvious density in the right lower zone has a well-defined upper edge due to the displaced major fissure.

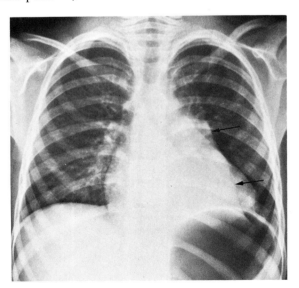

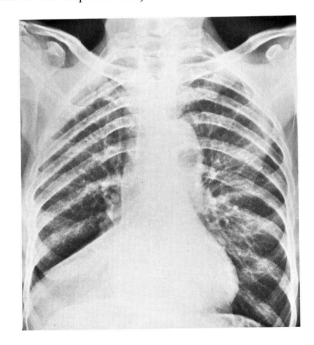

ance identical to that of pulmonary edema may be seen in widespread pneumonia (especially aspiration pneumonias, aspiration of gastric contents, inhalation of noxious gases, and pulmonary hemorrhage). A helpful feature in distinguishing cardiogenic pulmonary edema from widespread pulmonary exudates is the rapidity with which edema appears and disappears on treatment. Substantial changes in the severity of air-space filling in a 24-hour period strongly suggest pulmonary edema.

Pulmonary Consolidation

Consolidation and collapse (atelectasis) often coexist. It is, however, convenient to consider these two phenomena separately. Consolidation of a whole lobe is virtually diagnostic of pneumonia, usually bacterial. Lobar consolidation produces an opaque lobe, except for air bronchograms. Since the consolidated lobe is airless, the fissure between it and the normal lung does not appear as a line, but is seen as a clear-cut border to the opacity. Because of the silhouette sign, the boundary between the affected lung and the adjacent heart, mediastinum, and diaphragm will be invisible. The appearance of consolidation of the left lower lobe is shown in Figure 4–18.

Patchy consolidation (Fig 4–19), i.e., one or more patches of ill-defined shadowing up to the size of one or more segments, is usually due to infection, infarction, or, less commonly, eosinophilic pneumonia. There is no reliable way of telling from the films which of these possibilities is the cause but, in most instances, the clinical and laboratory findings point to one of these options. As discussed above, with very widespread patchy consolidation it may be difficult to decide whether one is dealing with exudates or pulmonary edema.

Consolidation may, in rare cases, be spherical (Fig 4–20), an appearance occasionally seen with pneumococcal and legionella pneumonia and rarely in other community-acquired infections. When a spherical consolidation is seen, it may be impossible to distinguish it from other causes of spherical shadows, particularly lung tumor. Spherical pneumonia is rarely misdiagnosed, however, because most patients have the typical symptoms of acute pneumonia. Serial films show a change over a short interval if the shadow is due to pneumonia, whereas no change will be apparent if it is due to a tumor.

The consolidated areas of lung may cavitate. The organisms particularly liable to produce cavitation are *Staphylococcus aureus*, *Klebsiella*, *Mycobacterium tuberculosis*, anaerobic bacteria, and various fungi. Cavitation or abscess formation is only recognizable once the ab-

scess communicates with the bronchial tree, allowing the liquid center of the abscess to be coughed up and replaced by air. The air, which may be visible only on tomography, is seen as a translucency within the consolidation. With the patient erect, an air-fluid level will be visible if enough of the fluid contents of the abscess cavity remain (Fig 4–21).

Pneumatoceles are another type of air space within an area of consolidation (Fig 4–22). They are associated with a number of processes; staphylococcal pneumonia and pulmonary contusion are the most common. The air cyst is believed to be the result of an air leak into the lung from a small airway. Pneumatoceles may rapidly increase or decrease in size or, alternatively, they may persist for many years after the original consolidation has resolved. They almost always disappear eventually.

Atelectasis

Atelectasis (collapse or loss of volume of a lung or a lobe) may be due to any of the following: bronchial obstruction, pneumothorax or pleural effusion, fibrosis of the lobe, bronchiectasis, or, rarely, pulmonary embolism. The plain radiographic signs are the shadow of the collapsed lobe and displacement of other structures to take up the space normally occupied by the collapsed lobe. As with any pulmonary shadow, the silhouette sign may be seen.

Consolidation almost invariably accompanies obstructive lobar collapse, so the resulting shadow is usually obvious. Occasionally, the loss of volume is very severe, and the lobe becomes so shrunken that, unless it is precisely tangential to the x-ray beam, the shadow may be difficult to see. It is in this situation that the silhouette sign is particularly helpful, since the mediastinal and diaphragmatic borders adjacent to the collapsed lobe will be ill-defined. The silhouette sign also helps in deciding which lobe is collapsed. Collapse of the anteriorly located lobes (upper and middle) obliterates portions of the mediastinal and heart outlines, whereas collapse of the lower lobes obscures the outline of the adjacent diaphragm and ascending aorta.

When a lobe collapses, other structures move to take up the space. The unobstructed lung on the side of the collapse expands; this process is reflected by displacement of fissures and the movement of the hilum toward the collapsed lobe. As with consolidation, the fissure in this condition is seen as a boundary to an airless lobe, not as a line between aerated lobes. The mediastinum and hemidiaphragm may move toward the collapsed lobe. The appearance of collapse of the various lobes is illustrated (see Figs 4–

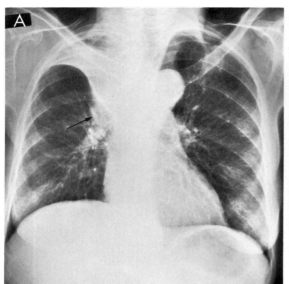

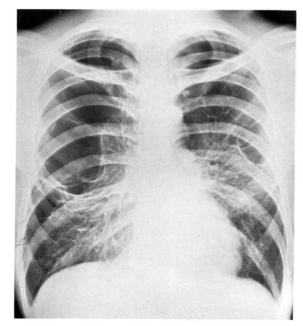

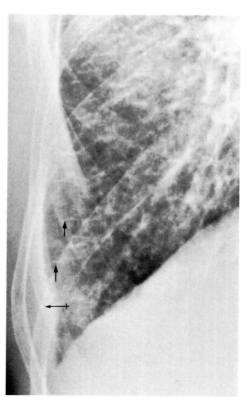

FIG 4–26.
A and **B,** collapse of the right upper lobe. The opaque right upper lobe shows elevation of both the minor and major fissures. There is an additional feature in this case; the fissures are bowed around a large intrapulmonary mass *(arrows).*

FIG 4–27 (left).
Long line shadows bounding and traversing bullae.

FIG 4–28 (right).
Septal lines (Kerley's B lines) in a case of pulmonary edema *(arrows).* A lamellar collection of subpleural pulmonary edema is also present *(crossed arrow).*

13 and 4–23 to 4–26). In collapse of the whole of one lung, the entire hemithorax is opaque, and there is substantial mediastinal and tracheal shift to the side of the collapse.

Collapse also occurs when air or fluid in the pleural cavity allows the lung to retract. Recognizing lower-lobe collapse in association with pleural effusion may be difficult. Even if the collapse is recognized, there may be difficulty in determining whether it is due simply to the presence of pleural fluid or whether both the collapse and the effusion are due to the same process, e.g., carcinoma of the bronchus.

When atelectasis is due to lobar fibrosis or bronchiectasis, the lobe usually remains aerated. The signs are, therefore, those of displacement of structures, and there may be little additional shadowing within the lobe. The fissure in this situation is seen as a line, since there is air on both sides of it.

Spherical Shadows (Lung Nodule or Mass)

If a spherical lung shadow is seen, it is important to review both lungs carefully to see whether the lesion is single or multiple. If multiple, well-defined, spherical shadows are seen, the diagnosis is almost always metastatic carcinoma or other widespread neoplasm. Occasionally, such a pattern is seen with multiple lung abscesses, e.g., septic emboli.

The usual causes of a solitary spherical shadow in the lung are primary carcinoma, metastasis, benign tumor of the lung, tuberculous or fungal granuloma, and lung abscess. Occasionally, pneumonia may present as round consolidation (see page 187).

The major question in a patient with an unexpected solitary pulmonary nodule is whether or not the patient has a malignant tumor. The investigation of a solitary pulmonary nodule falls outside the scope of emergency radiology, but two important points should be borne in mind by the emergency room physician: (1) extensive central calcification within a nodule excludes the diagnosis of bronchial carcinoma, and (2) review of old films to assess growth rate can be the single most helpful action in deciding whether or not a solitary pulmonary nodule is or is not a lung cancer. Lack of growth over a 2-year period excludes the diagnosis. A doubling time of between 1 month and 18 months is typical for primary lung carcinoma.

Line Shadows

Long line shadows, other than fissures, are usually due to pleuropulmonary scars from previous infection or infarction. They often reach the pleura and are associated with visible pleural thickening. They are of no significance to the patient. Emphysematous bullae

are often bounded and traversed by thin line shadows (Fig 4–27). Since they traverse an obvious bulla which contains no normal vessels, the interpretation of such lines is easy.

Another cause of line shadows are septal lines (Kerley's A and B lines). The pulmonary septae are connective tissue planes containing lymph vessels. They are normally invisible. Only when they become thickened can they be seen on the chest film (Fig 4–28). When these lines are seen in the middle and upper zones radiating toward the hila, they are known as Kerley's A lines. They are much thinner than the adjacent blood vessels and do not reach the lung edge. Kerley's B lines are the small horizontal septal lines, never more than 2 cm in length, best seen at the periphery of the lung bases. In contrast to the blood vessels, they often reach the edge of the lung. The most common causes of septal lines are pulmonary edema and lymphangitis carcinomatosa.

Widespread Small Shadows

Chest films with widespread 2- to 5-mm nodular or reticular densities present a common diagnostic problem. With few exceptions, it is only possible to give a differential diagnosis from the film alone. Many descriptive terms have been applied to these shadows, the most common being "mottling," "honeycomb," "fine nodular," "reticular," and "reticulonodular" shadows. In this discussion only two basic terms will be used: "nodular" to signify discrete small round shadows (Fig 4–29) and "reticular" to describe a net-like pattern of small lines (Fig 4–30). Often there are both nodular and reticular elements, and the pattern is then called "reticulonodular." All these patterns are due to very small lesions, no larger than 1 to 2 mm. Individual lesions of this size are invisible on the chest film. That these very small lesions are seen at all is explained by the phenomenon of superimposition: when numerous tiny lesions are present in the lungs, it is inevitable that some will be superimposed on one another. It follows that, when very small noncalcified shadows are visible, the lung must be diffusely involved by disease. It is worth noting that the size of the multiple small shadows seen on the x-ray film bears no relation to the true size of the responsible lesions, except to predict that they are small, nor can the shape of the lung shadows be reliably used to predict the shape of the responsible lesions.

How to Decide Whether Multiple Small Pulmonary Shadows are Present

Often the greatest problem is to decide whether

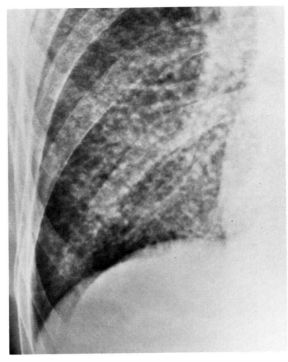

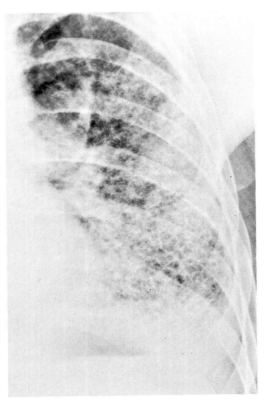

FIG 4–29 (near right).
Widespread nodular shadows. In this particular case, the diagnosis was coal-worker's pneumoconiosis.

FIG 4–30 (far right).
Widespread reticulonodular pattern. In this particular case, the diagnosis was diffuse interstitial pulmonary fibrosis.

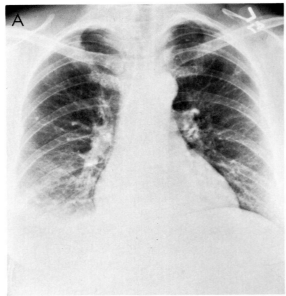

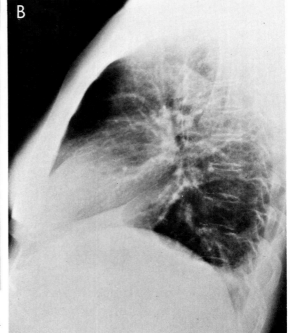

FIG 4–31.
Right pleural effusion. Note the hazy density on the frontal view **(A)** with a higher lateral than medial margin. The costophrenic angle is filled by this density. On the lateral view **(B),** the effusion can be seen rising up the posterior wall of the chest and running into the major fissure.

TABLE 4–1.

Radiologic Features of Diffuse Pulmonary Disease

Diagnosis	X-ray Pattern	Usual Distribution	Remarks
Infection			
TB and various fungi (coccidioidomycosis, cryptococcosis, blastomycosis, histoplasmosis)	Small well-defined nodules of uniform size	Uniform	May show mediastinal and/or hilar adenopathy, pleural effusion, and one or more patches of consolidation
Mycoplasmal and viral	Ill-defined nodules	Uniform	
Pulmonary fibrosis			
Idiopathic	Reticulonodular	Usually lower zone predominant and maximal at lung periphery	Hemidiaphragms often high and indistinct
Known causes, e.g., rheumatoid arthritis, scleroderma, extrinsic allergic alveolitis, drug reaction			
Sarcoidosis	Two patterns, usually not simultaneous Fine nodular Coarse reticulonodular	Uniform Middle and upper zone predominant	Often with hilar and paratracheal adenopathy
Pneumoconiosis			
Coal worker's silicosis	Nodular—variable size up to 1 cm or more	Upper zone predominant	Progressive massive fibrosis may be present; emphysema often visible
Asbestosis	Fine reticulonodular	Lower zone predominant	Usually shows pleural thickening and/or calcification
Neoplastic			
Lymphangitis carcinomatosa	Reticulonodular	No set pattern	Septal lines or bronchial wall thickening usually visible; hilar adenopathy frequent; other signs of metastatic cancer may be visible
Miliary metastases	Miliary nodules	Uniform	
Pulmonary edema	Ill-defined nodules	Perihilar predominance, often with relatively clear lung periphery	Septal lines are a major feature; cardiac enlargement and pleural effusion may be present

widespread abnormal shadowing is present at all, since normal blood vessels can appear as nodules and interconnecting lines. The normal pattern can only be established by looking carefully at many hundreds of films. The areas that should be particularly reviewed are the portions of the lungs seen between the ribs, where the lungs are completely free of overlying shadows. Normal vessels seen end-on appear as small nodules, but these nodules are no bigger than the vessels seen in the immediate vicinity, and their number corresponds to the expected number of vessels in that area. The normal linear pattern is a branching system that connects in an orderly way with more central larger vessels and no visible vessels in the outer centimeter of the lung.

The silhouette sign is useful in assessing diffuse pulmonary disease. Pathologic shadows will obscure the adjacent vessels, and the borders of the heart, mediastinum, and diaphragm may be less sharp than normal.

Once the presence and pattern of the abnormal shadowing has been determined, the next step is to decide on the distribution of shadowing. Associated findings should also be looked for. Having made all these observations, one is in a position to make the differential diagnosis. The common or more important conditions are described in Table 4–1.

The Pleura

Pleural Effusion

Fluid in the pleural cavity has the same appearance regardless of whether the fluid is a transudate, an exudate, pus, or blood. With rare exceptions this is true even for CT and ultrasound. Fluid that is free to move collects in the most dependent portions of the pleural cavities. Clearly, the dependent portions vary with the position of the patient and, therefore, on plain films the appearance of pleural effusion will vary between upright, supine, and decubitus films.

CT examinations are routinely conducted with the patient in the supine position, whereas ultrasound examination is carried out with the patient in any posi-

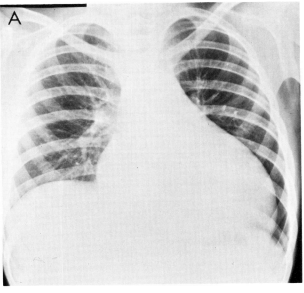

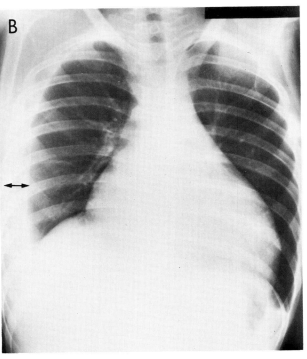

FIG 4–32.
Right subpulmonary pleural effusion, which has the same shape as the hemidiaphragm. The only way to suspect it on the frontal view **(A)** is to note that the apparent "hemidiaphragm shadow" is elevated. The lateral decubitus view **(B)** shows the fluid layered against the lateral chest wall *(arrows)*. The cardiac enlargement in this case is due to cardiomyopathy.

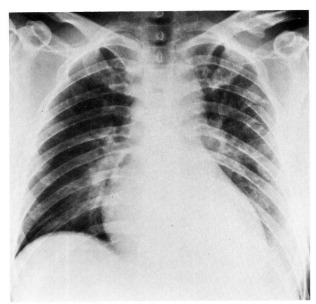

FIG 4–33.
Pleural effusion in patient in supine position. The left pleural effusion has a very ill-defined upper edge. The most obvious sign in this case is the complete lack of visibility of any portion of the left diaphragm. Note fractures of the left upper ribs.

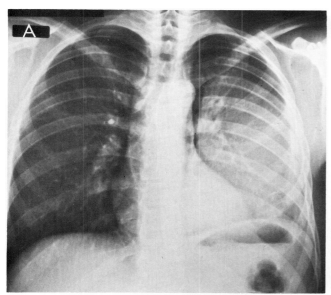

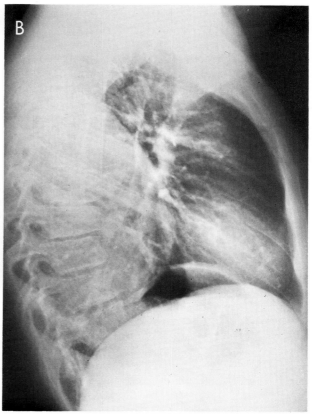

FIG 4–34.
A and **B,** loculated pleural fluid due to empyema posteriorly in the left thorax. Note how the differential diagnosis from lobar consolidation depends on appreciating the shape of the shadow in the lateral projection.

tion that seems desirable to the operator. It is important to take these variations in position into account when comparing the information from different modalities. Position becomes a very important issue in deciding where to place a thoracentesis needle or chest tube. The fluid may well be in a different position at the time of the procedure than it was when the diagnostic examination was being performed.

On plain chest radiographs free pleural effusions can be classified into two basic shapes, usually seen in combination with one another. The first of these shapes is similar to what would be seen if a large balloon were pressed down into a container of water. The water would be forced around the outer surface of the balloon up the sides of the container. Similarly, in most pleural effusions some of the fluid is seen running up the sides of the lungs and into the fissures (Fig 4–31). With large effusions, fluid may be seen extending over the lung apex. The smooth edge between the lung and the fluid can often be recognized on an adequately penetrated film, providing that the underlying lung is aerated. The fluid itself casts a completely homogeneous shadow in contrast with many pulmonary consolidations that show patchy air shadows or air bronchograms within them. In the upright position, all the fluid may lie in a subpulmonary location (Fig 4–32), so that the upper border of the fluid assumes a shape similar to that of the normal hemidiaphragm. Since the true diaphragm shadow is obscured by the fluid, it may be difficult and even at times impossible to tell from standard plain films that pleural fluid is present. Even the costophrenic angle may appear sharp, though fortunately it is usually less sharp than in the normal patient. On the left side it may be possible to suspect subpulmonary effusion because of the increase in the distance between air in the stomach and air in the lung.

If there is doubt about the presence or the amount of fluid, a lateral decubitus view can be of great help. The fluid, if free to move, will settle along the dependent lateral chest wall. It will then be possible to appreciate how much fluid is present by noting the distance between the ribs and the lung edge (see Fig 4–32,B).

Two mechanisms of pulmonary collapse may be seen in association with pleural effusion: compression collapse of the underlying lung, or, alternatively, both the pleural effusion and the pulmonary collapse can be due to the same basic process, e.g., carcinoma of the lung. Distinguishing between these two forms of pulmonary collapse can be very difficult. The position of the trachea is the most useful sign. If the trachea is displaced to the side of the effusion, there must be substantial collapse of the lung, more than could be accounted for by effusion alone. Very large effusions with little underlying pulmonary collapse will displace the mediastinum and trachea to the opposite side. If the trachea is central, it is then difficult to decide the mechanism of the pulmonary collapse.

It may be difficult to tell on plain chest radiographs whether an opacity at a lung base is due to pleural effusion or whether it is due to pulmonary consolidation or collapse. The shadow of pleural fluid is usually higher laterally than medially. It is homogeneous and lies outside the lung, being bounded by a sharp concave interface with the lung. No air bronchogram can be seen in a pleural effusion. Where the effusion runs into a fissure, both sides of the fissure are visible. The trachea and mediastinum are either central or are pushed to the opposite side. Conversely, with consolidation or collapse, the shape of the shadow conforms to that of a lobe or segment. An air bronchogram may be present and, where the consolidation abuts a fissure, the fissure is seen as an edge with only one side being visible. With consolidation or collapse, the trachea and mediastinum are either central or pulled toward the side of the shadow.

Free pleural effusions have a different appearance in supine films than on upright examinations (Fig 4–33). In the supine position the dependent portions of the pleural cavity are along the posterior chest wall and, therefore, the posteriorly-layered fluid causes ill-defined increase in density of a variable portion of the hemithorax, and the hemidiaphragm outline is often indistinct. Fluid may be seen over the lung apex, forming a well-demarcated band of density. With large effusions this band of density extends around the outer edge of the whole lung, and the entire hemithorax is denser than normal.

Loculated pleural effusions occur whenever the movement of pleural fluid within the pleural cavity is prevented by pleural adhesions. Loculation occurs in many types of effusions, but it is a particular feature of empyema (Fig 4–34). The loculations may be anywhere in the pleural cavity, including the fissures. If the fluid is loculated in an interlobar fissure, it may simulate a lung tumor in the frontal projection, but this misdiagnosis can be avoided by noting that, on the lateral view, the effusion is clearly lens-shaped and lies within the known position of one of the fissures (see Fig 4–12). Loculated effusions may resemble lung tumors or can be confused with dense pulmonary infiltrates (see Figs 4–11 and 4–34). The correct diagnosis of loculated fluid on plain chest radiographs depends on recognizing the clearly defined curved border of a pleural-based density.

The basic signs of pleural effusion on CT are similar

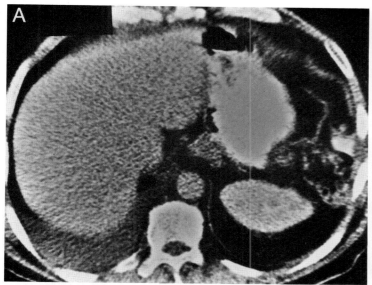

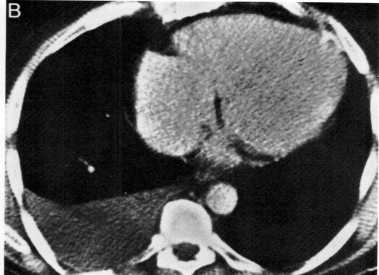

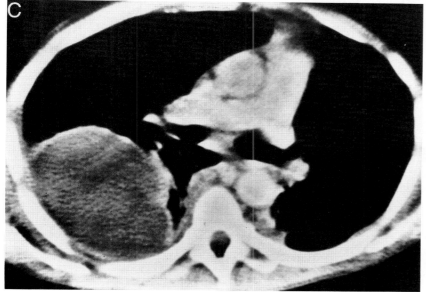

FIG 4–35.
CT scan of pleural fluid. A transudate in the right pleural cavity is shown in **A** and **B**. Two levels are illustrated: **A** shows pleural effusion lying behind right hemidiaphragm and liver; **B** shows a higher section where the fluid layers behind the right lower lobe. **C** is a case of empyema showing loculation of fluid within a layer of thickened fluid. Note the similar homogeneous nature of the fluid in both cases.

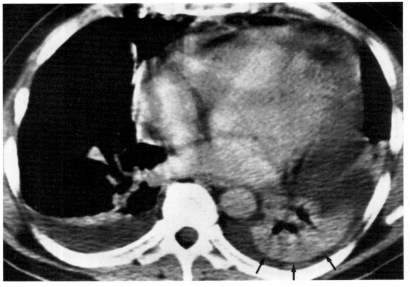

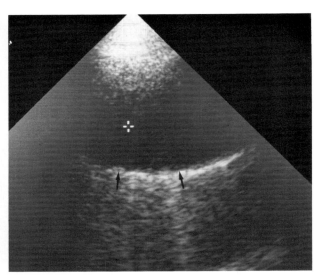

FIG 4–36.
CT scan showing collapse of left lower lobe within surrounding pleural effusion. The *arrows* point to the edge of the collapsed lung. There is also a right pleural effusion with a little streaky atelectasis in the right lower lobe. An adjacent section from this patient with widespread small cell carcinoma is shown in Fig 4–74.

FIG 4–37.
Ultrasound scan of pleural fluid. The *cross* is the center of the echo-free fluid. The interface between lung and fluid is well seen *(arrows)*. In this case the fluid was in an empyema.

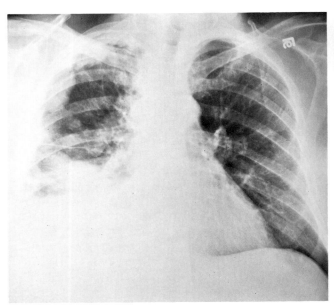

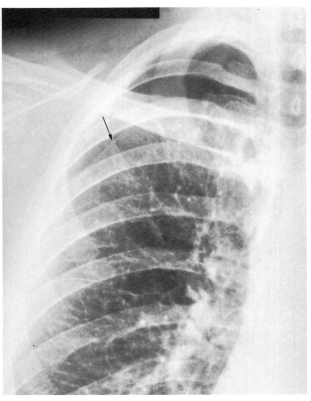

FIG 4–38 (left).
Lobulated pleural masses due to malignant pleural mesothelioma of the right thorax.

FIG 4–39 (right).
Pneumothorax clearly showing lung edge with air outside the visceral pleura *(arrow)*.

to those on plain film, with the additional information that the density of pleural fluid is homogeneous and, characteristically, pleural fluid is of lower density than most soft tissues (Fig 4–35). Distinguishing between pleural effusion and lobar collapse is very easy with CT, but CT is only occasionally needed because the lateral decubitus view is a simpler method. At CT, the density of the collapsed lobe is usually appreciably greater than that of the pleural effusion, even more so if intravenous contrast enhancement is used. Also, air within the bronchi can often be traced into the compressed lung (Fig 4–36). If contrast medium has been given, the blood vessels coursing through the collapsed lung can be identified. Pleural effusions are of uniform fluid density on CT and do not contain blood vessels or bronchi.

Ultrasound examination can be useful in investigating pleural effusion. As discussed above, loculated fluid can be very difficult to diagnose from plain films, and it is in this situation that ultrasound has a particular role to play. Because pleural effusion usually loculates against the chest wall, it is possible to place the ultrasound probe directly over the fluid collection, show its size and extent, and determine the best site for needle or chest tube placement (Fig 4–37). The other major role for ultrasound is diagnosing or excluding a subdiaphragmatic process, such as abscess or ascites, which could be responsible for the pleural effusion. The diaphragm and subdiaphragmatic regions are clearly visible on upper abdominal sonograms and ultrasound is, therefore, ideally suited to demonstrate fluid above or below the diaphragm.

Pleural Thickening

Pleural thickening can be due to fibrosis following previous pleural effusion or hemorrhage, pleural plaque formation in asbestosis or, on occasion, pleural neoplasm. Pleural fibrosis resembles pleural fluid, but the resulting shadow is always smaller (often much smaller) than the original pleural shadow. The costophrenic angle frequently remains obliterated, but the obliteration may be uneven, being greater in one projection than another. It may be impossible to distinguish pleural fluid from pleural fibrosis on conventional projections. Comparison with previous films may be necessary to show that the pleural shadow is not changing and is, therefore, fibrosis. Alternatively, the problem can be tackled by taking a lateral decubitus view, in which free fluid will lie along the lateral chest wall, whereas pleural thickening or loculated fluid will be unaltered in appearance.

Pleural fibrosis usually produces a smooth edge to the pleural shadow, whereas pleural tumors produce lobulated masses based on the pleura (Fig 4–38). Malignant pleural tumors, both primary and secondary, frequently cause pleural effusions, and the tumor itself may be partly or wholly hidden by the shadow of the fluid.

The distinction between pleural fibrosis/neoplasm and pleural fluid is readily made at CT and is particularly easy with ultrasound, since fluid and solid have such different characteristics at both CT and sonography.

Pneumothorax

The diagnosis of pneumothorax depends on recognizing the line of the pleura separated by air from the chest wall, mediastinum, or diaphragm. There will normally be no vessels beyond this line (Fig 4–39). Lack of vessel shadows alone is insufficient evidence on which to make the diagnosis, since there may be few or no visible vessels in emphysematous bullae. It is widely believed that the collapsed lung beneath the pneumothorax is more opaque than normal but, in fact, unless the pneumothorax is very large, there is no appreciable increase in the density of the lung.

The detection of a small pneumothorax can be very difficult. It is easy to confuse the pleural edge with the cortex of normal ribs and so fail to detect the presence of a pneumothorax. Sometimes a pneumothorax is more obvious on a film taken in expiration.

With tension pneumothorax, there is mediastinal shift, and one hemidiaphragm is often flattened (Fig 4–40).

In most cases of pneumothorax, whatever the cause, some fluid is present in the pleural cavity, and an air-fluid level will be visible. In spontaneous pneumothorax the amount of fluid, mostly blood, is often small.

A skin fold can, on occasion, be confused with a pneumothorax (Fig 4–41).

The Diaphragm

The position of the diaphragm may reflect disease. Both hemidiaphragms may be pushed up by abdominal distention, or they may be high as a result of lung disease.

Unilateral elevation of one hemidiaphragm occurs with loss of volume of the ipsilateral lung, or it may be due to an abdominal mass or a subphrenic abscess. In each of these situations, the cause of the elevated hemidiaphragm should be visible, or at least suspected, from the chest or abdominal film. Marked elevation of one hemidiaphragm with no other visible abnormality suggests either eventration or paralysis. It should always be borne in mind that subpulmonary effusion may mimic elevation of a hemidiaphragm.

The Mediastinum

Apart from the airway, the normal structures within the mediastinum all have the same radiographic density on plain chest radiographs. Even though they are surrounded by fat, it is usually not possible to identify fat planes other than the epicardial and pericardial fat. Therefore, the recognition of mediastinal disease on the chest radiograph depends on being able to identify widening of the mediastinum or noting either air or unusual calcification within it.

Acute mediastinal widening indicates the accumulation of blood or other fluid with bleeding from the arteries or veins in the mediastinum the most frequent cause. Bleeding may follow trauma or may be spontaneous from an aneurysm of the aorta or one of its branches. With leaking aneurysms, the aneurysm itself is frequently visible. In patients with transvenous lines, faulty positioning of the line may lead to extravasation of infused fluid into the mediastinum (Fig 4–42). Accumulations of pus or lymph are very rare causes of fluid in the mediastinum.

The plain film signs are similar, whatever the nature of the fluid. The fluid collection is maximal close to the site of any leak and often tracks through the mediastinum, leading to generalized widening and loss of clarity of the normal contours. The mediastinal space is continuous with the extrapleural space, and mediastinal fluid collections frequently track extrapleurally over the hemidiaphragms and over the lung apices, where they can be recognized as a cap of fluid density over the cupula of the lung (Fig 4–43). This capping of the pleura is not specific to extrapleural fluid collections. A similar appearance is seen with inflammatory or neoplastic pleural thickening and can even be seen, due to extrapleural fat, in normal patients. The features that should lead one to suspect hematoma or other fluid are the absence of adjacent disease and no similar shadow on the other side. The case for a fluid collection is strengthened if the interface with the lung is very smooth. As always, comparison with old films may be definitive in distinguishing acute from chronic changes.

Recognizing mediastinal widening can be very difficult on plain films because of the great variability in the configuration of the mediastinum in the normal population. The major reason for this variability is the shape of the thoracic aorta, which elongates and unfolds with increasing age, leading to substantial distortion in the outline of the right and left mediastinal contours. The degree of unfolding varies enormously. Therefore, a change in configuration compared to previous films is often more reliable evidence of mediastinal pathology than an evaluation based on a single film.

Computed tomography is the procedure of choice for evaluating the mediastinum since, with CT, it is possible to distinguish vascular from nonvascular widening and to confirm or exclude mediastinal bleeding.

Pneumomediastinum

Air in the mediastinum may result from a tear in the esophagus or tracheobronchial tree, either spontaneously or following trauma. Pneumomediastinum may also be due to air originating outside the mediastinum, such as subcutaneous emphysema or retroperitoneal air, which has tracked into the mediastinum. The most common reason for pneumomediastinum in a nontraumatized patient is air leaking from the bronchial tree during an asthmatic attack. It is also occasionally seen in a variety of disorders including diabetic ketoacidosis and leukemia, but the reason for the association with these disorders is not known; pneumomediastinum may be due to a forced Valsalva maneuver or it may be coincidental. Provided pharyngeal and esophageal perforation or traumatic leak from the tracheobronchial tree can be excluded, pneumomediastinum is, of itself, not of clinical significance.

Pneumomediastinum (Figs 4–44 and 4–49) is recognized on plain chest radiographs as a streaky translucency within the mediastinum, usually most obvious along the main pulmonary artery and adjacent left hilum, aortic knob, and left heart border. The air dissects up the perivascular areolar tissues and tracks into the neck, supraclavicular areas, and even into the axillae. It sometimes also tracks down into the retroperitoneum or extraserosally on either side of the diaphragm. In young children, the air often remains confined to the mediastinum. Mediastinal widening is usually absent or minor in benign pneumomediastinum. If the mediastinum is clearly wide, mediastinal fluid must be suspected and esophageal perforation becomes a possibility.

Pneumomediastinum may be difficult to distinguish from a medially located pneumothorax. The points to consider in the differential diagnosis are that pneumomediastinum is usually streaky and bilateral. Pneumomediastinum is readily and reliably detected by CT, but CT is reserved for those cases, such as suspected rupture of a major airway or the esophagus (see Fig 4–91), in which the presence of pneumome-

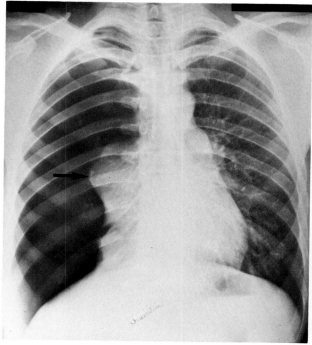

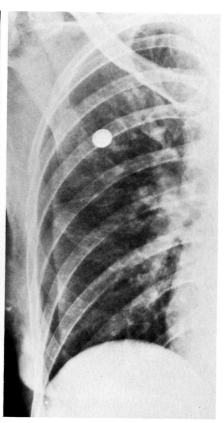

FIG 4–40 (left).
Tension pneumothorax. Note the collapsed right lung *(arrow)*, the low flat hemidiaphragm, and the mediastinal shift to the opposite side.

FIG 4–41 (right).
Skin fold mimicking pneumothorax. Note that here the edge of the skin fold is not a line as it is with pneumothorax, but the edge of a density with an ill-defined medial border.

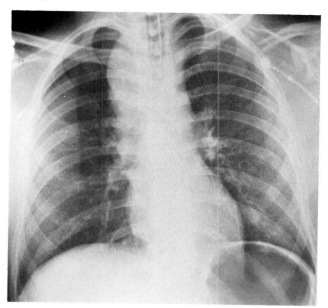

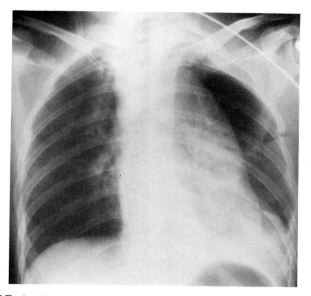

FIG 4–42.
Right superior mediastinal widening due to infused fluid following faulty positioning of an intravenous line.

FIG 4–43.
Aortic rupture leading to fluid (blood) capping the left upper lobe. There is also mediastinal widening and a large left subpulmonary pleural fluid collection.

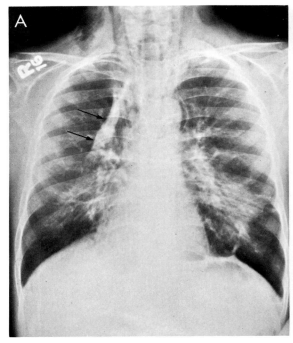

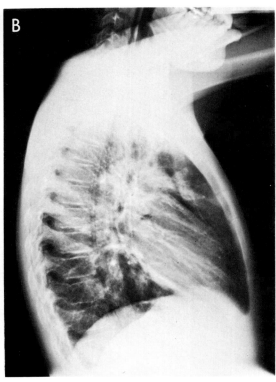

FIG 4–44.

A and **B**, pneumomediastinum in an asthmatic patient. Air is seen adjacent to the ascending aorta and aortic knob and has tracked into the neck. The thymus *(arrows)* has been lifted off the aorta. The air between the thymus and the great vessels must lie within the mediastinum and should therefore not be confused with pneumothorax. Note also the patchy atelectasis in both lungs due to mucous plugs.

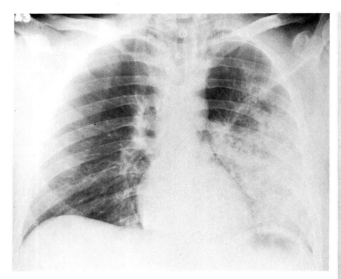

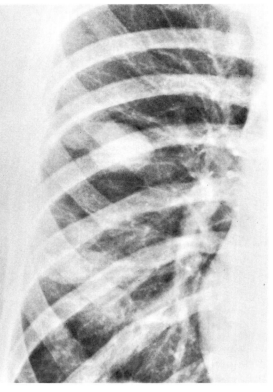

FIG 4–45 (left).

Large pulmonary contusion in the left lung. Note that the density due to the contusion cannot be distinguished from pneumonia or other causes of pulmonary infiltrate.

FIG 4–46 (right).

Pulmonary hematomata. Note the oval configuration and the well-defined edge of the upper of the two lesions.

diastinum leads to a significant change in management.

Trauma to the Chest

Rib Fracture

Recognizing a rib fracture depends on noting the loss of continuity of the cortex of the rib. There is usually a step-down across a fracture site, and the bone ends may appear dense because of overlap. Occasionally, there is no inferior displacement, and the only radiographic sign is increase in density caused by the overlapped portions of rib. The hematoma that accompanies a rib fracture is frequently visible as an extrapleural soft tissue swelling. This swelling may be the most obvious, or sometimes the only, sign of the fracture in any particular view.

The best view to demonstrate a fracture varies with the location of the fracture. The ribs are curved structures and therefore, whatever the view, some portions will be well seen and others poorly demonstrated. The standard chest film, which provides information about intrathoracic injury as well as chest wall damage, serves as the frontal view of those ribs above the diaphragm which are not obscured by the heart. Oblique views of symptomatic ribs can be added. For ribs below the domes of the diaphragm and behind the heart, penetrated frontal and oblique views are necessary. It is essential that the physician inform the technologist precisely which ribs are to be evaluated because the exposure factors for optimal visualization are determined by the rib to be demonstrated.

Rib fractures can be difficult to diagnose. Not infrequently, they are invisible because there is no displacement, or they are seen only in foreshortened projection and cannot be recognized. Fractures through costal cartilage or costochondral junctions are not diagnosable with conventional radiographic techniques.

Ribs four through nine are the most frequently fractured. In otherwise healthy patients, simple fractures of these ribs without accompanying pleural or pulmonary injury are usually innocuous. Flail chest is a clinical diagnosis, but the fractures causing the flail segment can, of course, be recognized.

Fractures of the upper three ribs indicate severe trauma and require a careful evaluation for bronchial or aortic injury. Similarly, fracture of the lower two ribs should raise suspicion of damage to the liver, spleen, and kidney. Serious intrathoracic injury can, however, occur without rib fracture. Indeed, owing to the pliability of the ribs in children, fractures may not occur despite considerable trauma.

Lung Contusion and Laceration

Lung contusion appears on plain chest radiograph within 6 hours of injury as a nonsegmental patchy or homogeneous consolidation, usually, but not invariably, on the traumatized side of the thorax (Fig 4–45). Clearing begins within 48 hours and is complete within 3 to 24 days. If the consolidation does not clear within 72 hours, an alternative diagnosis for the infiltrate should be considered, e.g., continued bleeding, pneumonia, or atelectasis. The contusion may not be visible for 4 to 6 hours after the injury. Rib fracture and pleural fluid (hemothorax) are frequently present. Many patients with clinically significant and even life-threatening pulmonary contusion do not have rib fractures.

Lung laceration may be seen with both blunt and penetrating trauma. The tear in the lung may fill with hematoma or may expand with air to become a pneumatocele. Lung laceration is frequently accompanied by hydropneumothorax. Pneumatoceles often contain an air-fluid level due to blood in the air space. The lung laceration is usually surrounded by contusion and, unless a pneumatocele is present, the laceration will be hidden on chest x-ray by the contusion. As the contusion clears, the hematoma may persist as a fairly well-defined rounded or oval density (Fig 4–46) that may take many weeks to resolve, eventually leaving a scar. The average clearing time is 5 weeks, but large hematomas may take a year to resolve. Pneumatoceles (Fig 4–47) are seen as rounded air lucencies that appear soon after the injury and usually disappear quickly. Their rapid appearance after injury distinguishes them from lung cavitation.

The CT features of lung contusion and laceration are similar to the plain film findings discussed above. There is little practical information to be gained from evaluating these lesions by CT, even though CT, as always, shows their extent more accurately.

Pleural and Chest Wall Abnormalities Following Trauma

Fluid in the pleural cavity following trauma is usually blood or, very rarely, chyle from thoracic duct injury. The radiology of hemothorax and chylothorax is identical to that of pleural effusion (see page 171).

Hemothorax after trauma may be caused by laceration of the lung, intercostal vessels, great vessels, or diaphragm or may accompany a lung contusion. Hemothorax from pulmonary injury is usually self limiting. Massive or persistent bleeding suggests serious mediastinal blood vessel or intercostal artery injury.

Pneumothorax following trauma can be due to lung

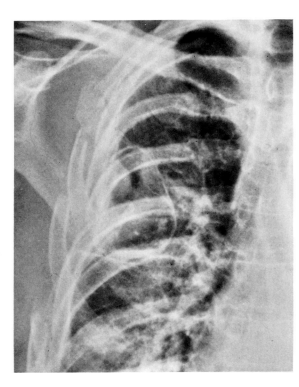

FIG 4–47 (top left).
Pneumatocele 6 days after severe chest injury. The thin-walled air cyst contains a small amount of fluid. The pneumatocele was present at the time of admission to the emergency room but was surrounded by pulmonary contusion at that time. Numerous rib fractures are also present.

FIG 4–48 (middle and bottom left).
Illustration of the sensitivity of CT in detecting pneumothorax in trauma. The chest film was taken supine **(A)** owing to the patient's poor condition. The pneumothorax is very difficult to see and was not seen prospectively. The CT scan **(B)** shows a large right pneumothorax.

FIG 4–49 (bottom right).
Fractured bronchus leading to pneumomediastinum. Note that the only indication of a bronchial tear in this patient is the presence of a pneumomediastinum.

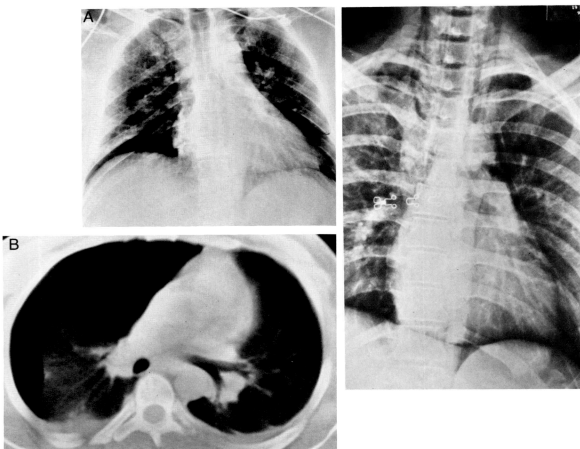

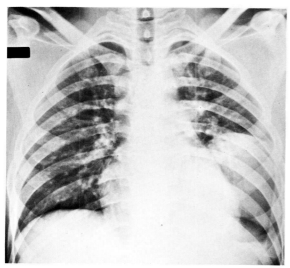

FIG 4–50.
Rupture of the left hemidiaphragm. The stomach is herniated through the tear, and gas in the stomach is seen above the predicted position of the hemidiaphragm.

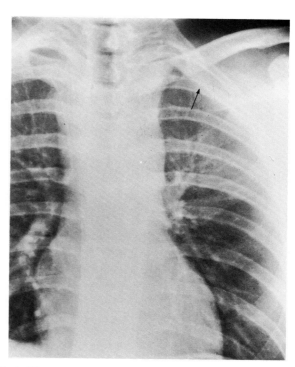

FIG 4–51.
Traumatic rupture of the aorta. The mediastinum is wide due to hematoma, and there is blood surrounding the left lung producing an apical cap *(arrow)*.

FIG 4–52.
Traumatic rupture of aorta. Aortogram showing an intimal flap and widening of the aorta distal to the origin of the left subclavian artery, both of which are typical of the immediate post-trauma appearances of aortic rupture.

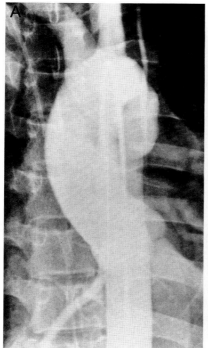

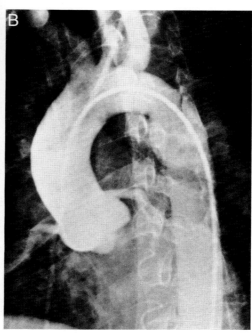

laceration from penetrating injury or from the sharp end of a rib fracture. When seen in cases of blunt trauma, it may be due to shearing or compression forces. Occasionally, the air in the pleural space is consequent to pneumomediastinum from bronchial tear. The radiology of pneumothorax has been described on page 177. Hemopneumothorax is frequently present and is recognized by noting an air-fluid level in the pleural space. Pneumothoraces that are life-threatening are obvious radiographically. Small pneumothoraces should be looked for with particular care in patients on positive-pressure ventilation.

In trauma victims CT scan will show many more pneumothoraces than plain chest radiographs. This is partly because of the inherent advantages of CT, but also because chest radiographs in a trauma setting are so often single views in the supine position exposed with mobile machines. CT examinations are, by comparison, hardly compromised because the procedure is much the same as in the nontraumatized patient.

The substantially higher sensitivity of CT in detecting pneumothorax in patients with major trauma was first discovered on abdominal CT examinations, since these invariably include the lung bases. In pneumothorax, the air rises to the upper-most portion of the pleural cavity which, in the supine patient, is just above the diaphragm. Thus, if an abdominal CT is obtained, the images will show any significant pneumothorax that may have been overlooked or invisible on plain chest radiograph (Fig 4–48). Chest CT is almost never required exclusively to look for pneumothorax.

Chest Wall Emphysema

Subcutaneous emphysema of the chest wall is usually, in itself, of no significance, but its recognition may lead to the finding of significant abnormality. It occurs when a fractured rib punctures the lung. Subcutaneous emphysema of the chest wall and neck should always lead to careful evaluation of the chest film to exclude pneumomediastinum, which could indicate a tear of a major bronchus.

Tracheobronchial Tear

Tracheobronchial tears occur only with major thoracic trauma, usually an anterior chest wall deceleration injury. They are associated with intracranial or great vessel injury in 50% of patients and are usually in the main stem bronchus just distal to the carina. The major problem with bronchial tear is the late complication of significant bronchostenosis.

Pneumomediastinum (Fig 4–49), lobar collapse, and

pneumothorax, particularly one that does not respond to chest tube suction, are the important signs on imaging examinations. It should be remembered, however, that 10% of patients will have no physical or radiographic evidence of intrathoracic injury, probably because the integrity of the bronchial sheath is maintained.

Ruptured Diaphragm

Ruptured diaphragm is usually the result of blunt trauma to the lower chest and upper abdomen; 95% of cases involve the left hemidiaphragm. Rib fracture and ruptured spleen are commonly associated.

The radiologic signs are pleural effusion and herniation of abdominal contents through the diaphragm (Fig 4–50). The tear itself is never visualized, even at CT. The diagnosis is frequently difficult, since it is often impossible to be sure of the position of the diaphragm, especially if pleural effusion develops. Therefore, it is not easy to say if bowel shadows are above or below the diaphragm. Consequently, the chest radiograph or CT scan of any patient with an "elevated hemidiaphragm" following trauma should be very carefully analyzed to ensure that this is not a pseudoelevation with the upper edge of hernial contents mimicking an elevated diaphragm. If a nasogastric tube has been inserted, the course of the tube may give valuable information regarding the presence of herniated stomach. In clinical practice, many cases of ruptured diaphragm are missed initially.

Fat Embolism

Fat embolism produces respiratory failure with diffuse pulmonary opacification and is now considered to be one of the precipitating factors in adult respiratory distress syndrome (see page 196).

Traumatic Rupture of the Aorta

Traumatic rupture of the aorta is usually due to sudden deceleration injury, which produces severe shearing stresses. In almost all patients who survive the initial accident, the rupture is at the aortic isthmus just beyond the origin of the left subclavian artery. The next most common site of injury is the origin of the brachiocephalic artery.

In almost all cases, the chest radiograph is abnormal (Fig 4–51). The plain film signs are purely those of the resulting hematoma. Post-traumatic aneurysms only occur several weeks after the initial injury and, therefore, immediately after the accident the contours of the aorta itself are not recognizably abnormal. The hemorrhage results in mediastinal widening and lack

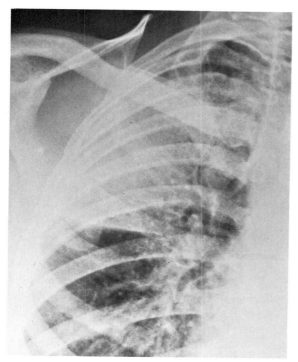

FIG 4–53.
Right upper-lobe pneumonia. Note that the infiltrate is densest in the most dependent portion of the upper lobe, and its boundary is sharp where it contacts the minor fissure. The upper margin of the infiltrate is ill defined.

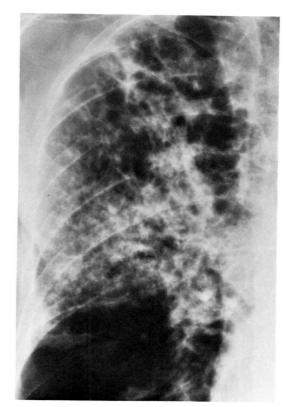

FIG 4–54.
Right upper-lobe pneumonia in a patient with severe emphysema.

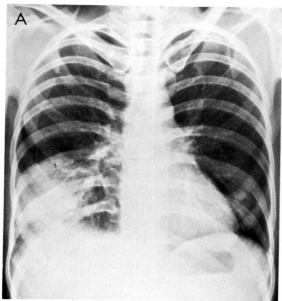

FIG 4–55.
A and **B,** pneumococcal pneumonia causing dense consolidation of most of the right lower lobe.

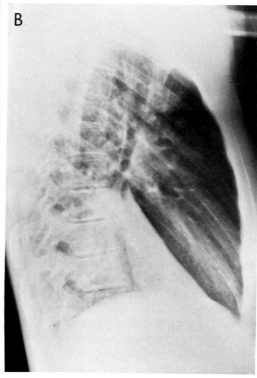

of clarity of the aortic knob. The trachea and left main bronchus may be displaced away from the bleeding site. The mediastinal hematoma may dissect extrapleurally and can be recognized over the lung apex, almost invariably the left. Free pleural fluid will be noted if the hematoma has ruptured into the pleural space. Because the initial injury is severe, other signs of chest trauma, such as fractured ribs and pulmonary contusion, are frequently seen. In the appropriate clinical setting, these findings may be diagnostic of aortic rupture, but each by itself is nonspecific.

Whenever the possibility of traumatic rupture of the aorta is being seriously considered on combined clinical and plain film grounds, aortography should be undertaken (Fig 4–52). It is the most sensitive and the most specific test available. The use of chest CT remains controversial. The chief problem with using CT when an urgent decision is needed is that a normal CT scan, even with intravenous contrast opacification, does not rule out a laceration of the aorta in which the bleeding is confined by the adventitia. Thus aortography will be indicated whatever the CT findings in cases where the clinical suspicion of aortic rupture is high. The findings on CT are mediastinal hemorrhge, which may be diffuse mediastinal hemorrhage, an intramural hematoma, or a focal hematoma close to the laceration. Mediastinal hemorrhage alone is not enough to establish the diagnosis of laceration of the aorta or great vessels since the hemorrhage may be from damage to smaller branches of the aorta or rupture of mediastinal veins. When any of the above signs are found at CT, aortography should be undertaken. The laceration itself is rarely demonstrated on CT, but may, on occasion, be seen as a small pseudoaneurysm of a linear lucency caused by the torn edge within the lumen of the aorta—always providing intravenous contrast opacification has been used. If a traumatic dissecting hematoma occurs, then the two lumens may be seen separated by an intimal flap.

There is one situation in which CT may obviate aortography, namely in a patient in whom the clinical probability of a ruptured aorta is very low, but in whom the plain chest radiographs show nonspecific mediastinal widening. CT scanning may then be able to demonstrate an alternative, clinically unimportant, reason for the plain film findings such as fat deposition or aortic unfolding. The appearances at CT depend on how much mediastinal bleeding has occurred from the aortic tear. When still confined by the adventitia, the hematoma will be small in amount and could easily be overlooked. Once hemorrhage into the periaortic tissues occurs, the resulting blood will be visible as soft tissue density tracking through the mediastinum and extrapleural space, often with accompanying pleural fluid. The density of blood is usually indistinguishable from the density of soft tissue, e.g., muscle. Retracted blood clot may show recognizable high density.

Pneumonia and Lung Abscess

The primary purpose of the chest radiograph in patients with suspected chest infection is to establish whether or not pneumonia is present. Diagnosing the infective agent is more problematic because there is considerable overlap in the appearances of the various pneumonias. Clearly, the chest radiograph cannot replace bacteriologic and laboratory information. The principal radiographic features of pneumonia are one or more areas of pulmonary consolidation, which may show cavitation and may be accompanied by pleural effusion. The appearance of individual consolidations within the lung varies from a small, ill-defined density to a large shadow involving the whole of one or more lobes, the pattern depending on the infecting organism and the integrity of the host defenses. Although the term "segmental infiltrate" is commonly used, an infiltrate that conforms precisely to segmental anatomy is rarely seen. Infective consolidation can readily cross segmental boundaries since there are no anatomical barriers to prevent such spread, but it is usually held up by the interlobar fissures. The infiltrate is usually densest in the most dependent portions of a given lobe. Where it lies against a pleural fissure, it has a well-defined edge, but otherwise its margin is hazy (Fig 4–53). Occasionally, a well-defined, round infiltrate is seen (see Fig 4–20). Lobar atelectasis may result from pneumonia, particularly in children. The atelectasis is the result of obstruction of multiple small airways by inflammatory exudate and mucus.

The diagnosis of cavitation depends on recognizing an air space or an air-fluid level within the infiltrate (see Fig 4–21). If an air-fluid level is recognized, providing one is certain that it is in the lung, the diagnosis of cavitation is certain. However, if the only sign is the air space, it can be difficult to be sure that cavitation is present. Patchy consolidation with intervening normal areas of lung is commonly seen, and these normal areas can be mistaken for cavities. Also, pneumonia in bullous areas will show air spaces caused by bullae, which may resemble cavities (Fig 4–54).

The appearances of pneumonia may be modified if the underlying lung is diseased. Emphysema, generalized pulmonary fibrosis, or focal scarring all distort the lung and may alter the radiologic appearance of superimposed pneumonia.

Certain generalizations can be made regarding the radiographic features of pneumonia. These comments will be limited to community-acquired infection in the noncompromised host in order to make them more relevant to the emergency physician.

1. Lobar consolidation or consolidation involving the greater part of one lobe is almost always due to pneumonia (Fig 4–55); it is rarely due to the other causes of pulmonary infiltrate. The pneumonia is usually either bacterial or mycoplasmal in origin. The usual organism is Streptococcus pneumonia; occasionally it is Klebsiella, S. aureus, or Legionella. Expansion of the lobe caused by intense exudate is virtually diagnostic of pneumococcal or Klebsiella pneumonia (see Fig 4–60).

2. Cavitation within the consolidation suggests bacterial rather than viral or mycoplasmal pneumonia. The organisms that commonly cause cavitation are gram-negative or anaerobic organisms associated with aspiration pneumonia, Streptococcus pyogenes, Pseudomonas, S. aureus, Klebsiella, or Escherichia coli. Neither the number nor the size of the cavities is of diagnostic importance.

3. Spherical pneumonia is usually due to pneumococcal infection or Legionnaire's bacillus. Multiple spherical pneumonias are frequently due to Legionnaire's disease. Spherical pneumonia can be confused radiographically with a lung mass, particularly primary carcinoma. However, spherical pneumonia expands to involve the adjacent lung over the next few hours or days and is associated with obvious clinical features of acute bacterial pneumonia (see Fig 4–20).

4. When widespread, small, ill-defined shadows with or without septal lines (Kerley's lines) are due to infection, the infection is likely to be due to a virus or to Mycoplasma pneumoniae (Fig 4–56). Fungal and tuberculous disease may give a similar appearance (Fig 4–57).

5. Miliary nodulation in the lungs has many causes. When due to infection, the usual organisms are Mycobacterium tuberculosis and fungi. The nodules in these infections are well defined, uniformly distributed, and equal in size, usually 2 to 4 mm in diameter (Fig 4–58). The nodules are usually present in the first film taken, but if the film is taken early in the course of the disease it may be normal. The entity that radiologically most closely resembles miliary infection is pneumoconiosis, and the chest x-ray appearances of the two may be totally indistinguishable. The clinical differences are, however, so great that true confusion almost never occurs.

6. When hilar adenopathy and pleural effusion accompany pulmonary consolidation, three entities should be seriously considered: carcinoma of the lung, anaerobic bacterial infection, and chronic infection such as tuberculosis and fungal disease.

7. Patchy upper lobe infiltrates suggest tuberculous or fungal infection.

8. Empyemas may be indistinguishable from pleural effusions on plain chest radiographs. The possibility of empyema should be considered if the effusion accompanies a pneumonia in which empyema is known to be common, e.g., pneumonia due to anaerobic bacteria or Staphylococcus aureus. Other indications of possible empyema are effusions that are large, appear rapidly, or loculate early in the course of the disease.

Lung Abscess

The infectious agents most frequently responsible for lung abscess are Staphylococcus aureus, Klebsiella, mixed anaerobic organisms, Mycobacterium tuberculosis, and various fungi. A lung abscess is seen as a spherical shadow containing central lucency due to air within the cavity (Fig 4–59). This air may be difficult to appreciate without tomography. The air is often accompanied by fluid, in which case an air-fluid level will be visible on erect films.

It may be difficult or impossible to distinguish lung abscess due to infection from the other causes of a cavitary mass, including cavitary malignant neoplasm, infarction, and granulomas due to collagen vascular disease. Most infective lung abscesses are in the posterior portions of the lung, and caution should be exercised when diagnosing an anterior cavitary mass as a lung abscess. Very irregular cavity walls are an important sign that the lesion is something other than lung abscess and is probably a lung carcinoma. Tomography can play a role in determining the thickness and regularity of the cavity wall. Uniformly thin smooth cavity walls are usually benign, whereas a cavity in which any portion of the wall is thicker than 2 cm is usually a malignant neoplasm.

Pneumonia Due to Underlying Disease

BRONCHIAL OBSTRUCTION.—Bacterial pneumonia may be secondary to obstruction of the bronchus. In a patient over 35 years of age, the obstruction is likely to be neoplastic, usually carcinoma. In children, the common cause of obstruction in a major bronchus is an inhaled foreign body. Lesions that cause obstructive pneumonitis are usually in a lobar bronchus and occasionally in a segmental bronchus. More peripheral lesions do not produce obstructive pneumonitis

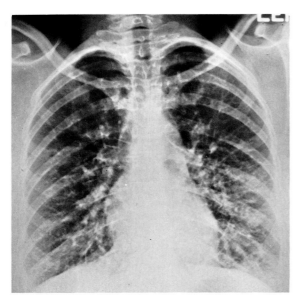

FIG 4–56.
Mycoplasma pneumonia, showing widespread ill-defined small shadows with numerous septal lines.

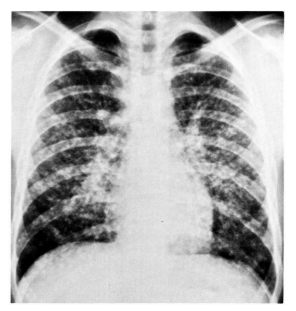

FIG 4–57.
Acute inhalational histoplasmosis, showing diffuse ill-defined small nodules throughout the lungs.

FIG 4–59.
Lung abscess, showing a slightly irregular, relatively thin-walled cavity and an air-fluid level. An identical radiographic appearance could be seen with a malignant tumor or, very rarely, with a lung infarct or granuloma due to collagen vascular disease.

FIG 4–58.
Miliary nodulation in the lungs due to miliary tuberculosis.

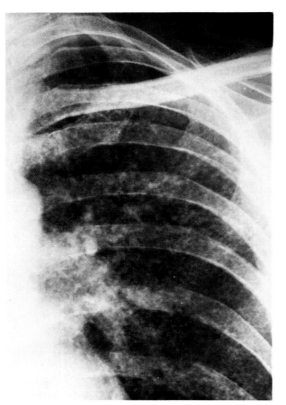

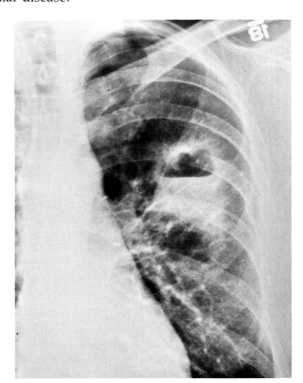

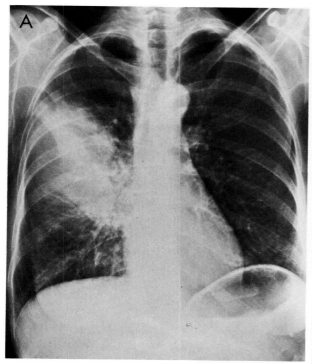

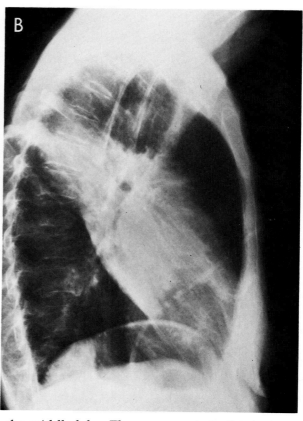

FIG 4–60.
A and **B,** expansion of a consolidated lobe due to Klebsiella pneumonia. The major fissure is bulged backward due to the intense exudate in the middle lobe. The pneumonia in this instance also involves the right upper lobe.

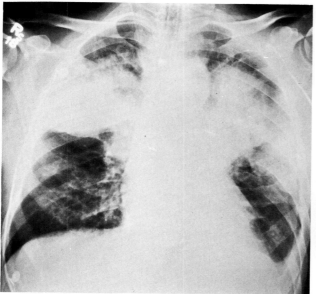

FIG 4–61 (left).
Pneumonia due to *S. aureus* with multiple dense consolidations in both lungs.

FIG 4–62 (right).
Pulmonary tuberculosis, showing a patchy infiltrate in the right upper lobe together with adenopathy at the right hilum and in the right paratracheal area. This combination is known as the primary complex.

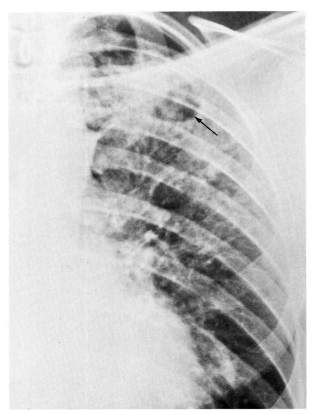

FIG 4–63.
Postprimary pulmonary tuberculosis, showing multiple ill-defined small consolidations in the upper lobe together with cavitation *(arrow)*.

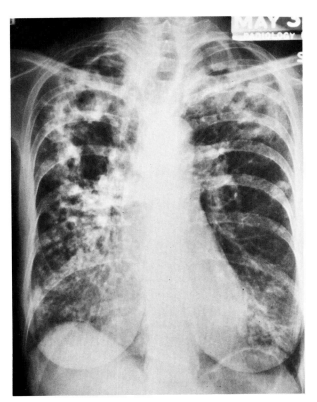

FIG 4–64.
Tuberculous bronchopneumonia, showing widespread patchy consolidation predominantly in the upper zones with multiple large cavities.

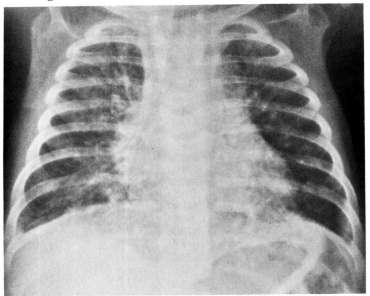

FIG 4–65.
Bronchiolitis and interstitial pneumonia in a 2-month-old child. Note the widespread streaky infiltrate and the low flat diaphragm.

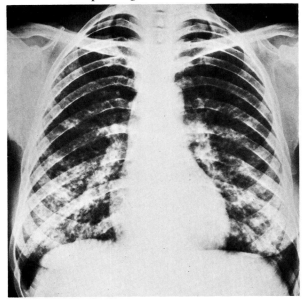

FIG 4–66.
Viral pneumonia, in this instance due to chickenpox, showing multiple small consolidations throughout the lungs.

because of collateral air drift within and between segments. The importance of this knowledge is that, if pneumonia is due to an underlying bronchial obstruction, the responsible lesion should be easily visible at bronchoscopy.

Postobstructive pneumonitis is usually confined to one lobe but, if more than one lobe is involved, the two lobes will usually share a common bronchus; e.g., the right lower and middle lobes can be involved from a lesion in the bronchus intermedius. The lobe will almost invariably show some loss of volume, and an air bronchogram will almost never be visible within the area of consolidation. Typically, the pneumonia will not resolve radiologically on antibiotic therapy, although partial improvement is frequently seen.

It should be remembered that, even if a mass is present, it is usually surrounded by pneumonia and cannot be separately identified. Occasionally, the central mass is so large that it deforms the outline of the affected lobe (see Fig 4–26).

BRONCHIECTASIS.—It is possible, although frequently difficult, to recognize bronchiectasis as the underlying pathology in pneumonia. The air in the dilated, thick-walled bronchi can occasionally be identified on plain film. When the bronchi are infected, air-fluid levels may be seen within the dilated airways. The affected areas always lose volume to a recognizable degree if much of the lobe is involved.

Specific Infections

Although it is rarely possible to determine accurately the precise infectious agent, it is frequently necessary to begin treatment guided by the combination of the clinical impression and the chest radiographic pattern. This section will therefore briefly review the radiographic features of some of the more common community-acquired infections.

Pneumococcal Pneumonia

Pneumococcal pneumonia (see Fig 4–20) usually causes homogeneous consolidation that begins in the periphery of a lobe. As it spreads, it crosses segmental boundaries and, if untreated, usually involves the whole lobe to become lobar pneumonia. Nowadays, true lobar pneumonia is rare. If seen early in its course, before any of the pleural boundaries have been reached, the pneumonia may appear spherical in shape.

The infection is purely alveolar in location, and the absence of bronchial obstruction means that loss of volume is unusual and that air bronchograms are frequent. The infiltrate usually involves just one lobe, but on occasion more than one lobe may show consolidation.

With appropriate treatment, the consolidation usually clears within 10 to 14 days. Cavitation is rare.

Pleural effusion is seen in at least 10% of cases and, occasionally, the effusion becomes an empyema.

Staphylococcus Aureus

Pneumonia due to S. aureus produces a patchy segmental consolidation, often with loss of volume. The infiltrates frequently involve several lobes and may be bilateral (Fig 4–61). Irregular abscess cavities are common. Pleural effusion is seen in about half of adult cases and may develop rapidly. The consolidations in the lung may spread rapidly in both adults and children. Pneumatoceles are a particular feature of childhood disease and may lead to pneumothorax (see Fig 4–22).

Anaerobic Organisms

Pneumonia due to anaerobic organisms usually involves the posterior segments of the upper lobes or the superior segments of the lower lobes. One or more irregular infiltrates are seen in the lungs, and these frequently cavitate, producing thick-walled irregular cavities. Pleural effusions are common and are usually infected, forming empyemas. Hilar adenopathy is seen in about half the cases that develop lung abscesses and may be so prominent as to lead to a misdiagnosis of malignant neoplastic adenopathy.

Gram-Negative Bacterial Pneumonia

Most gram-negative pneumonias show bilateral patchy lower lobe predominant bronchopneumonia. Patchy atelectasis is common and air bronchograms are unusual. Cavitation is a particular feature as are pleural effusions which may convert to empyema. *Klebsiella* pneumonia may give a similar picture, but sometimes the consolidations are confined to one lobe and appear as homogeneous nonsegmental shadows that spread rapidly to become lobar pneumonia. The appearances may, therefore, with one exception closely resemble pneumococcal pneumonia: Klebsiella pneumonia frequently cavitates, whereas cavitation in pneumococcal pneumonia is rare.

Legionella pneumophila is another gram-negative bacterium which causes pneumonia with somewhat distinctive features (Legionnaire's disease). It gives rise to patchy dense areas of consolidation in one or more lobes, often involving both lungs. The consolidations may coalesce to resemble lobar pneumonia. A spherical shape just like that in pneumococcal pneumonia is sometimes seen. Cavitation is unusual, and pleural effusions are usually small.

Tuberculosis

Pulmonary tuberculosis is often divided into primary and postprimary forms, even though these divisions are not clear-cut. Primary tuberculosis follows the initial infection with *Mycobacterium tuberculosis* and usually occurs in childhood. Postprimary tuberculosis is the usual form seen in adults. It is believed to be a reinfection in a patient who has developed relative immunity.

Primary tuberculosis appears radiographically as an area of consolidation in the lung, usually in the middle and upper zones, together with enlarged hilar or mediastinal nodes. This combination is known as the primary complex (Fig 4–62). Sometimes one or the other of the components is difficult or impossible to see on plain chest radiograph. In most cases, whether treated or not, the primary complex heals and frequently calcifies.

The disease may progress, giving rise to tuberculous bronchopneumonia, which looks just like any other bacterial bronchopneumonia but frequently involves more than one lobe, including one or both upper lobes, and cavitates readily.

Miliary tuberculosis is the result of spread through the bloodstream which produces innumerable small pulmonary nodules on chest x-ray (see Fig 4–58). The nodules are all much the same size and fairly evenly distributed. They are usually well defined, but in severe cases may coalesce and be difficult to appreciate as individual nodules. Early in the clinical course the chest radiograph may be normal.

Pulmonary involvement in postprimary tuberculosis is usually greatest in the upper portions of the lungs, the apical and posterior segments of the upper lobes, and the apical segments of the lower lobes. Multiple small areas of consolidation are seen initially. As the infection progresses, the consolidations enlarge and frequently cavitate (Fig 4–63). Widespread bronchial spread may occur, giving rise to multilobar bronchopneumonia, usually including one or both upper lobes, cavitation being a frequent phenomenon (Fig 4–64). Healing occurs with fibrosis and calcification, but signs of healing may be seen despite continuing activity. Occasionally, tuberculosis takes the form of lower- or middle-lobe bronchopneumonia and may even resemble lobar pneumonia. As with the primary form, the infection may spread via the bloodstream to give rise to miliary tuberculosis.

Pleural effusions are frequent in both primary and postprimary tuberculosis and may be the only manifestation of the disease.

Deciding whether pulmonary tuberculosis is active can be very difficult. Valuable radiographic signs of activity are the development of new lesions on serial films and the demonstration of cavities. Lack of change over a long period is useful evidence of inactivity, but the changes may be very subtle, even with active disease. A single examination cannot exclude activity, nor does the presence of calcification.

Many routine chest films in asymptomatic patients show evidence of tuberculosis. In a few, the diagnosis of active disease will be readily apparent from the presence of cavities or comparison with previous films. In the remainder, it can be a considerable problem to decide which patients to investigate further and which to accept as having old, inactive infection. The better defined the shadows and the greater the calcification, the less the likelihood of activity. Ill-defined shadows, even if partially calcified, suggest active disease. However, the decision is based largely on the clinical findings and on the results of sputum examination.

Mycoplasmal Pneumonia

There are two basic patterns seen with mycoplasmal pneumonia. It may resemble many other pneumonias with one or more segmental consolidations, occasionally involving a whole lobe. Small pleural effusions may be present. Alternatively, a reticulonodular pattern with septal lines may be seen throughout both lungs (see Fig 4–56).

Viral Infections of the Lower Respiratory Tract

Inflammation of bronchi and bronchioles in adults does not produce any radiologic signs, but in children bronchiolitis has important radiographic features. The airway inflammation may extend into the peribronchial interstitial tissues, producing streaky perihilar reticulonodular shadows (Fig 4–65). With more extensive disease, patchy consolidations may be seen; these are usually multiple and small (Fig 4–66), but may be large and indistinguishable from a host of bacterial bronchopneumonias. In severe cases, the infiltrates are extensive and may be identical to the pattern seen with pulmonary edema. Pleural effusion is common and is often associated with pleuritic pain.

Fungal Pneumonias

A variety of radiographic patterns too numerous to discuss in detail are seen with fungal diseases. In general, the signs are similar to tuberculous, mycoplasmal, or viral infections.

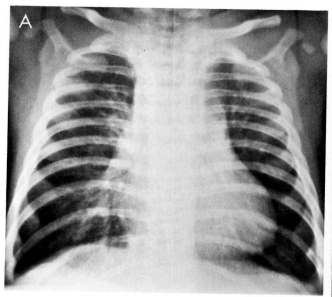

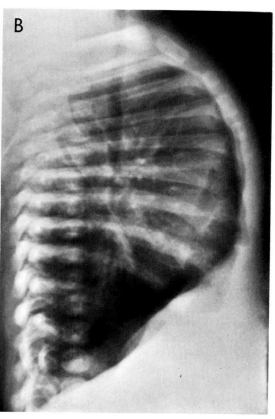

FIG 4–67.
A and **B,** acute bronchiolitis in a young child showing severe overinflation of the lungs with extremely low flat hemidiaphragms.

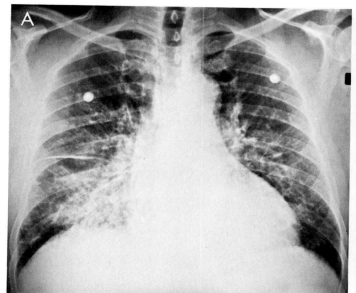

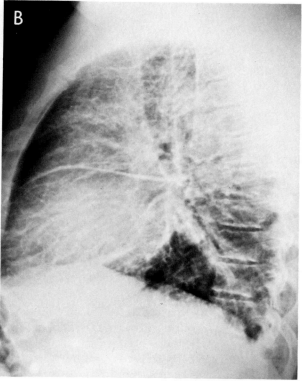

FIG 4–68.
A and **B,** interstitial pulmonary edema. There are widespread septal lines, and the fissures appear thickened due to edema in the lung against the pleural surfaces.

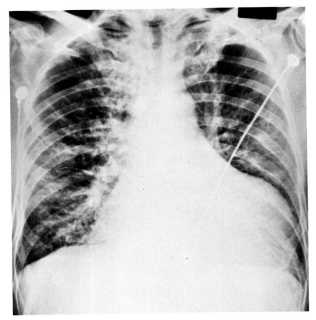

FIG 4–69.
Raised pulmonary venous pressure resulting in enlargement of the upper-zone vessels. Note also the greatly enlarged heart.

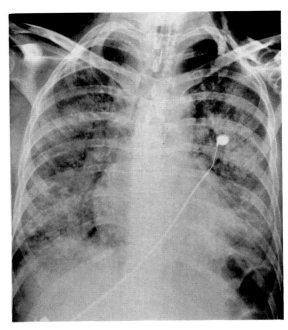

FIG 4–70.
Adult respiratory distress syndrome in 43-year-old man. Note widespread, fairly uniformly-distributed pulmonary shadowing.

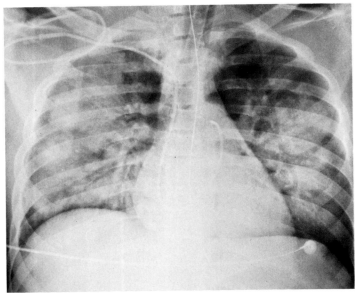

FIG 4–71 (left).
Near drowning. In this instance, the near drowning occurred in fresh water. There is florid bilateral pulmonary edema. The appearance is identical to that seen with either acute cardiogenic pulmonary edema or adult respiratory distress syndrome.

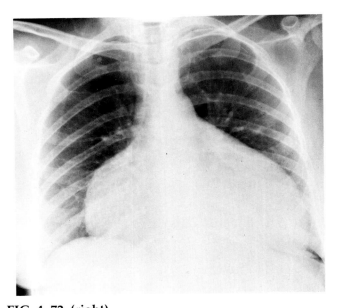

FIG 4–72 (right).
Typical large pericardial effusion showing smooth oval enlargement of the heart. Note the well-defined outline.

Differences Between Adults and Children

Even trained radiologists can be uneasy when asked to interpret a chest radiograph of an infant or young child with possible pneumonia. Often the definition of anatomical detail is poorer because of the technical problems encountered in radiographing children. The signs of pneumonia are the same regardless of age, but disturbances of aeration such as atelectasis or air trapping are much more frequent in small children because the airways in infancy are relatively small and collateral air pathways are less effective. When generalized, as in bronchiolitis, inflammatory narrowing of the smaller airways causes two major radiologic signs: irregularity of aeration and generalized hyperinflation. The presence of low flat hemidiaphragms—the best indication of hyperinflation—is often best appreciated on the lateral view (Fig 4–67).

The question most frequently asked regarding children with suspected chest infection is, "Does this child have bacterial pneumonia?" If there is no visible infiltrate, bacterial infection is unlikely. There are two provisos to this statement. First, the chest x-ray may have been taken too early; in rare instances the infiltrate only becomes visible a few hours after the patient first presents with symptoms. Second, the pneumonia may be difficult to identify if it is hidden behind the heart or mediastinum or is below the levels of the domes of the diaphragm. These areas should therefore be viewed with particular care on both PA and lateral projections before declaring the lungs normal.

If there is an infiltrate on the film, deciding its cause can be a problem since both viral and bacterial pneumonias, as well as atelectasis without pneumonia, may look identical. A large infiltrate without signs of volume loss usually indicates pneumonia rather than noninfective atelectasis.

Inhalation of Noxious Gases and Smoke

Many forms of lung disease result from inhalation of gases and other noxious substances. Only the more common acute disorders will be considered here.

Inhalation of Toxic Gases

The initial radiologic effect seen in the lungs following inhalation of a variety of toxic gases (including carbon monoxide, nitrous dioxide, sulfur dioxide, ammonia, and chlorine) is the appearance of pulmonary edema within 4 to 24 hours of the injury. This edema will often clear, even though the bronchi or bronchioles have suffered severe structural damage. The effects of bronchial damage will be seen later in the patient's course, often following a latent interval without clinical or radiographic abnormality.

Soon after injury, smoke inhalation may also produce a pattern resembling pulmonary edema, but this may not develop for up to 96 hours after exposure. Other patterns seen with smoke inhalation include focal collapse and/or consolidation or irregular patchy infiltrates. The average time of appearance of these abnormalities is 24 to 36 hours after injury. It is important to realize that there is no correlation between the chest x-ray findings and the degree of hypoxemia or carboxyhemoglobinemia. Significant hypoxemia and carboxyhemoglobinemia can coexist with a film that remains normal throughout the patient's hospital stay.

Hydrocarbon Pneumonia

Children who ingest petroleum distillates such as kerosene frequently develop patchy consolidations at the lung bases. The severity of the pulmonary change is related to the volume ingested. The pulmonary consolidations usually appear within an hour of ingestion. They resolve slowly, taking up to 2 weeks or more to clear, and their resolution usually lags well behind the clinical improvement. Pneumatoceles may develop, as may pleural effusion.

Pulmonary Edema, Adult Respiratory Distress Syndrome, and Circulatory Disorders

The radiographic appearance of a patient in heart failure varies with the cause. Although there are radiologic signs of right heart failure—cardiomegaly with dilatation of the right atrium, superior vena cava, and azygos vein, together with pleural effusions—the diagnosis of right heart failure is made primarily on clinical grounds. By contrast, left heart failure produces radiographic signs that may be pathognomonic even when the clinical features are absent or nonspecific. The plain film signs can be divided into two categories: those due to the effects of raised pulmonary venous pressure, including pulmonary edema, and those due to alterations in cardiac shape, including dilatation of the left ventricle and/or left atrium. Other features that indicate the specific cause may be present, e.g., valve or pericardial calcification.

Raised Pulmonary Venous Pressure and Pulmonary Edema

Pulmonary edema occurs in many situations. Whatever the cause, both cardiac and noncardiac pulmonary edema show the same radiographic signs. The more severe the changes, the more likely the edema is to be acute. Pulmonary edema occurs when the pulmonary venous pressure is above 24 to 25 mm Hg (the oncotic pressure of plasma). Initially, pulmonary edema is seen in the interstitial tissues but, when more severe, the edema is also visible in the alveoli. Both interstitial and alveolar pulmonary edema can be recognized on chest radiographs.

Interstitial edema (Fig 4–68) causes thickening of the interstitial tissues of the lungs. When thickened, the interstitial septae are seen as line shadows, known as Kerley's A and B lines. The B lines are short, horizontal, 1 to 2 cm lines at the extreme edge of the lungs, best appreciated at the bases. Unlike the blood vessels, the B lines can be seen to reach the pleural edge. A lines are 3 to 6 cm long and radiate from the hila mainly in the middle and upper zones. They are much thinner than the adjacent blood vessels and show fewer branches.

Septal lines are the hallmark of interstitial pulmonary edema. Edema may also be recognized as thickening of the bronchial walls which is best appreciated where bronchi are seen end-on. Normally the lung and hilar vessels are moderately well defined but, when surrounded by edema, the vessels may be fuzzy and indistinct. This is a very difficult sign to evaluate. Interstitial edema also collects subpleurally to produce an extremely useful sign, uniform thickening of the fissural lines (see Fig 4–68), together with the so-called lamellar pleural effusion. This term is a misnomer, since the dense stripe is due to subpleural pulmonary edema, not fluid in the pleural cavity. The radiological features of alveolar edema are discussed on page 163.

It is possible to recognize raised pulmonary venous pressure even in the absence of visible pulmonary edema. Normally, blood flow is greatest to the most dependent portions of the lungs. Therefore, in the upright chest film, the blood vessels in the lower zones are larger than those in the upper zones. In raised pulmonary venous pressure, the vessels in the upper zones enlarge and, if this enlargement is obvious, the diagnosis of raised pulmonary venous pressure can be made (Fig 4–69). The diagnosis needs to be made with caution, however, since it may be difficult to decide whether the vessels are truly enlarged. Also, other causes of redistribution of blood flow to the upper zones, e.g., basal pulmonary emboli and basal emphysema, need to be considered.

The heart usually enlarges in a nonspecific way with prolonged left ventricular failure. Left atrial enlargement often accompanies left ventricular enlargement but, if the left atrium is selectively enlarged, the probable explanation is mitral valve disease. In acute left ventricular failure, e.g., myocardial infarction, the heart is usually normal in size and shape.

Noncardiogenic Pulmonary Edema (Adult Respiratory Distress Syndrome)

Adult respiratory distress syndrome is characterized by unexpected or severe respiratory distress in patients whose lungs were previously normal. There are many precipitating disorders, including hypotension, septic shock, aspiration of gastric contents, hemorrhagic pancreatitis, near drowning, ingestion of drugs, fat embolism, and severe trauma. The common feature appears to be damage to the pulmonary capillaries which leads to increased permeability and consequent proteinaceous edema. A second component is widespread alveolar atelectasis due to surfactant deficiency.

Radiologically, the edema of adult respiratory distress syndrome is initially identical to cardiogenic alveolar edema. Cardiac enlargement and pleural effusions are not features of the disorder. The pulmonary edema seen on the chest radiograph may sometimes only be identified a few hours after the onset of hypoxemia, in contrast to cardiogenic pulmonary edema, which is visible coincident with the development of hypoxemia. With time, the patient develops increased lung density involving the whole of both lungs with little variation in severity in the different portions (Fig 4–70). Such patients invariably require artificial ventilation and are therefore liable to such complications as interstitial emphysema, pneumothorax, and pneumomediastinum.

Near Drowning

The major chest radiographic feature of near drowning is the development of pulmonary edema (Fig 4–71). The mechanism of the excess alveolar fluid varies according to the circumstances of the drowning episode. It may be totally due to capillary damage leading to adult respiratory distress syndrome, or it may be compounded by inhaled water. Pulmonary edema is seen with near drowning in both fresh water and sea water. The presence or absence of pulmonary edema on the initial chest film is of prognostic importance in that a fatal outcome is unlikely for a patient with a normal plain chest radiograph on admission. But a normal chest film does not exclude the subsequent development of life-threatening pulmonary edema. Indeed, the pulmonary edema may not become manifest for up to 48 hours following the drowning accident.

Pneumonia may supervene and can be very diffi-

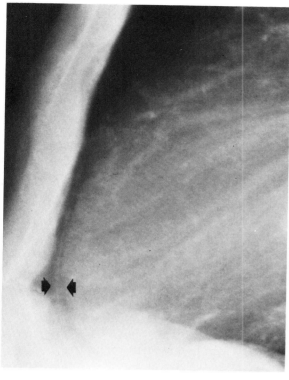

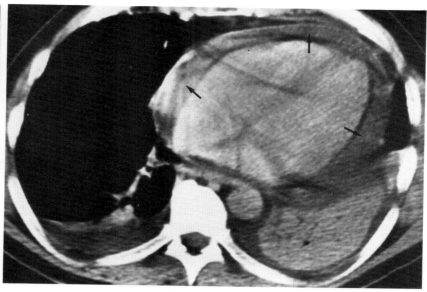

FIG 4–73 (top left).
Normal pericardium visualized on the lateral view. The fine line with fat on either side *(arrows)* represents the thickness of both layers of the pericardium.

FIG 4–74 (top right).
CT of pericardial effusion *(arrows)*. The water density encasing the heart is readily recognized, even without intravenous contrast opacification. There are also bilateral pleural effusions and underlying collapse of the left lower lobe. The patient had widespread small cell carcinoma of the lung.

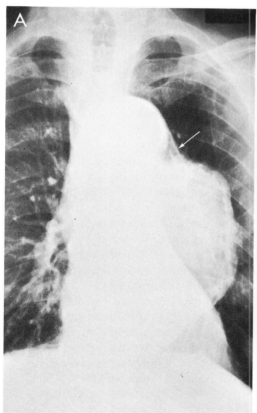

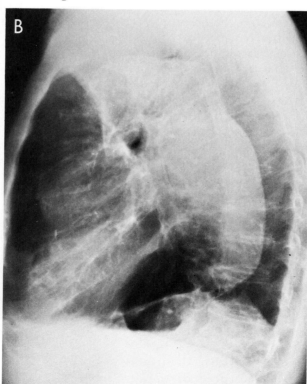

FIG 4–75.
A and **B,** atherosclerotic aneurysm of the descending aorta. There is fine curvilinear calcification in the wall of the aneurysm *(arrow).*

cult to diagnose if it does since the density due to the pneumonia may not be noticeably different from that due to the underlying edema.

Pericardial Disease

Pericardial effusion leads to a generalized increase in the size of the heart. With large effusions, the cardiac silhouette becomes globular in shape, with a smoothing out of the bumps and indentations normally seen in the region of the aorta and the main pulmonary artery (Fig 4–72). The cardiac outline also becomes well defined, since movement of the pericardium is reduced because of the cushioning effect of the fluid. An identical appearance may occasionally be seen with cardiomegaly due to chamber dilatation (see Fig 4–32). A specific feature is separation of the epicardial and pericardial fat planes by widening of the pericardial space. These fat planes are, for practical purposes, seen only on the lateral projection. This popular sign is of limited value since it is so frequently not visible in patients with pericardial effusion. The fat planes are perhaps of greater value in showing that the pericardium is of normal thickness (Fig 4–73).

Echocardiography is more sensitive and accurate than plain film in diagnosing pericardial effusion, so plain film radiology usually has little to offer except in cases where rapid change in cardiac size allows a definite diagnosis of pericardial effusion.

Pericardial effusion is readily diagnosed at CT (Fig 4–74). It is often recognized in patients being examined for other reasons. The examination is rarely recommended specifically to detect pericardial effusion since echocardiography is a quicker and easier method of diagnosis, particularly in an emergency setting. When pericardial thickening or tumor is suspected, CT and magnetic resonance imaging (MRI) may provide more information than echocardiography.

Thoracic Aortic Aneurysm

The most common causes of thoracic aortic aneurysms are atherosclerotic disease and medionecrosis; these two conditions may coexist. In patients with medionecrosis, blood may leak into the media of the aortic wall and cause dissecting aneurysm, perhaps better called dissecting hematoma. Any aortic aneurysm may rupture, resulting in leakage into the media and subsequently into the pleura and even the lung. A dissecting aneurysm is particularly prone to leak, often with a fatal outcome. Rarer causes of aortic aneurysms include trauma, noninfectious aortitis, syphilis, mycotic aneurysm, and, on occasion, congenital aneurysm. (Traumatic aortic rupture is discussed on page 184.)

The chest radiographic signs can be conveniently divided into the signs due to the aneurysm itself and those due to leakage of blood beyond the wall of the aorta. The aneurysm is frequently seen as widening of the aorta on standard PA and lateral films. This is particularly true of aneurysms of the distal arch and descending aorta. When the aneurysm is caused by arteriosclerosis, curvilinear calcification of the wall of the aneurysm is frequently identified (Fig 4–75). This calcification is an important sign, since it enables one to exclude the alternative diagnostic possiblity of a neoplasm in contact with the aortic wall. The configuration of the aortic widening varies with the cause. Degenerative aneurysms are usually fusiform and are largest in the descending aorta, often sparing the ascending aorta. Saccular arteriosclerotic aneurysms do occur, but they are less common.

Aneurysms of the ascending aorta are more difficult to diagnose on plain chest radiography, since the first third to half of the ascending aorta is not border-forming, and dilatations of this portion of the aorta may be completely invisible on plain films, whatever the projection. This is not a limitation for CT which, particularly when done with intravenous contrast enhancement, will provide a very accurate picture of the diameter of the aorta at all levels. Echocardiography can visualize the intrapericardial portion of the aorta (roughly the proximal one third of the ascending aorta) and therefore offers a good means of assessing aneurysms of the aortic root. The root of the aorta is a particular site of predilection for medionecrosis aneurysms, which may cause aortic regurgitation and may be complicated by dissecting hematoma.

Dissecting aneurysm is a particularly difficult diagnostic problem on plain chest radiography. The affected aorta is usually uniformly widened, but not necessarily dramatically so (Fig 4–76). The appearances may be very difficult to distinguish from the common, and clinically insignificant, aortic unfolding with mild dilatation. A completely normal-appearing aorta is extremely unusual in patients with dissecting aneurysm. Therefore, a normal chest radiograph is fairly reliable in excluding the diagnosis.

The patients in whom the diagnosis can be made with confidence are those in whom progressive widening of the aorta can be appreciated on serial films. However, the comparisons must be made from technically comparable films. Portable AP films taken with poor inspiration may show spurious widening when compared with routine PA films taken on good inspiration.

Leakage of aortic aneurysms initially causes a mediastinal hematoma, the signs of which are discussed on page 184. Blood may also leak into the pleural cavity, causing a pleural effusion indistinguishable from transudative and exudative effusions. The hemorrhage in the pleural cavity is often exclusively on the left. When bilateral, it is much greater on the left than the right. With severe bleeding, pulmonary infiltrate due to hemorrhage into the lung may be seen.

In practice, the diagnosis of dissecting aneurysm always requires confirmation by one or more additional tests. Chief among these are CT, angiography, and ultrasound, but MRI may, in the future, partially or completely replace all these modalities. Ultrasound examination of the root of the aorta is routine in echocardiography and is an excellent initial test in suspected dissection of the ascending aorta. It confirms or excludes pericardial hemorrhage, a major complication of the disease, and may also show the double lumen and intimal flap of the dissection itself. This combination of signs may be adequate information with which to proceed directly to surgery in a severely ill patient. A normal echocardiographic examination cannot, however, be used to exclude the diagnosis.

CT and angiography both have excellent sensitivity and specificity for aortic dissection. Aortography is still regarded as the most reliable diagnostic test, in that it effectively demonstrates the condition, if it is present, or excludes the diagnosis when negative (Fig 4–77). It also provides excellent information about the extent of the dissection, particularly by demonstrating details of which branches of the aorta are compromised. For this reason, some surgeons recommend aortography at an early stage, arguing that they need the study in any patient who requires surgery and, in the sick patient, the delay and the additional contrast requirements of a CT scan mitigate against using CT as a preliminary test. CT is, however, an equally sensitive test. It demonstrates the extent of the lesion well enough to permit a clear-cut decision between medical and surgical treatment. In cases which require surgery, some surgeons are willing to operate on the evidence of the CT scan without an angiogram; others insist on aortography.

The technique of CT is partly determined by the equipment being used and also by the radiologist's preferences. Intravenous contrast is required and is injected while the sections are being exposed. Sections from the origins of the great vessels down to the midleft atrial level suffice to cover the relevant portions of the aorta. The advantage of limiting the study to the portions of the aorta at risk is that the total intravenous contrast load can be correspondingly reduced. The signs at CT are (Fig 4–78):

1. Dilatation of the aorta. If the whole thoracic aorta is of normal diameter, the chances of dissection are low.

2. Double lumen sign. The true and false lumen are separated by an intimal flap, which is seen as a band of low density crossing the aorta. Frequently the two lumens show different concentrations of contrast medium, a helpful feature in determining that they are truly separate lumens. Artifact needs to be borne in mind when the diagnosis is based solely on the presence of an intimal flap. Streak artifacts from very dense objects in the section, particularly if they are moving, may create linear streaks of low density (Fig 4–78,B). These streaks are straight and can be traced to the responsible density. Also, they are not consistently seen on adjacent sections. Clearly, if the streak is an artifact, there will be no difference in the concentration of contrast medium on either side of the streak.

Pulmonary Embolism and Infarction

Although many chest radiographic abnormalities are described in pulmonary embolism and infarction, they are all nonspecific; hence it is impossible to decide from the plain chest radiograph alone whether the patient has or has not had a pulmonary embolus. Signficant, even life-threatening, pulmonary embolism may occur in patients with perfectly normal chest radiographs. The simplest way to consider pulmonary embolism is to divide the signs into embolism with or without infarction.

Pulmonary embolism without infarction usually produces no recognizable abnormality. Reduction in size of occluded pulmonary blood vessels may be seen, but this is usually so difficult to evaluate that, unless one has identical comparison films, the sign has little use. A major problem is that it is usually impossible to distinguish a reduction in size of the blood vessels due to pulmonary embolism from that due to emphysema or old infections. Enlargement of a major arterial trunk at the hilum is another well known, but very rarely seen, sign. Discoid atelectasis may be seen, but this phenomenon occurs with numerous disorders and is frequently a reflection of poor diaphragmatic excursion rather than vascular occlusion. Elevation of one hemidiaphragm is very common in pulmonary embolism. It is, however, seen in a variety of other intrathoracic conditions, and its significance is usually uncertain since, in many patients without pulmonary embolism, the height of the diaphragm varies slightly from day to day without obvious explanation.

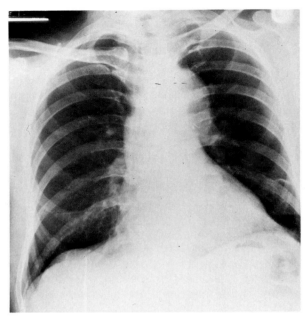

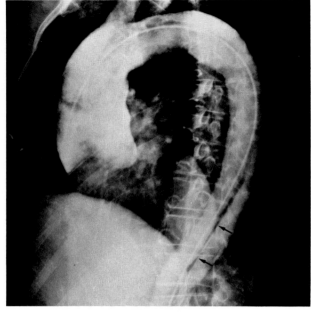

FIG 4–76.
Dissecting aneurysm of the descending aorta. The widening of the descending aorta is due to the dissecting hematoma. Without previous films for comparison, it would be difficult to distinguish widening due to aortic dissection from aortic unfolding.

FIG 4–77.
Aortic dissection. Aortogram showing type A dissection originating in ascending aorta. Both true and false lumens opacify showing the intimal flap (*arrows*) separating the lumens.

FIG 4–78.
A, aortic dissection of the descending aorta. CT scan with intravenous contrast opacification shows two aortic lumens separated by an intimal flap (*arrow*). **B,** streak artifact in descending aorta mimics an aortic dissection.

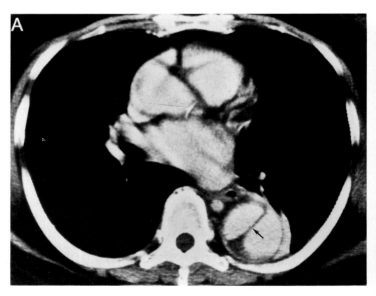

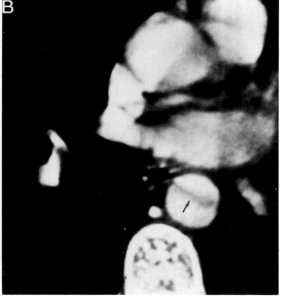

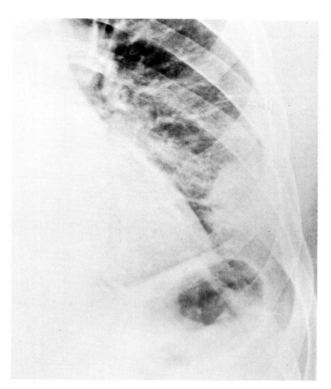

FIG 4–79.
Infiltrate in the left costophrenic angle due to a pulmonary infarct. The rounded medial edge of the infarct is the so-called Hampton's hump.

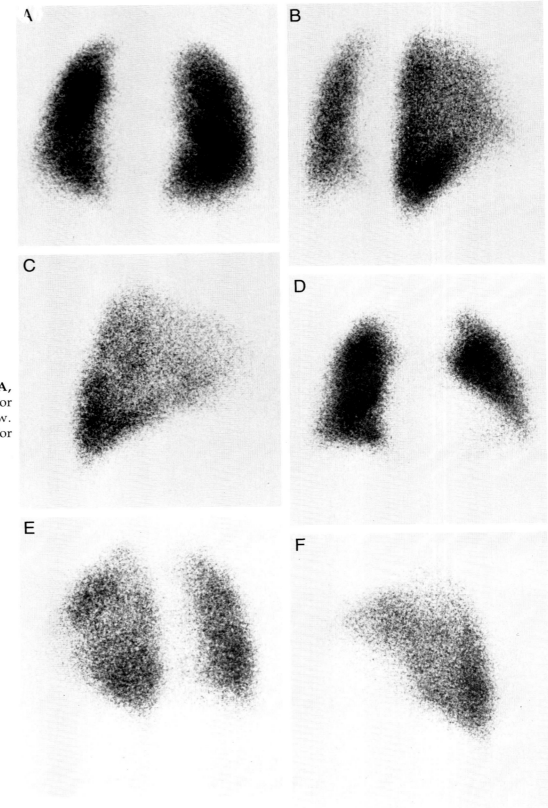

FIG 4–80.
Normal ^{99m}Tc perfusion scan. **A,** posterior view. **B,** right posterior oblique view. **C,** right lateral view. **D,** anterior view. **E,** left posterior oblique view. **F,** left lateral view.

Pulmonary embolism causing infarction gives rise to a radiographically-visible consolidation. The resulting infiltrate tends to be wedge-shaped and based on the pleura, but many patterns are seen. The infiltrate may have a round medial edge (Hampton's hump) (Fig 4–79). This sign is uncommon and, although very suggestive of pulmonary infarction, is also seen with other infiltrates, particularly pneumonia.

Since plain film radiology is so nonspecific in diagnosing pulmonary embolism, further investigation with radionuclide imaging is often needed. One of the principal values of the chest radiograph is to exclude clinically similar diseases that may show radiographic abnormalities, e.g., pneumothorax or dissecting aneurysm.

Diagnosing pulmonary embolism by radionuclide techniques depends on recognizing a perfusion defect on images of the lungs following the injection of radioactive particles into a peripheral vein. The particles, usually 200,000 to 500,000 in number, have a diameter of approximately 10 to 60 microns. They travel in the blood stream to lodge in the pulmonary arterials or capillaries. Imaging their distribution reflects regional blood flow, provided there is uniform mixing of the particles in the right side of the heart. High resolution gamma camera images of the lungs are obtained in multiple projections. The safety of the technique depends on the fact that there are approximately three hundred million pulmonary arterioles with a small enough diameter to trap the particles, and therefore only a small proportion of the pulmonary arterial bed is occluded by the particles. As discussed below, there are many causes for perfusion defects, pulmonary embolism being just one. Increased specificity can be obtained by adding a ventilation scan to the procedure. The most widely used method of performing ventilation scanning is the inhalation of a gas mixture containing ^{133}Xe. There is, however, one technical problem that must be understood. When both ^{99m}Tc and ^{133}Xe are present within the lungs, the image will reflect radioactivity from both the technetium and the xenon. The best ^{133}Xe examinations are, therefore, obtained either before the ^{99m}Tc perfusion scan or after a delay of several hours during which the radioactivity of the ^{99m}Tc will have decayed. But if the ^{133}Xe scan is routinely done before the perfusion scan, the ventilation scan will have been an unnecessary additional examination in those patients where the perfusion scan turns out to be normal. Also, it will not be possible to obtain the best projection for the ventilation scan, since this depends on knowing the results of the perfusion scan. Thus, some compromise is inevitable. In many centers, the ^{133}Xe ventilation scans are performed immediately after the ^{99m}Tc perfusion scans, and the inevitable degradation of the images due to the overlap of information from the xenon and the technetium is accepted.

The ^{133}Xe ventilation study usually consists of one image taken after a single breath inhalation, followed by serial images at intervals during a rebreathing period of 3 to 5 minutes. A final series of images is taken while the patient breathes room air/oxygen, allowing the tracer to wash out of the lungs so that areas of retention caused by partial airway obstruction can be identified. A single projection is chosen for the entire exam. The projection is the one that shows the perfusion defect to advantage. If the ventilation scan is done before the perfusion scan, then a posterior projection is chosen.

Interpretation of Radionuclide Lung Scanning

The cardinal sign of pulmonary embolism on radionuclide lung scanning is a perfusion defect. Perfusion defects are usually segmental in shape and extend to the pleural surface. A normal perfusion scan excludes the diagnosis of pulmonary embolism (Fig 4–80), but the presence of a perfusion defect is nonspecific. There are many disease processes besides pulmonary embolism that can cause focal reduction in blood flow. The list includes obstructive airway disease, either acute or chronic; pneumonia; atelectasis; pulmonary edema; and vasculitis. The likelihood of a perfusion defect being due to pulmonary embolus depends on the findings on plain chest radiographs and on radionuclide ventilation studies. The major patterns are:

1. Mismatched ventilation/perfusion defects (Fig 4–81):
- Perfusion defects in an area with normal ventilation strongly suggest pulmonary embolism without infarction.
- Perfusion defects which are larger than the corresponding ventilation defects suggest pulmonary infarction. Such cases will often show consolidation on plain chest radiograph.
2. Matched ventilation/perfusion defects may be seen with pulmonary infarction, pneumonia, pulmonary edema, or airway disease. These findings are, therefore, usually classified as indeterminate.

Abnormal ventilation-perfusion scan results are expressed in terms which indicate the probability that the diagnosis of pulmonary embolism is correct, but the radionuclide scan findings alone cannot provide a reliable estimate of likelihood without factoring in the clinical probability of pulmonary embolism. Unfortu-

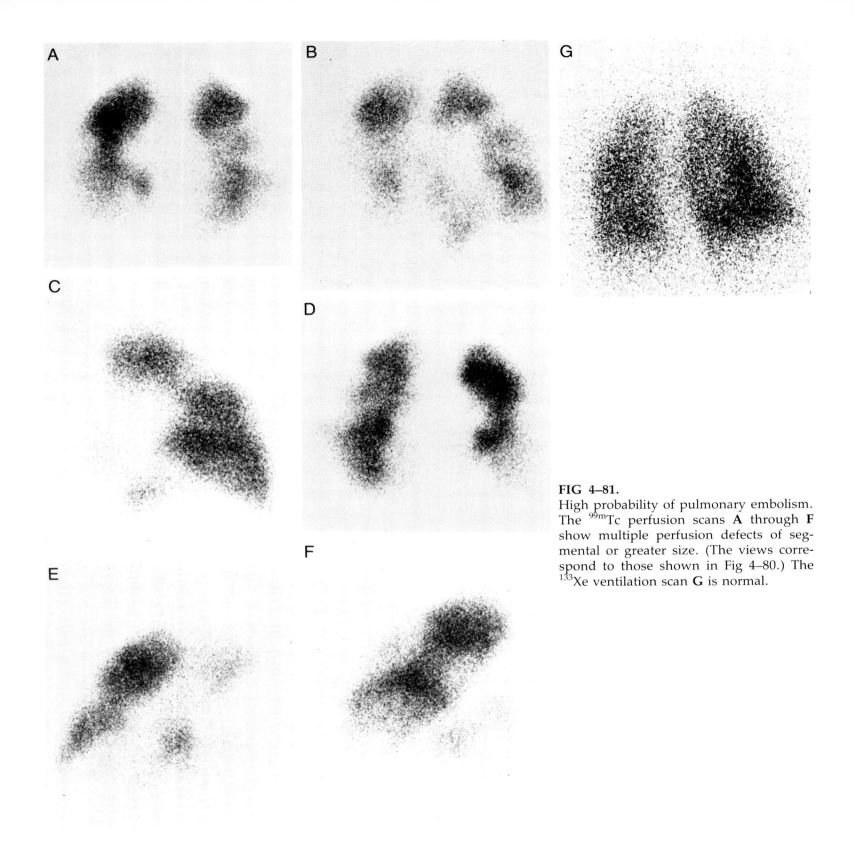

FIG 4–81.
High probability of pulmonary embolism. The ^{99m}Tc perfusion scans **A** through **F** show multiple perfusion defects of segmental or greater size. (The views correspond to those shown in Fig 4–80.) The ^{133}Xe ventilation scan **G** is normal.

nately, this important concept is often overlooked, and the radionuclide scan findings in isolation are used to predict the probability of pulmonary embolism. The criteria for classifying the VQ images as low, intermediate, indeterminate, or high probability for pulmonary embolism vary from center to center. Even if the criteria are agreed upon, there is still difficulty in deciding what proportion of a segment has reduced perfusion. The following definitions are provided as a guideline only.

A. Low probability.
1. Perfusion defects that are small regardless of their number and regardless of the ventilation or the chest x-ray findings.
2. Perfusion defects that are smaller than, or are equivalent in size to, the corresponding ventilation defect with no corresponding radiographic abnormality.
3. Perfusion defects that are substantially smaller than the radiographically demonstrated abnormalities.
4. Perfusion defects that are readily accounted for by structures such as a large hilum, a large aorta, or previous surgery.

A VQ study interpreted as low probability is associated with a 10% to 15% incidence of pulmonary embolism.

B. Intermediate probability.
Any abnormality that is not defined by either "high" or "low" probability is categorized as intermediate in probability. In essence, the probability of thromboembolism in patients who fall into this category is likely to be very similar to what it was prior to the test.

C. High probability.
1. Perfusion defects that are substantially larger than any visible radiographic abnormalities.
2. Two or more moderate or large defects which are not matched by a corresponding ventilation defect or by an abnormality on the plain chest radiograph.

The term "high probability," in general, means a likelihood greater than 85%. It is worth noting that when the diagnosis is clinically likely and there are multiple segmental or larger defects in the presence of a normal ventilation scan, the probability of pulmonary embolism exceeds 90%.

Differential Diagnosis of Pulmonary Thromboembolism on Radionuclide Scans

There are a number of conditions that can cause perfusion defects without disturbing ventilation and without producing recognizable abnormality on the chest radiograph. These include previous pulmonary emboli, obstruction to pulmonary arteries by vasculitis, neoplasm or inflammation, primary pulmonary arterial hypertension, systemic arterial blood flow to a portion of the lung, and intrathoracic hernia. This long and varied list highlights the lack of specificity of matched defects.

Pulmonary Angiography

Pulmonary angiography is the most sensitive and the most specific available test for pulmonary embolism (Fig 4–82). Accurate morbidity and mortality statistics for pulmonary angiography are difficult to obtain. In many large series there are no deaths; in others, deaths and serious complications are recorded, but mortality is rare, usually well under 0.5%. Pulmonary hypertension is a major predisposing factor to serious complications. In one review of 4,209 patients, 10 deaths were recorded; 9 of these patients had proven or presumed pulmonary hypertension.[1] The only specific sign of pulmonary embolism on angiography is an intraluminal filling defect within the opacified arterial tree on two or more films. Occlusion of an artery is frequently found. Occlusion is, however, a less specific sign and may be seen in a variety of conditions including previous embolus or occlusion due to direct involvement by neoplasm or inflammatory disease. Focal reduction in blood flow, the equivalent of the perfusion defects seen at radionuclide imaging, is an even less specific sign.

Given that pulmonary angiography is the gold standard for the diagnosis of pulmonary embolism, but also carries the risk of complications, the question arises, which patients should undergo pulmonary angiography? There are no generally agreed-upon recommendations. It has been argued that physicians should realize that, the risks of pulmonary angiography, when performed by experienced operators, though not negligible, are often less than those of anticoagulant therapy, particularly in patients whose ventilation/perfusion scan findings are nonspecific. The following could be considered indications for pulmonary angiography in patients suspected of having pulmonary embolus:

1. When the VQ scan result is significantly at variance with the clinical probability of pulmonary embolism.
2. When long-term anticoagulation is comtemplated or when drug therapy would carry a high risk.
3. Prior to embolectomy, vena caval interruption, or filter insertion.
4. When the VQ scan is abnormal, but cannot be

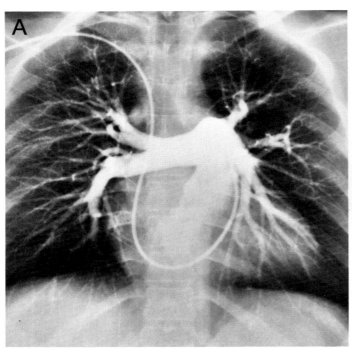

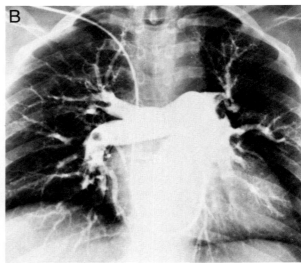

FIG 4–82.
A, normal pulmonary angiogram. **B,** pulmonary emboli demonstrated by pulmonary angiography. There are large intraluminal filling defects surrounded by opacified blood in all the lobar and segmental branches of the pulmonary artery.

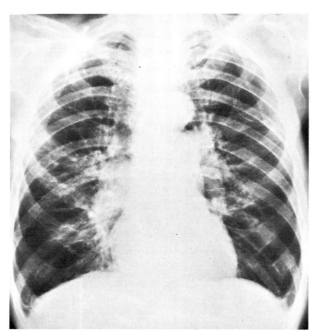

FIG 4–83.
Cor pulmonale. The signs of emphysema are apparent. In addition, the hilar arteries and the main pulmonary artery are markedly enlarged due to the pulmonary arterial hypertension.

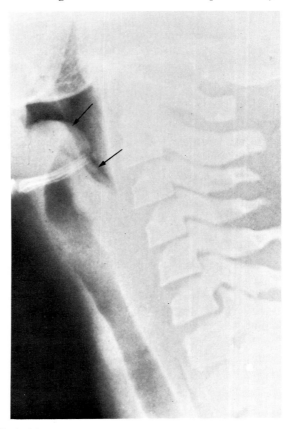

FIG 4–84.
Acute epiglottitis. The epiglottis and the adjacent aryepiglottic folds are markedly swollen *(arrows)*. The region of the vocal cords and the subglottic trachea show a hazy density.

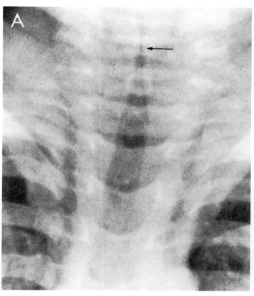

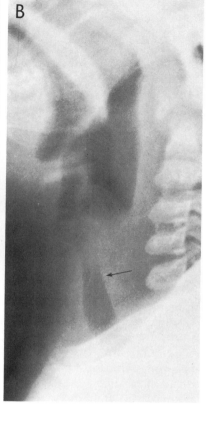
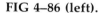

FIG 4–85.
Croup. **A,** the major finding in the AP view is narrowing of the subglottic trachea *(arrow).* **B,** the aryepiglottic fold and the epiglottis are only slightly thickened in this lateral view from another patient. Note the clearly visible subglottic narrowing *(arrow).*

FIG 4–86 (left).
Aspirated foreign body in the left main bronchus. The left lung shows substantial air trapping.

FIG 4–87 (right).
Bronchial asthma. There are numerous patchy atelectases in both lungs, particularly adjacent to the left hilum. There is also air in the upper mediastinum, the neck, and the supraclavicular areas.

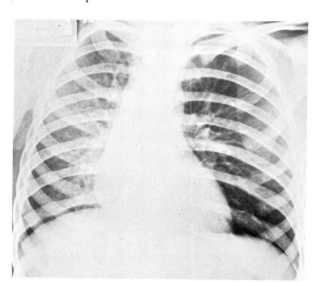

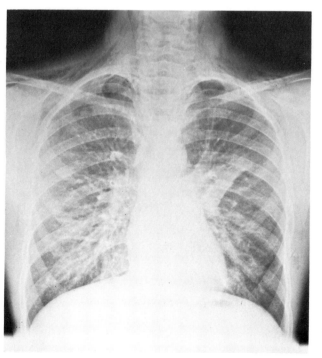

placed into either high or low probability categories. This is a fairly common situation in patients with underlying chronic obstructive lung disease.

It was originally hoped that digital subtraction angiography would prove to be a less invasive alternative to conventional pulmonary angiography for detecting pulmonary emboli. Unfortunately, a number of technical problems have prevented this method from becoming sufficiently sensitive or specific. Both CT with intravenous contrast and MRI can detect pulmonary emboli but, currently, only large emboli in central vessels can be visualized and there is no reliable data on sensitivity and specificity. At the present time, therefore, none of these techniques are used routinely.

Cor Pulmonale

Right heart failure due to lung disease manifests itself radiologically by cardiomegaly with dilatation of the right atrium, superior vena cava, and azygos vein and by the signs of pulmonary arterial hypertension. The responsible lung disease may be visible, e.g., emphysema or pulmonary fibrosis. But, when chronic bronchitis is the major cause, the chest x-ray may provide no reliable indication of lung disease despite a clinical story that points overwhelmingly to chronic bronchitis. Pulmonary arterial hypertension is recognized by dilatation of the main pulmonary artery and the central pulmonary arteries (Fig 4–83). There is disparity between the size of the enlarged hilar vessels and the vessels in the lungs. In emphysema, the lung vessels may be truly decreased in size, and then the disparity is accentuated. In cor pulmonale due to chronic bronchitis, the vessels in the lungs may be larger than normal, leading to an appearance that has been labeled "increased markings emphysema." The central vessels are usually disproportionately large, and it may be difficult to distinguish this appearance from increased pulmonary blood flow due to left-to-right shunts such as atrial or ventricular septal defects.

Many patients with cor pulmonale have left ventricular failure, which may manifest itself as upper-zone vessel dilatation and pulmonary edema.

Airway Obstruction

Acute Epiglottitis and Croup

Acute epiglottitis is a rapidly progressive bacterial infection of the epiglottis and surrounding mucosa. The usual infecting organism is Hemophilus influenzae, but group A streptococci may produce an identical disease. The common form of croup is an acute viral pharyngotracheobronchitis. These two conditions differ in their clinical presentation, treatment, and the seriousness of the airway obstruction. In acute epiglottitis, the maneuvers involved in laryngoscopy may lead to life-threatening obstruction of the larynx. Therefore, plain film examination of the neck may be indicated to distinguish the two disorders. In acute epiglottitis, the epiglottis and adjacent aryepiglottic folds are very swollen (Fig 4–84). The epiglottis is best visualized in the lateral projection. It is normally a thin structure, projecting upward and slightly backward into the airway from the base of the tongue. The aryepiglottic folds are very delicate and difficult to identify. In acute epiglottitis, the epiglottis becomes oval or round, and the aryepiglottic folds are thick and easily identified. The subglottic trachea appears normal or, at most, slightly narrowed. In viral croup, the epiglottis and aryepiglottic folds are normal or slightly thickened. The diagnostic feature is subglottic narrowing (Fig 4–85) which can be visualized in both projections, but is often best appreciated in the AP view. In the normal individual, shape of the airway beneath the true vocal cords can be likened to a rounded archway whereas, in croup, edema of the vocal cords and subglottic trachea produces an appearance more like a church steeple.

Bronchial Foreign Bodies

Opaque foreign bodies in the respiratory tract are usually readily visualized and localized radiographically. Teeth fragments, however, may be difficult to recognize. Most foreign bodies, e.g., nuts, candies, and small plastic objects, are not radiopaque. It is unusual to directly visualize the shadow of a nonradiopaque foreign body lying in the air column of the major airway. The radiographic signs are, therefore, those of the effects of the foreign body on the lungs—namely, the signs of major airway obstruction. In children, the obstruction is usually of the ball-valve type, and evidence of air trapping is the commonest sign. A minority show atelectasis or postobstructive pneumonia. A significant proportion of children with proven foreign body in the trachea or bronchi have normal plain chest radiographs.

Air trapping is rarely great enough to be appreciated on standard films taken on full inspiration. The signs are always more obvious on expiration. Indeed, the inspiratory film may be completely normal in cases where the diagnosis is obvious on expiration. The signs are increased radiolucency of the affected lung with a decrease in the size of the vessels within that lung, together with the signs of increased or fixed volume flat hemidiaphragm and mediastinal shift to the opposite side (Fig 4–86). If the foreign body is in a lobar bronchus, the affected lobe shows increased transradiancy, but the air trapping leads to displacement of the corresponding interlobar fissure rather than mediastinal shift.

Chest fluoroscopy is useful in detecting air trapping. The changing volume density of the normally-aerated lung contrasts sharply with the fixed volume and unchanging density of the lung with air trapping. When fluoroscopy is not available, plain film techniques are a possible, though less accurate, alternative. Lateral decubitus films normally show decreased aeration of the dependent lung, whereas gas trapped behind an aspirated foreign body may be detected by equal aeration of the two lungs in the decubitus position. Another plain film technique that may be successful in demonstrating air trapping is a forced expiratory view. A supine chest film is exposed while firm manual compression of the upper abdomen is applied by the physician, whose hand is protected by a lead glove.

Fluoroscopy is the most sensitive radiographic technique for detecting an inhaled foreign body and will be abnormal in over 90% of cases. Plain film techniques are much less sensitive. The radiologic diagnosis of laryngeal or tracheal foreign body is more difficult, even fluoroscopy being normal in up to half of the patients.

Bronchial Asthma

The chest radiographic findings in asthma vary with the age of the patient. In children, the lungs may be overexpanded between attacks and show bronchial wall thickening with prominent hilar vasculature. Although adults may show the same signs, they usually have normal chest radiographs. Usually, none of these signs are striking, and the chest radiograph plays no part in the diagnosis of asthma. Its purpose is to diagnose the complications of an attack or to demonstrate a pneumonia that may have precipitated the attack.

During an asthmatic attack, the lungs are often recognizably overexpanded. Atelectasis of the whole lobe, or part of one or more lobes, is fairly common (Fig 4–87). Atelectasis is usually due to retained secretions, but may be due to a pneumonia that precipitated the asthmatic attack. Distinguishing between these two processes can be impossible. In general, the less the loss of volume, the more likely the atelectasis is due to pneumonia, and the greater the loss of volume, the more likely the atelectasis is due to a mucus plug. Tenacious mucous plugs may be a repetitive

problem, leading to persistent or recurrent atelectasis. In older children and adults, they may be part of the syndrome of allergic bronchopulmonary aspergillosis.

Both pneumothorax and pneumomediastinum may be seen. Pneumomediastinum is more common and is, in itself, of no extra clinical significance to the patient.

Airway Obstruction Due to Extrinsic Compression

Acute airway obstruction is occasionally due to extrinsic compression by a mass or by a congenital vascular anomaly.

When due to a mass, the mass is usually large and may have been asymptomatic up to the time of presentation. Acute obstruction may occur because a critical degree of narrowing has been reached, or it may be precipitated by a sudden increase in the size of the mass following bleeding or infection. The mass in such cases usually appears as focal mediastinal widening with displacement or compression of the trachea. It is important to remember that the tracheal narrowing may be visible only in the lateral projection. It is rarely possible to predict the nature of the mass from the chest radiograph alone.

Tracheal obstruction from a congenital vascular ring, such as a double aortic arch, is very difficult to diagnose from plain chest films. Since it usually presents in young children in whom the thymus is still large, it is frequently difficult to recognize the aortic arch and to define the tracheal airway. The diagnosis is easily made on barium swallow, where indentations of the barium-filled esophagus are readily apparent.

Chronic Obstructive Pulmonary Disease

Chronic obstructive pulmonary disease is an imprecise, but convenient, term covering several airway disorders: chronic bronchitis, emphysema, bronchiectasis, and cystic fibrosis. These disorders may coexist.

Uncomplicated chronic bronchitis produces no abnormality on plain chest radiographs. Indeed, patients may succumb to respiratory failure due to chronic bronchitis and have normal chest films throughout their course. If the chest film is abnormal, a complication or a coexisting abnormality is present, e.g., emphysema, pneumonia, or cor pulmonale. If chronic bronchitis is combined with emphysema or leads to cor pulmonale, the abnormal radiographic signs are the signs of those disorders.

Centrilobular emphysema is not recognizable radiologically unless cor pulmonale is present. It is pan-

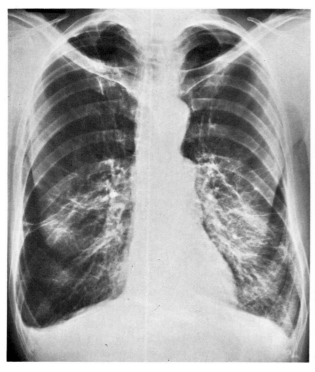

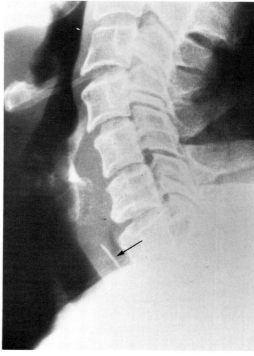

FIG 4–88 (far left).
Widespread severe emphysema. The large-volume lungs leading to low, flat diaphragms and an elongated, narrow heart are well shown. The pulmonary blood vessels in both upper lobes and in the right lower lobe are markedly narrowed. The relatively normal areas of the lung show increased vascularity, since most of the pulmonary blood flow goes through these regions.

FIG 4–89 (near left).
Swallowed piece of bone (*arrow*) stuck in the upper esophagus.

FIG 4–90 (bottom left).
Rupture of the esophagus. There is an extensive infiltrate in the left lower lobe and a moderate-size left pleural effusion. Mediastinal emphysema, predominantly on the left side, is also present. The air has tracked from the mediastinum into the neck and the supraclavicular areas.

FIG 4–91 (bottom right).
Rupture of the esophagus. CT scan shows bilateral pleural effusions plus mediastinal emphysema (*arrows*). Patchy pneumonia/atelectasis is also present in the lungs (bilateral chest tubes and a nasogastric tube are in position).

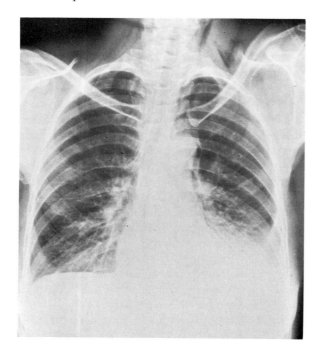

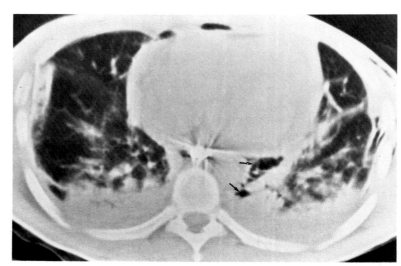

acinar emphysema that produces the signs (Fig 4–88) that are so commonly labeled "COPD" in x-ray reports. The lungs are increased in volume due to chronic airway obstruction with compliant lungs. The diaphragm is pushed down and appears low (below the seventh anterior rib or the twelfth posterior rib) and flattened. The heart is narrow, partly because the low diaphragm leads to elongation of the heart shadow. The increased lung volume causes widening of the ribs and herniation of the lungs behind and in front of the heart. Attenuation of blood vessels is a more specific sign of emphysema than overinflation of the lung. The reduction in the size and number of the pulmonary vessels can be generalized or localized. In the latter case, the area is labeled a bulla. The margins of bullous areas can vary greatly; occasionally they are bounded by a sharp line and may resemble a pneumothorax, but more commonly there is an almost imperceptible change to normal lung.

Pharyngeal and Upper Esophageal Foreign Body

Most swallowed foreign bodies that lodge do so in the pharynx or upper esophagus—usually just beyond the origin of the esophagus. Bones, meat, and disc-shaped objects such as coins are the most common foreign bodies. Their detection on plain films of the neck is almost entirely dependent on the radiopacity of the swallowed object. Man-made objects of high radiodensity are no problem to identify. Meat without bone cannot be visualized. Whole bones or slivers of bone that are small enough to be swallowed can be difficult to identify. The major problem centers around distinguishing a swallowed bone from calcifications in the laryngeal, cricoid, and hyoid cartilages (see pages 217–219). These normal calcifications lie within the expected anatomical position of the cartilages, whereas the swallowed bone may be anywhere in the pharynx or esophagus. Clearly, there are times when the anatomical location will not be helpful because the swallowed object will project over the larynx. The pattern of density will then be the deciding factor (Fig 4–89). Swallowed bone usually has an orderly structure with visible cortex, whereas cartilage calcification is irregular with no discernible organization. If perforation and abscess formation have occurred, a soft tissue swelling, possibly containing air, may be seen in the neck films.

Where the clinical suspicion is high and no radiopaque foreign body can be identified on plain film, it is best to proceed directly to barium swallow. A technique that is occasionally helpful, but does not require fluoroscopy, is to get the patient to swallow a small cotton ball that has been soaked in barium. This radiopaque ball may get caught on the foreign body, thereby revealing its presence even though the object itself cannot be identified.

Rupture of the Esophagus

Rupture of the esophagus usually presents as severe chest pain following an episode of vomiting. The diagnosis is difficult, which is particularly unfortunate since the condition has a high mortality.

The usual site of rupture is the left aspect of the distal esophagus just above the diaphragm. The plain chest film (Fig 4–90) shows mediastinal emphysema and mediastinal widening, which may be subtle early on. Left pleural effusion and left lower lobe atelectasis frequently develop.

The diagnosis can be rapidly and easily confirmed by barium or gastrografin swallow, when the contrast will leak outside the esophagus into the adjacent mediastinal tissues. CT scanning offers an alternative method of diagnosis. The tear itself will not be visualized, but the leakage of air and fluid into the mediastinum is readily recognized (Fig 4–91). Once abscess formation has occurred, fluid collections with enhancing walls will be seen within the mediastinum. Oral contrast agents may be seen outside the lumen of the esophagus, just as with conventional barium or gastrografin swallow.

Intrathoracic Manifestations of Abdominal Disease

The chest radiograph can be revealing in acute abdominal disorders. Chest disease, particularly pneumonia and pleurisy, can clinically resemble or totally mimic acute abdominal disorders. Conversely, upper abdominal problems such as subphrenic abscess, liver abscess and acute pancreatitis can cause pleural effusion and lung consolidation. In particular subdiaphragmatic abscesses frequently, although by no means always, result in ipsilateral pleural effusion often accompanied by basal pneumonia. The hemidiaphragm in such situations is invisible on plain chest radiograph; therefore, even if it were elevated, this finding would not be appreciated on plain films. Sometimes elevation or immobility of one hemidiaphragm is seen without accompanying pleural or pulmonary changes. Since most subdiaphragmatic abscesses cannot be visualized directly on plain abdominal films, the chest radiographic findings may be the only plain film abnormalities.

CT and ultrasound examination are both good methods of further investigation when the clinical features point to upper abdominal abscess as a cause for the chest film findings. Ultrasound is a quick and easy method of diagnosing intra- or extrahepatic fluid collections under the diaphragm. It has the advantage over CT that the diaphragm is directly visualized and thus the relative position of any fluid can be readily established. CT, on the other hand, is a better modality for general survey because it shows all structures without interference by bowel; gas in the bowel may significantly interfere with abdominal ultrasound images. CT is particularly useful for demonstrating fluid collections in or tracking from the pancreas in patients with pancreatitis.

Abdominal ascites, whatever its cause, is frequently accompanied by pleural effusions, which are usually bilateral.

It is easier to identify a pneumoperitoneum on chest film than on an abdominal film because the x-ray beam is tangential to the high point of the diaphragm and the standard exposure for a chest radiograph is optimal for seeing air without the aid of a bright light. The air is recognized as a translucency beneath the dome of the diaphragm. A few words of caution are needed here. Most gastrointestinal tract perforations lead to a visible pneumoperitoneum, but in a small number of patients this sign is not found, presumably because adhesions prevent the free passage of air. The yield of positive cases increases if the patient stays in the upright position for a few minutes since the air may take time to accumulate beneath the diaphragm. Fat beneath the diaphragm or lobulation of the diaphragmatic surface may simulate air and lead to a mistaken diagnosis of pneumoperitoneum.

Reference

1. Goodman PC: Pulmonary angiography. Clin Chest Med 1984; 5:465–477.

Normal Variants

Theodore E. Keats, M.D.

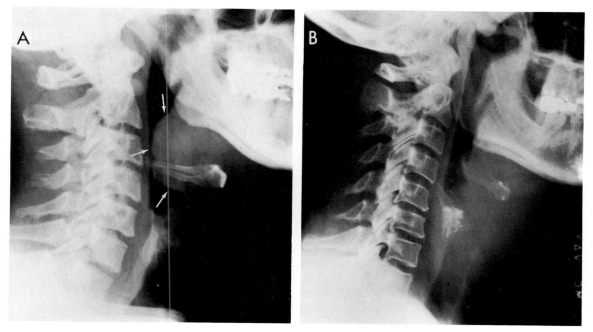

FIG 4–92.
A, pseudomass of the pharynx produced by the base of the tongue, filmed during the act of swallowing. **B,** normal configuration of soft tissues at rest in another patient for contrast with **A.**

FIG 4–93.
Two examples of large pharyngeal tonsils which may simulate a tumor of the pharynx.

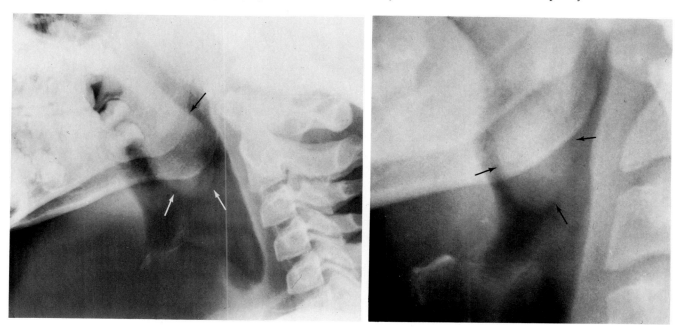

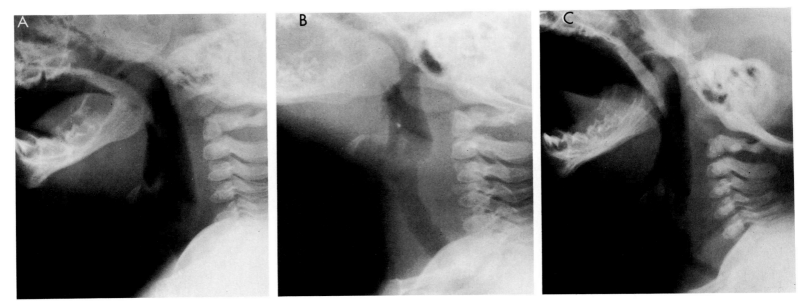

FIG 4–94.

Normal alterations of the retropharyngeal soft tissues with respiration in infancy. **A,** quiet breathing; **B,** in- spiration; **C,** expiration. The expiratory film resembles the changes of retropharyngeal abscess and is a po- tential source of misinterpretation.

FIG 4–95.

Two examples of normal prom- inence of the retropharyngeal soft tissues in expiration, mis- diagnosed initially as retro- pharyngeal abscesses.

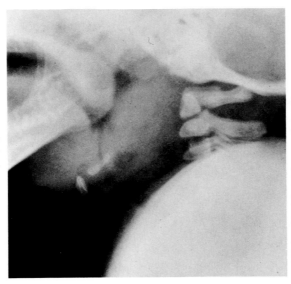

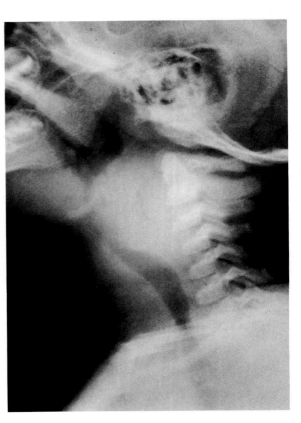

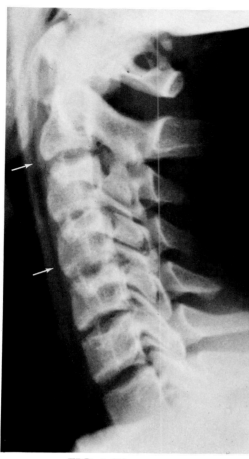

FIG 4–96.
Prominent prevertebral fat stripe, not to be mistaken for gas in the soft tissues. (Ref: Whalen JP, Woodruff CL: The cervical prevertebral fat stripe. A new aid in evaluating the cervical prevertebral new soft tissue space. *Am J Roentgenol* 1970; 109:445.)

FIG 4–97.
Calcified stylohyoid ligaments in lateral **(A)** and oblique **(B)** projections.

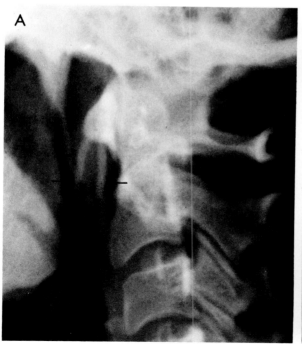

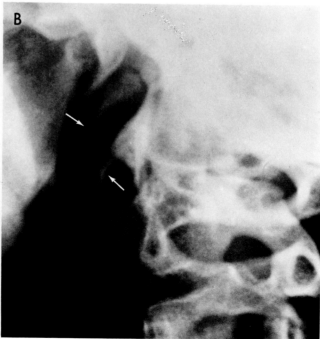

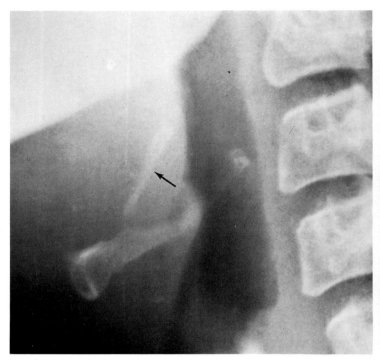

FIG 4–98.
Partial calcification of the stylohyoid ligaments, simulating a foreign body.

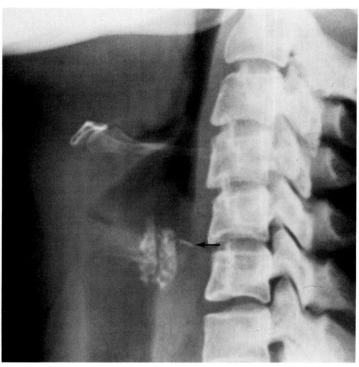

FIG 4–99.
Calcification in the arytenoid cartilage.

FIG 4–100.
Calcification of the superior cornua of the thyroid cartilage, which might be mistaken for a foreign body.

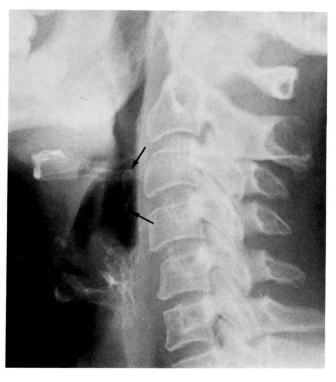

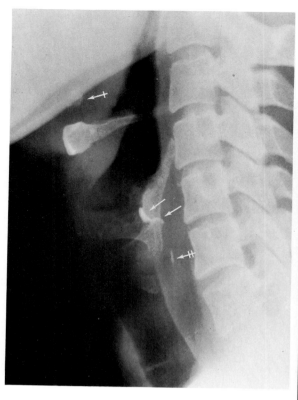

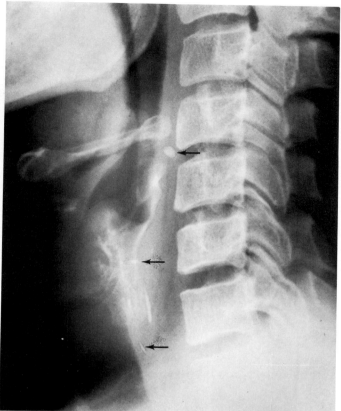

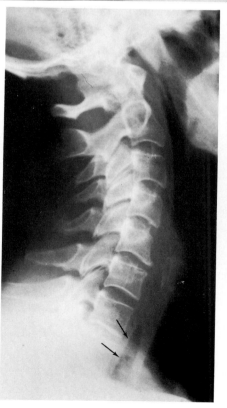

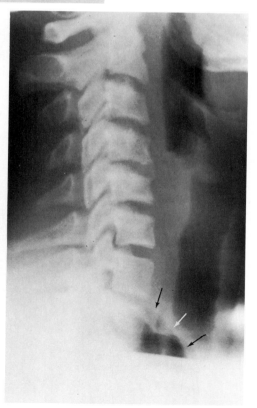

FIG 4–101 (top left).
Calcification in the arytenoid cartilages (*arrow*). Note also a submaxillary gland calculus (*notched arrow*) and calcifications in the posterior plate of the cricoid cartilage (*double-notched arrow*).

FIG 4–102 (top right).
Physiologic calcification of the soft tissues of the neck. The *upper arrow* indicates calcification in the thyrohyoid ligament (cartilago triticea). The *middle arrow* shows calcification in the arytenoid cartilage. The *lower arrow* indicates calcification in the tracheal cartilage.

FIG 4–103 (bottom left).
Air in the cervical esophagus.

FIG 4–104 (bottom right).
The apex of the lung seen in lateral projection.

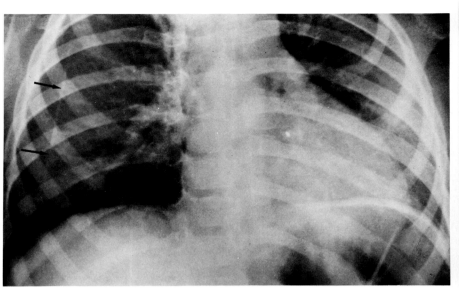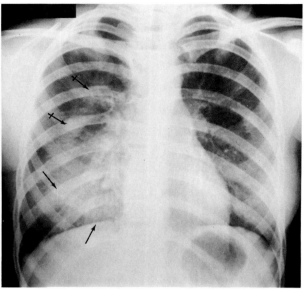

FIG 4–105 (left).
Simulated pneumothorax in a 3½-year-old child due to a skin fold.

FIG 4–106 (right).
The dense juvenile breast may cast shadows simulating parenchymal density (*arrow*). Note also shadows cast by hair braids (*notched arrows*).

FIG 4–107 (left).
Folds of lax skin in the elderly may also simulate a pneumothorax.

FIG 4–108 (right).
The floor of the supraclavicular fossa may be very well defined and simulate an air-fluid level in the lung. (Ref: Christensen EE, Dietz GW: The supraclavicular fossa. *Radiology* 1976; 118:37.)

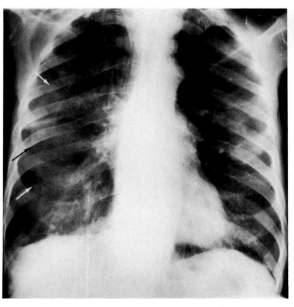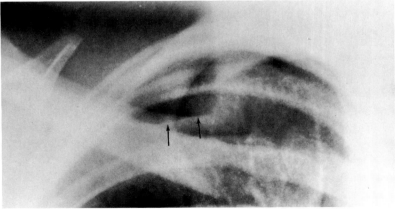

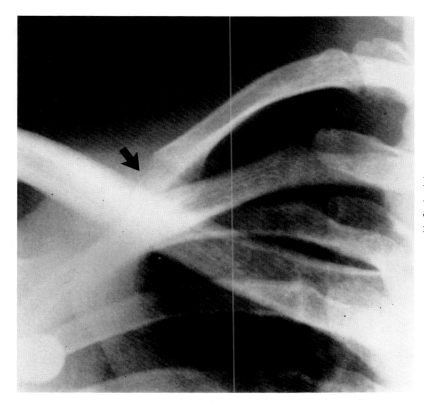

FIG 4–109.
Anomalous articulations in the first ribs (*arrow*) are more common on the right side and may be mistaken for a fracture or mass.

FIG 4–110.
Two examples of the shadows of the subcostal muscles that produce an appearance simulating pleural thickening or small pneumothorax.

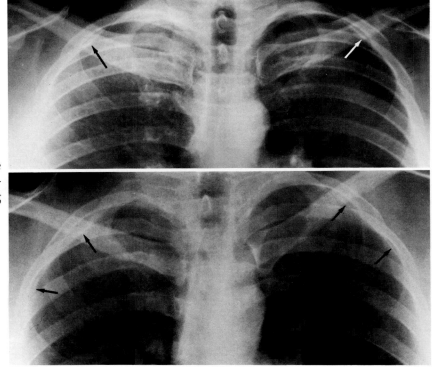

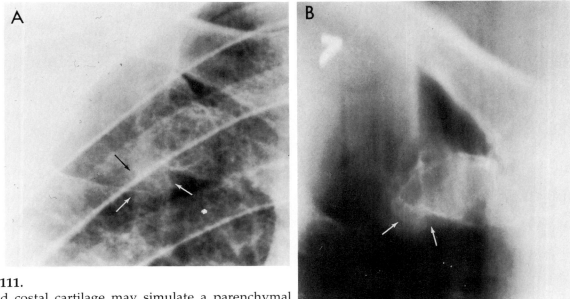

FIG 4–111.
Calcified costal cartilage may simulate a parenchymal lesion. **A,** plain film; **B,** laminography.

FIG 4–112.
In an improperly positioned chest film, the spine of the scapula may overlap the lungs and produce a shadow which may be mistaken for a pneumothorax.

(Ref: Harbin WP, Cimmino CV: The radiographic innominate lines of the scapular spine. *Va Med* 1974; 101:1050.)

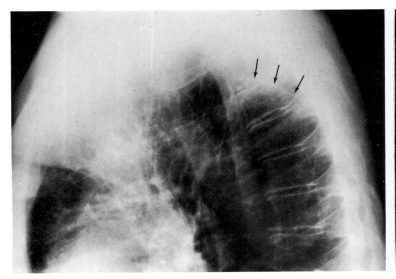

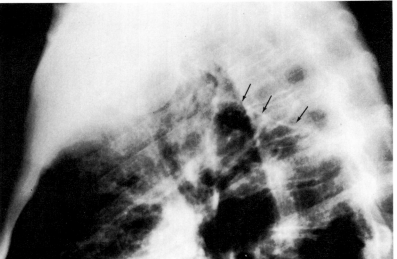

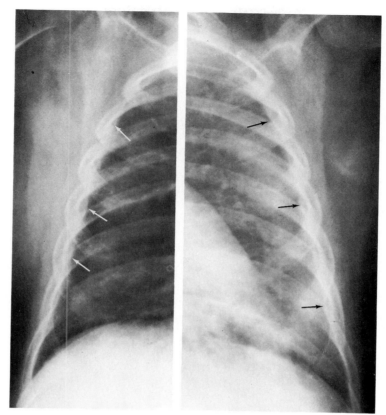

FIG 4–113.
Additional example of extrapleural fat deposits in
a very obese patient, simulating pleural thickening.

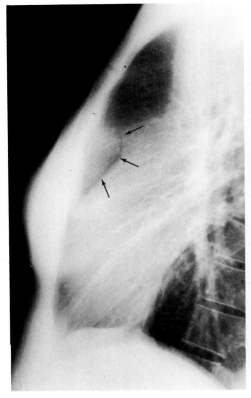
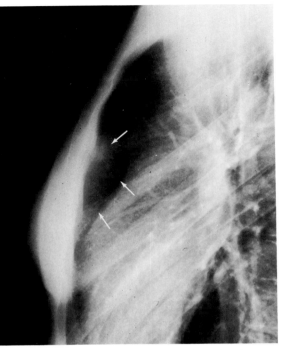

FIG 4–114.
Two examples of the mammary anterior mediastinal pseudotumor. The lateral aspects of the dense, small breasts in young women may project into the anterior mediastinum in the lateral projection and simulate a mediastinal mass. (Ref: Keats TE: Mammary anterior mediastinal pseudotumor. *J Can Assoc Radiol* 1976; 27:262.)

FIG 4–115.
The manubrium of a 2½-year-old boy, simulating a soft tissue mass.

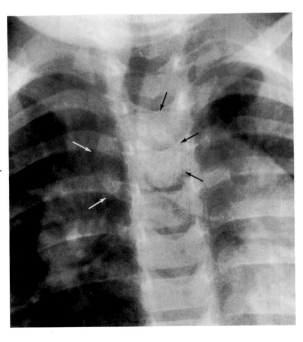

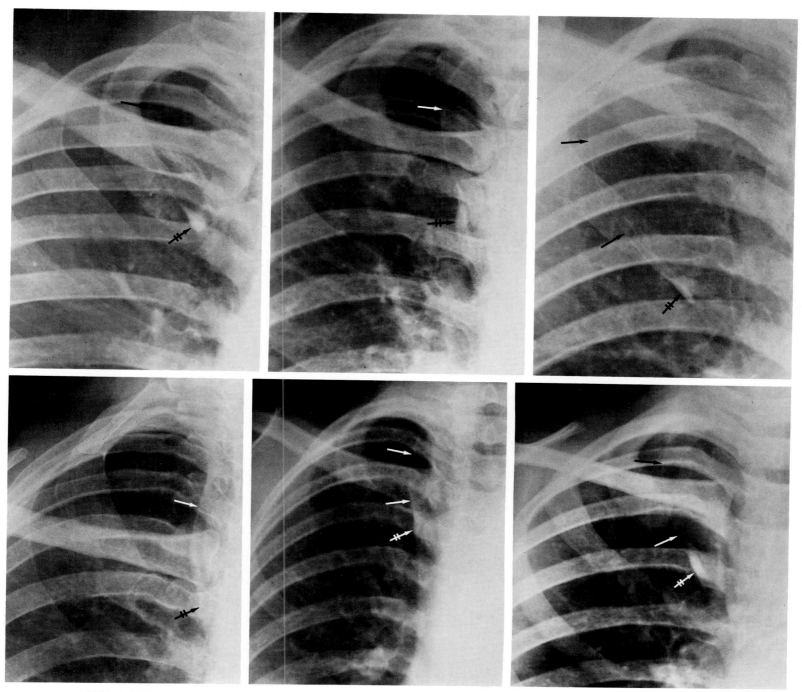

FIG 4–116.
Six examples of azygos lobes to demonstrate the variation in configuration of the pleural line (*arrows*) and the position and size of the azygos vein (*notched arrows*).

FIG 4–117.
The vertical fissure line. This line represents the caudal end of the major interlobar fissure. It may be seen in films of healthy children when it is ectopic and lies forward so part of it is in axial projection. It should not be mistaken for a pneumothorax. (Ref: Davis LA: The vertical fissure line. *Am J Roentgenol* 1960; 84:451.)

FIG 4–118.
Two examples of hair braids, simulating parenchymal abnormality.

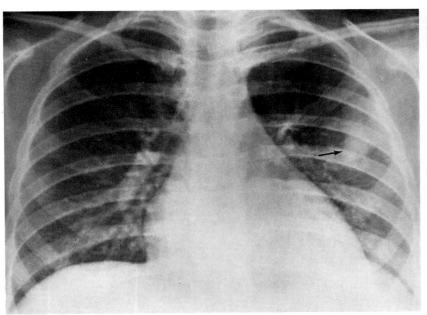

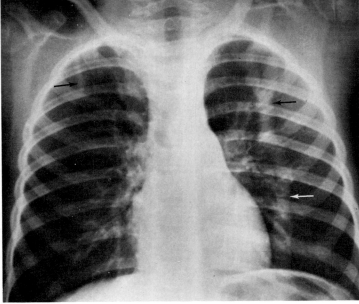

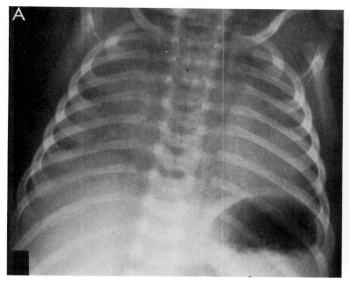

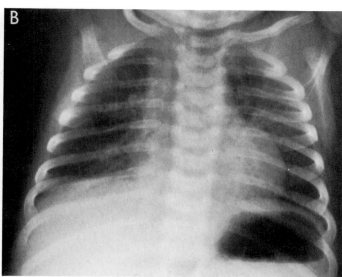

FIG 4–119.
Filming infant chests in even minor degrees of expiration may result in misinterpretation due to the marked opacity of the parenchyma which results, as illustrated in this normal infant. **A,** expiration; **B,** inspiration.

FIG 4–120.
Lateral buckling of the trachea at the thoracic inlet occurs normally in infants and children up to 5 years of age. The displacement is to the side opposite the aortic arch and is best seen in expiration. (Ref: Chang LWM, et al: Normal lateral deviation of the trachea in infants and children. *Am J Roentgenol* 1970; 109:247.)

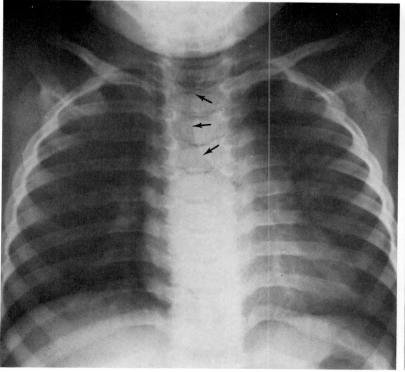

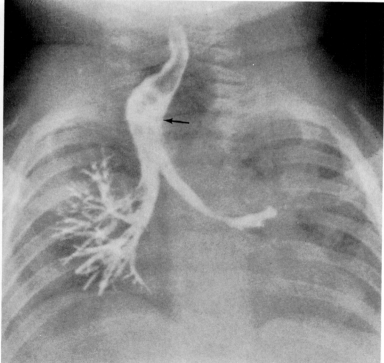

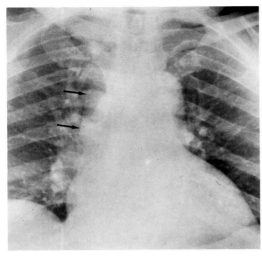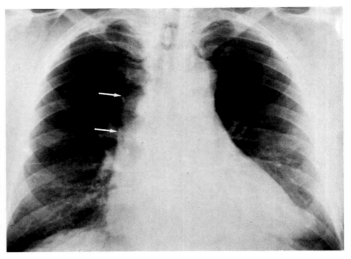

FIG 4–121.

Two examples of mediastinal fat, producing widening of the mediastinum. This may be seen in obesity, in Cushing's disease, and in patients receiving steroids. (Ref: Price JE, Jr, Rigler LG: Widening of the medias-tinum resulting from fat accumulation. *Radiology* 1970; 96:497.) Seen in the lateral projection, such fat may simulate the thymus. (Ref: Steckel RJ: Mediastinal pseudotumors associated with exogenous obesity. *Radiology* 1976; 119:74.)

FIG 4–122.

Examples of the spurious posterior mediastinal mass seen in infants as a result of the overlapping shadow of the scapula and the trachea and the air-filled esophagus. (Ref: Balsand D, et al: The scapula as a cause of spurious posterior mediastinal mass on lateral chest films of infants. *Am J Roentgenol* 1972; 116:571.)

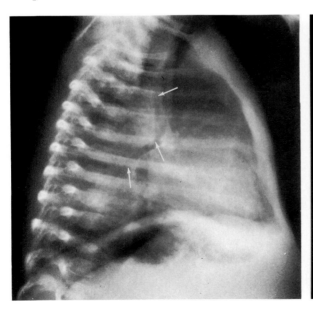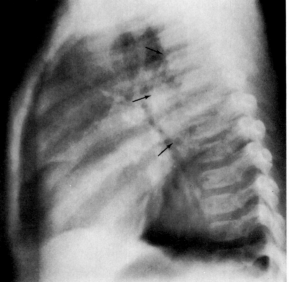

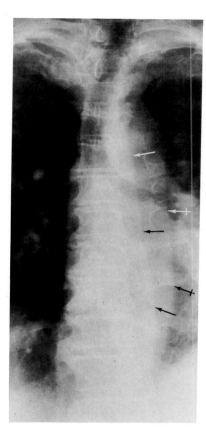

FIG 4–123.
The left paramediastinal stripe (*arrows*), representing the reflection of the pleura against the spine, may be deviated laterally by ectasia of the thoracic aorta (*notched arrows*) and is, therefore, not necessarily an indication of vertebral or mediastinal abnormality.

FIG 4–124.
Marked obesity will also result in displacement of the paravertebral stripe, presumably due to fat deposition. **A,** 300-lb 14-year-old boy; **B,** 250-lb 46-year-old man.

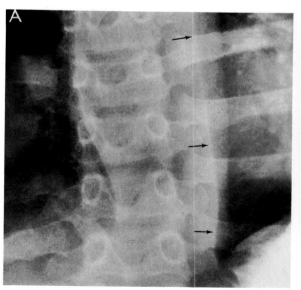
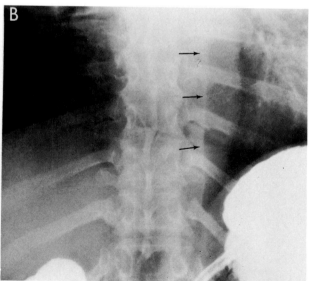

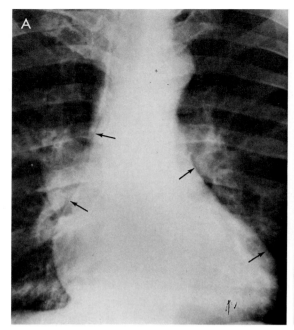

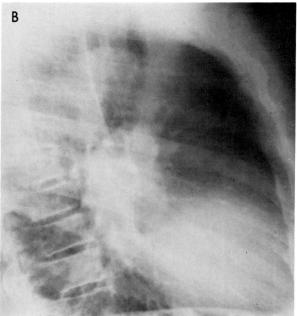

FIG 4–125.
A, simulated pneumomediastinum evidenced by a lucent halo around the heart due to the Mach effect. **B,** no evidence of pneumomediastinum in lateral projection. (Ref: Lane EJ, et al.: Mach bands and density perception. *Radiology* 1976; 121:9.)

FIG 4–126.
Air in the esophagus producing a lucency beneath the aortic arch (*arrow*). This is seen where the esophagus is displaced to the left by adhesions to a tortuous aorta. Barium may be retained in this pocket as well. Note position of pleural esophageal reflection (*notched arrow*). (Ref: Cimmino CV: A roentgenologic study in mediastinal anatomy affected by air in the mid-esophagus. *Am J Roentgenol* 1965; 94:333.)

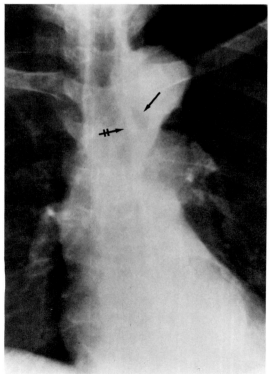

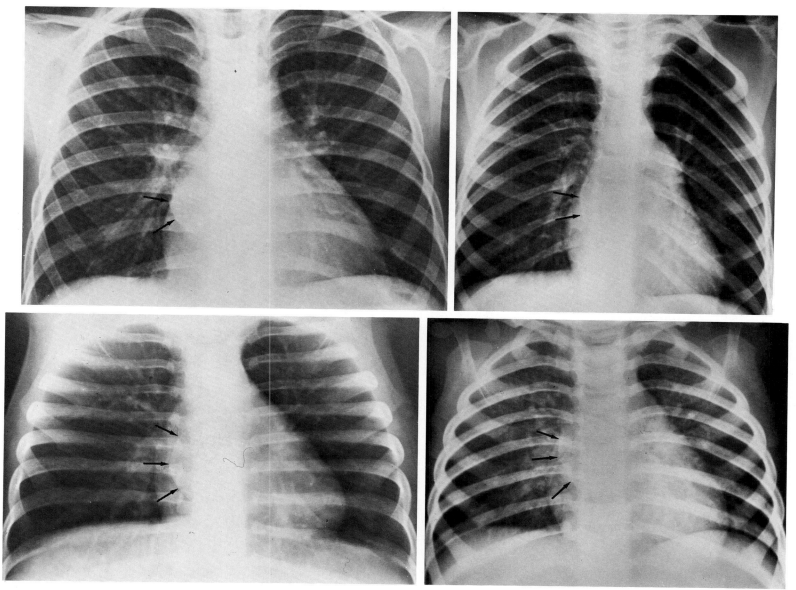

FIG 4–127.

Four examples of the visualization of the right border of the left atrium in normal children. This may be seen also in adults and should not be taken as evidence of left atrial enlargement in itself, unless correlative evidence is present in the other projections. (Ref: Burko H, Gyepes MJ: Radiologic assessment of left atrial size in infants. *Radiology* 1965; 85:1099.)

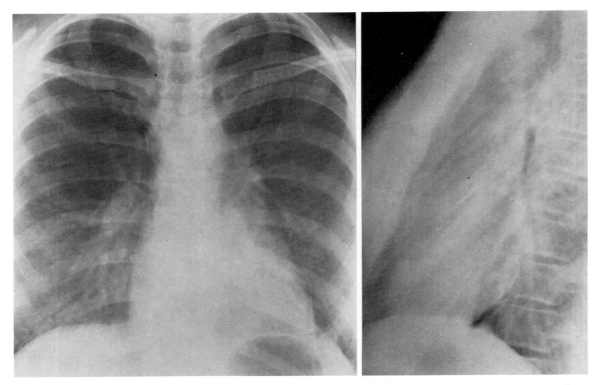

FIG 4–128.
The straight back syndrome, producing flattening of the heart and prominence of the pulmonary artery. Individuals with congenital absence of the normal dorsal kyphosis and narrow sagittal diameter of the chest present striking alteration in cardiac contour compounded by the coexistence of physical findings that may mimic organic heart disease. (Ref: de Leon A, et al: The straight back syndrome. *Circulation* 1965; 17:197.)

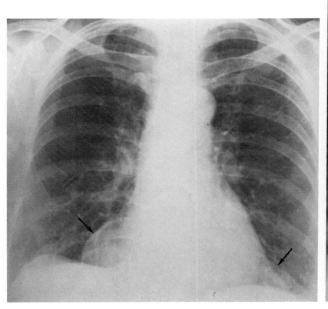

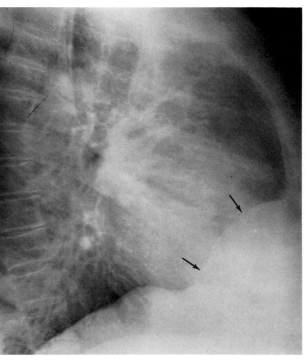

FIG 4–129.
Normal epipericardial fat pads. These fat collections may be confused with cysts and neoplasms. They vary in size with the weight of the patient. (Ref: Holt JF: Epipericardial fat shadows in differential diagnosis. *Radiology* 1947; 48:472.)

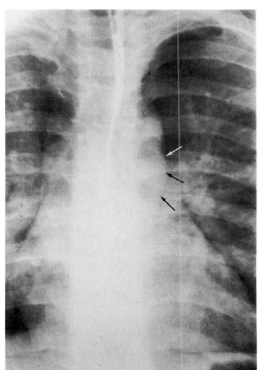

FIG 4–130.
The infundibulum of the ductus, the point of insertion of the ductus in early life. Its presence does not indicate patency of the ductus. (Ref: Keats TE, Steinbach HL: Patent ductus arteriosus: A critical evaluation of its roentgen signs. *Radiology* 1955; 64:528.)

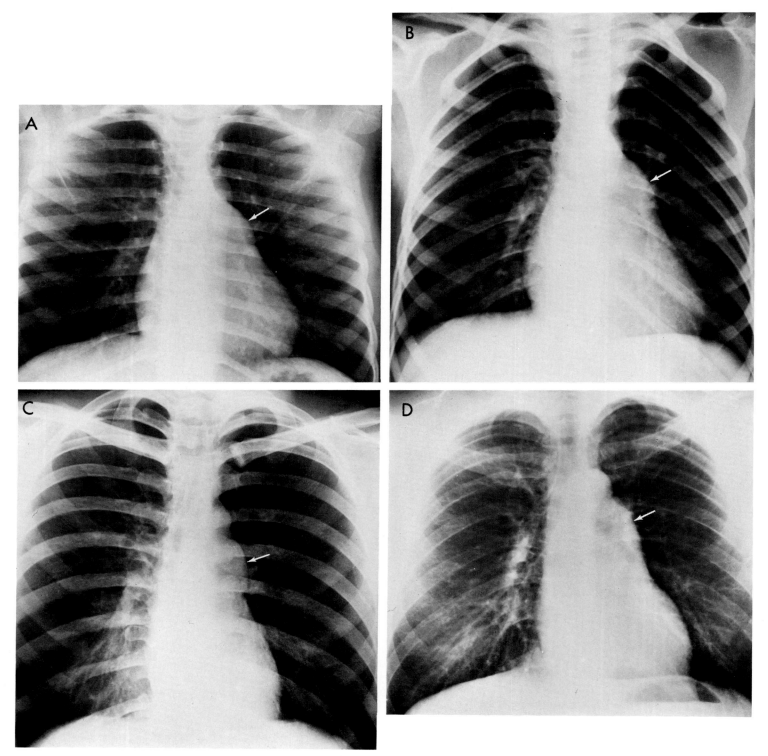

FIG 4–131.
Four examples of normal variation in size of the pulmonary artery in children and young adults. The pulmonary artery is extremely variable in size and its prominence in youth is a common finding. It should not be a source of concern in itself. **A,** 5-year-old boy; **B,** 8-year-old boy; **C,** 9-year-old girl; **D,** 18-year-old man.

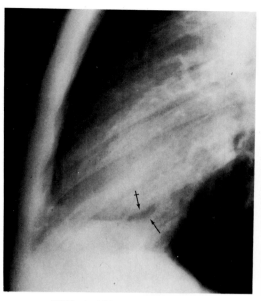
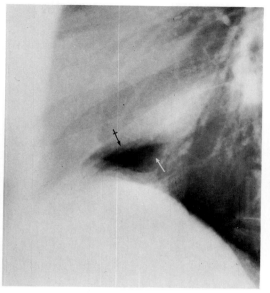
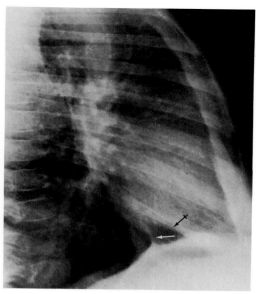

FIG 4–132.

Three examples of confusing radiolucencies produced by the inferior vena cava. With maximum inspiration, it is possible to clear a portion of the diaphragmatic surface of the heart and expose the anterior wall of the inferior vena cava (*arrow*). This results in a triangular area of radiolucency (*notched arrow*), which may be confusing if its origin is not appreciated. (Ref: Tonkin IL, et al: Radiographic isolation of the inferior vena cava. *Am J Roentgenol* 1977; 129:657.)

FIG 4–133.

Two examples of unilateral presentation of the thymus to the right side.

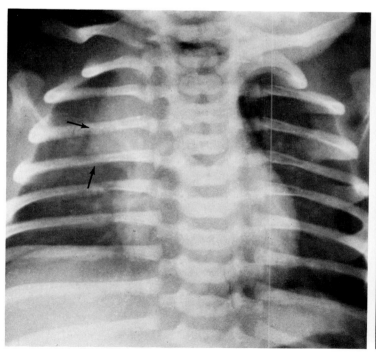
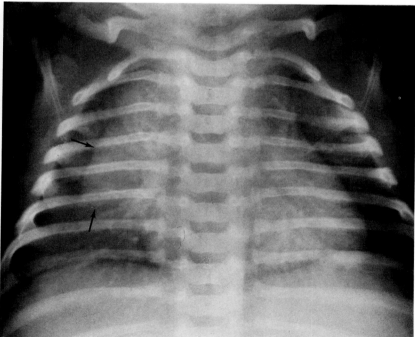

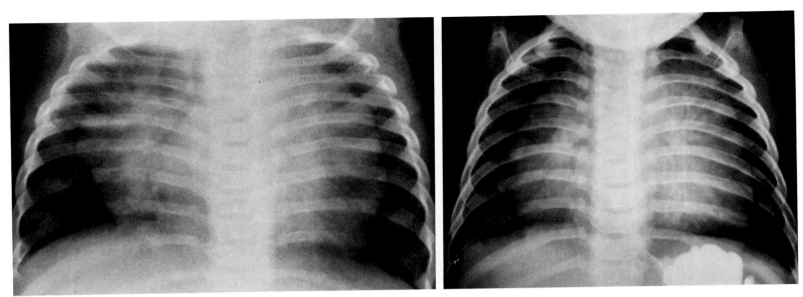

FIG 4–134.
Two examples of very large thymuses, simulating cardiomegaly.

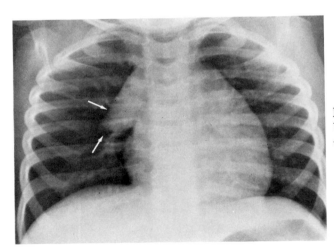

FIG 4–135.
Unilateral "sail" configuration of the right lobe of
the thymus.

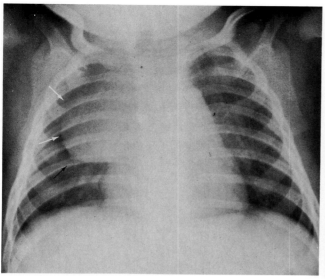

FIG 4–136.
Unusually rounded configuration of the thymus.

FIG 4–137 (left).
The thymus does not always regress in early childhood and may persist into early adolescence. Its presence in late childhood, therefore, should not be construed as evidence of abnormality. Note residual thymus in a 4-year-old boy. (Ref: Oh KS, et al: Normal mediastinal mass in late childhood. *Radiology* 1971; 101:625.)

FIG 4–138 (right).
Residual thymus in an 11-year-old boy.

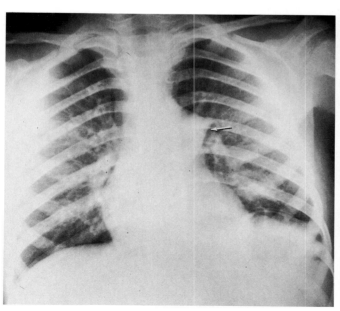

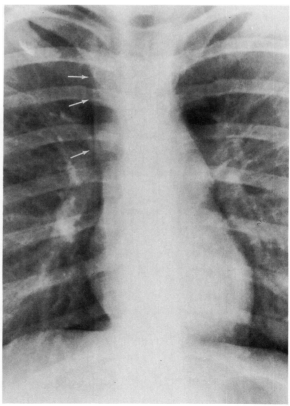

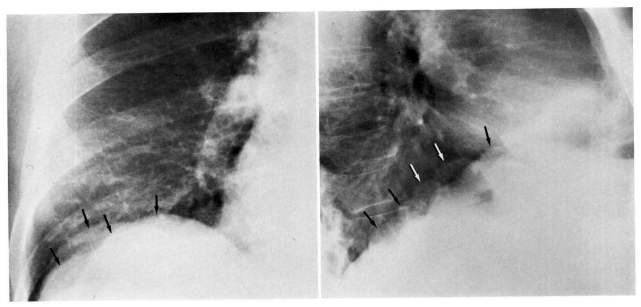

FIG 4–139.
"Scalloping" of the diaphragm is caused by hypertrophy and contraction of individual muscle bundles in the diaphragm. This case shows multiple small convexities.

FIG 4–140.
Localized eventration of the diaphragm in a child. Without benefit of the lateral projection, this variation could be mistaken for a mass lesion.

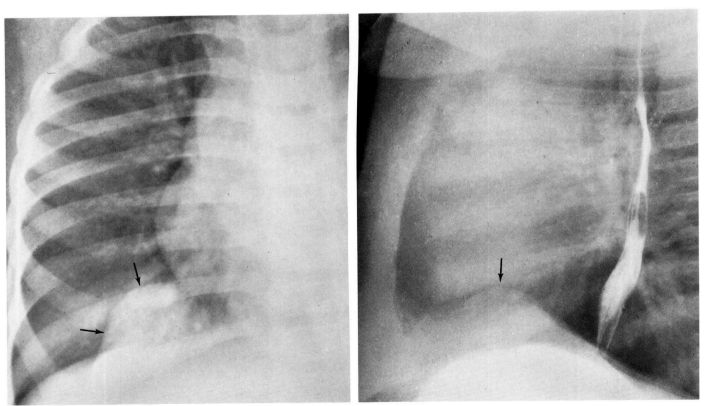

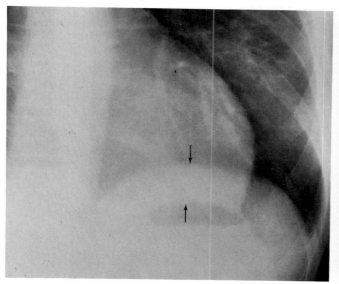 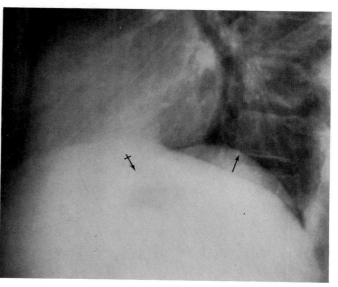

FIG 4–141.
The increased distance between the stomach gas bubble and the diaphragm suggests a subpulmonic effusion. The lateral projection indicates that this appearance is due to the fact that the posterior portion of the left hemidiaphragm (*arrows*) is higher than the anterior portion (*notched arrow*), which is adjacent to the gas bubble.

.

5

Abdomen

Paul A. Mori, M.D.
Kurt W. Mori, M.D.

This chapter is written for the physician who has not had substantial experience in abdominal film interpretation. It is intended to simplify and condense material contained in many excellent texts on the subject.

The abdomen is a neglected area in emergency radiology, probably because interpretation of abdominal radiographs is considered difficult or unrewarding. Some even advocate omitting films of the abdomen because they provide "little useful information." This chapter is intended to dispel such notions. With a simple knowledge of anatomy and a systematic approach to film interpretation, the physician will find that abdominal films often provide definitive diagnosis and are always useful in assessing the acute abdomen or abdominal trauma.

The material emphasizes frequently encountered conditions. It is presented in a format designed for first analysis of common diagnostic problems. Where more definitive work-up is required, some guidelines to further evaluation are included. Computed tomography, ultrasound, nuclear medicine, and angiography often contribute to evaluation of the emergency abdomen. Several selected illustrations are included. A reading list to assist performance and interpretation of these examinations is appended to the chapter.

All of the information in this chapter has appeared in the radiologic literature through the years. No attempt has been made to cite a specific reference for each concept. For simplicity's sake, theoretical concepts and details of mechanisms have been eliminated. Rather, an effort has been made to extract from a large body of complex information that which is most applicable clinically. It is hoped that this approach will make the information more rapidly assimilable and therefore more useful to the physician who must be prepared to make quick decisions. The material has been subjected to exhaustive clinical evaluation in the emergency setting and has been amalgamated into a practical step-by-step approach to abdominal film interpretation.

The material is presented sequentially, beginning with basic anatomy. Each case has been selected to emphasize one or more important signs or diagnostic points with reference to a specific patient condition.

The material may be useful as reference if, on the basis of clinical findings, the reader wishes to review or clarify specific points regarding film interpretation.

Radiographic findings are often minimal, even in the presence of significant disease; therefore, these findings should always be correlated with clinical evaluation of the patient. The major objective in radiologic service in the emergency setting is to offer comprehensive and competent radiologic examination leading to effective diagnosis and prompt patient treatment.

Perception of disease is dependent on sensory input. One must see the lesion before it can be analyzed. Examine Figure 5–1. Note that perception of one image suppresses awareness of the other. This interesting phenomenon explains why people miss things when they look at radiographs. If there is something obvious on a film, one's attention tends to be drawn to it and diverted from other images. Therefore, it is extremely important that the observer train himself to look at all x-ray films systematically. Particularly, one should learn to look at the obvious or the area of special interest last. It is important to go over the entire film systematically and then zero in on the point of interest. In particular, absence of a normal structure is more difficult to detect than anatomical distortion. Therefore, a conscious effort should be made to identify each normal structure. Perception depends on a logical system of film analysis. By following a strict search pattern, significant findings will not be overlooked.

Perception is also dependent on prior learning. Experience is an important asset in film interpretation. If you were to go to the airport to meet my Aunt Minnie, not having seen her before, you might ask how to recognize her. I might describe her as a little old lady of 85, wearing certain distinctive clothing. With those descriptive characteristics, you would, of course, immediately recognize her. If you were to meet her at the airport on her return one year later, it would not be necessary for you to ask how to recognize her. Having seen her before, you would know her instantly.

The Aunt Minnie concept is important in radiology. Film interpretation is fundamentally a process of pat-

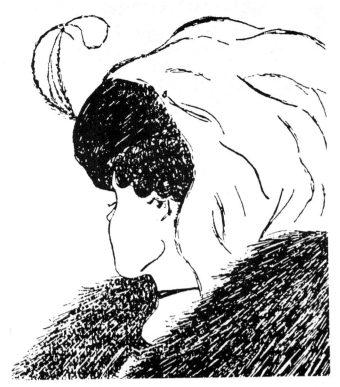

FIG 5–1.
Image perception. W. E. Hills' drawing "My Wife and My Mother-in-Law" contains the face of a young woman and the face of an old woman. The young woman's chin is the old woman's nose. Note how the images spontaneously shift when they are looked at steadily. (From *Curr Probl Diagn Radiol* 1974; vol 4: Mar/Apr. Reprinted with permission of Year Book Medical Publishers, Inc.)

tern recognition. If you are seriously interested in becoming proficient at film interpretation, each time you order a radiograph, challenge yourself to make the interpretation. Then follow up by talking to the radiologist or reading his report.

Anatomical Approach

The most effective method for systematic film analysis is to subdivide the information on the film into its simplest components using an anatomical outline (Fig 5–2). The outline should prove useful in your approach to abdominal films until sufficient experience has been gained to interpret anatomically by habit. This section will include normal anatomy and a few examples of frequently encountered minor pathology. More normal anatomy and variants are included in the section on normal variants, calcifications, oddities, and "Aunt Minnies."

Bones: ribs, lumbar spine, pelvis, hips, upper femurs
Lung bases (if included)
Opacities
    Calcifications: rib cartilages, vessels, soft tissues, mesenteric nodes
    Concretions: gallbladder, kidney, ureter, bladder, pancreas, appendix, phlebolith
    Metallic densities, barium, etc.
Major organs: liver edge, splenic tip, renal outlines, urinary bladder
Flank stripes, psoas margins
Gas in bowel: colon, small intestine, stomach
Gas outside bowel: under liver, diaphragm, in bile ducts, pockets, intestinal wall, retroperitoneal
Masses

FIG 5–2.
Outline for evaluation of abdominal films.

Refer to Figure 5–3. Survey the bone structure systematically, noting ribs, lumbar spine, pelvis, and hips. Bone abnormality may at times be related or give a clue to what is happening in the abdomen. A common finding is slight scoliosis of the lumbar spine. This is nearly always positional, but may at times be related to retroperitoneal infection, hemorrhage, or pain.

Evaluate the lung bases if they are included on the films. Basilar pulmonary infiltrates or pleural fluid may be related to abnormality in the abdomen. Visualization of lung bases on abdominal films usually requires use of a bright light.

Search for calcifications, concretions, and other opacities. In Figure 5–3, note the calcified hepatic granuloma in the right upper quadrant and the phlebolith in the pelvis. There are many normal or insignificant calcifications (costal cartilage, calcified lymph nodes, phleboliths) that should be recognized and distinguished from pathologic findings. Recognizing the presence of atherosclerotic vascular calcifications, soft tissue calcifications, concretions, and various other opacities may at times make a significant contribution to diagnosis (Fig 5–4).

Evaluate the four major organs (liver, spleen, kidneys, and urinary bladder).

The liver is generally visible in the right upper quadrant as a triangular shadow with an oblique lower edge (Fig 5–5). Apparent size varies greatly for a number of reasons. The clarity with which you see the liver edge is substantially affected by bowel content. In addition, because the posterior edge is higher than the anterior edge, the angle of projection of the

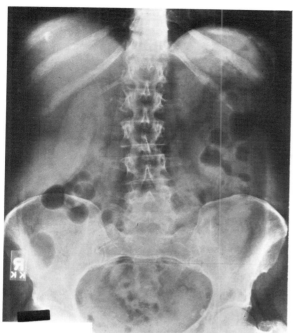

FIG 5–3.
Abdominal anatomy.

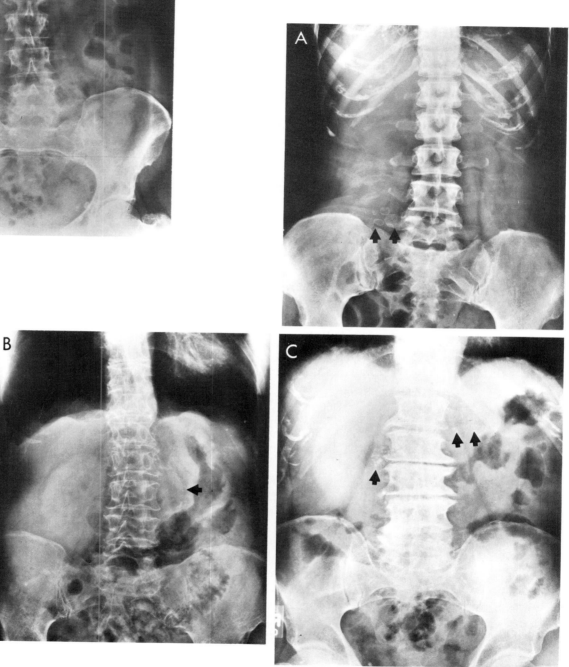

FIG 5–4.
Calcific densities (normal and abnormal). **A,** there is extensive calcification of costal cartilage. In addition, gallstones are seen in the right lower quadrant *(arrows).* **B,** note the thin shell of calcification in the wall of an abdominal aneurysm *(arrow).* **C,** there are calcifications in the head and tail of the pancreas *(arrow).* Also note costal cartilage calcification and phleboliths in the pelvis.

x-ray beam may be a factor in apparent magnification of the liver shadow. Additionally, position of the diaphragm is greatly influenced by the patient's age, pulmonary inflation, and body habitus. Plain film determination of liver size is relatively unreliable. You should depend more on your clinical sense and palpating hand.

The spleen is a posterior organ usually not visible in the adult on plain abdominal films unless it is at least slightly enlarged (see Fig 5–5). The spleen lies behind the splenic flexure of the colon and the stomach, close to the upper edge of the left kidney. As it begins to enlarge, you may recognize the splenic edge displacing any of these organs.

How well the renal outlines are seen depends principally on two factors. One of these is the amount of gas in the bowel. Bowel gas tends to obscure renal shadows. The other factor is the amount of retroperitoneal fat, which is usually related to the patient's total body fat. Kidneys surrounded by fat are much more easily seen.

The urinary bladder is an extraperitoneal organ. It is identified as an arcuate soft tissue shadow projected above the pubic symphysis (Fig 5–6). Size varies with degree of distention. The bladder may not be visible at all or may appear as a huge mass filling the central pelvis and lower abdomen. In most patients, the urinary bladder can be readily distinguished from other pelvic masses because the dome of the bladder is almost always covered by a thin layer of fat. In addition, a thin fat line in many patients may be traced along the inferior and lateral margins of the pelvic rim (see Fig 5–6). This fat shadow is of great importance in recognizing extraperitoneal rupture of the urinary bladder and pelvic hematoma following trauma. In the female, the bladder may be indented by the uterus.

Flank stripes are useful structures because they can help one to recognize intraperitoneal bleeding. They are referred to in the literature under a variety of names (peritoneal fat lines, properitoneal fat, retroperitoneal fat, medial stripe, etc.). Flank stripes are identified as fat shadows extending inferiorly from the lateral rib margins on both sides and gradually fading out over the iliac crests (Fig 5-7,A). The lateral margins are often well defined; the medial margins may be less well defined. The medial margin is extremely important because it delineates the peritoneal surface. The lateral gutter on each side is a potential space between this peritoneal surface and the colon.

Free blood in the peritoneal cavity tends to accumulate in the lateral gutters. It can be identified as a soft tissue shadow between the fat density of the flank stripe and the fecal content in the cecum and ascending colon on the right, or between the flank stripe and the descending colon on the left. The flank stripes are generally more prominent in adults than in children. They may be broader in fat people. They are not clearly visible in every normal patient and tend to be indistinct in older persons with little fat. They may not be included on the films in large patients or in those with protuberant abdomens. Absence of the flank stripes, therefore, may be of no particular significance. Peritonitis or retroperitoneal infection may obliterate the flank stripes as well.

The psoas shadows are generally identified on both sides of the lumbar spine, extending obliquely outward from the first lumbar vertebra and fading out over the iliac crests (Fig 5–7,B). The psoas shadows are important only if you see them. Delineation of the psoas shadows is evidence against retroperitoneal infection, abscess, hematoma, or lymphoma. However, absence of either or both psoas shadows may be a normal variation in as many as one third of patients. Psoas shadows may be obliterated by slight obliquity of the patient. Absence of the psoas shadow on one side accompanied by scoliosis and flank tenderness suggests possible retroperitoneal infection. Identification of both psoas shadows militates against any retroperitoneal abnormality.

Identification of stomach gas is generally not crucial to abdominal evaluation. Stomach gas varies in amount. On supine films, it is usually visible as an oblique gas collection projected upward from the central abdomen toward the left upper quadrant. In upright films, stomach content forms an air-fluid level beneath the left hemidiaphragm. Following ingestion of a meal, gas fluid and solid content in the stomach may be substantial. Some gas and fluid in the stomach are nearly always present in the normal patient. Stomach content may be minimal or absent in a patient who has recently vomited.

Distinguishing between small-bowel and large-bowel gas is generally easy and is crucial to evaluating for bowel obstruction. Look for large-bowel gas first.

The large bowel has three characteristics: (1). *Location.* Anatomically, the large bowel is peripheral in the abdomen. Its position has been likened to that of a picture frame. (2). *Haustrations.* The bowel is characterized by large, deep indentations. These are generally eccentric but at times may match or cross the lumen (Fig 5–8). (3). *Fecal content.* Any loop of bowel with solid content is unequivocally colon. Small-bowel content is always liquid. Fecal content is readily recognized as masses of gas intermixed with solid material. (Fig 5–9).

The small bowel has three anatomical characteris-

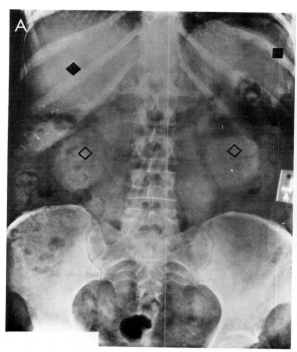

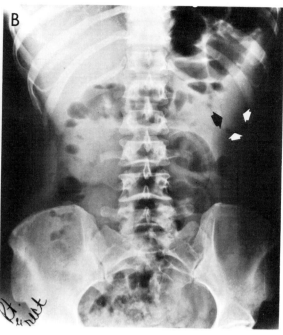

FIG 5–5.
Anatomy: normal liver and kidneys, enlarged spleen. **A,** obese patient. Liver and spleen *(closed diamonds)* are partially obscured by overlying bowel. The kid-

neys are well defined *(open diamonds).* **B,** thin patient. The spleen is moderately enlarged. The edge is obscured *(arrows).* The renal margins are less well defined than in the obese patient.

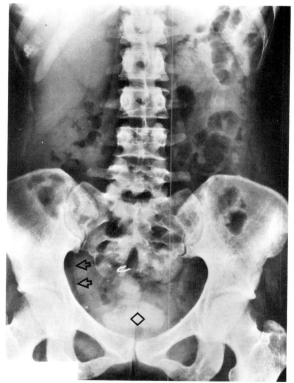

FIG 5–6.
Normal anatomy. The urinary bladder is clearly delineated *(diamond).* The fat along the right margin of the pelvic rim is marked with *arrows.* This extraperitoneal fat over the obturator internus muscle is continuous with the extraperitoneal fat over the dome of the bladder. In the presence of fracture, this fat shadow is obliterated by extraperitoneal hematoma or ruptured urinary bladder. An incidental finding is a metal surgical clip projected over the sacrum.

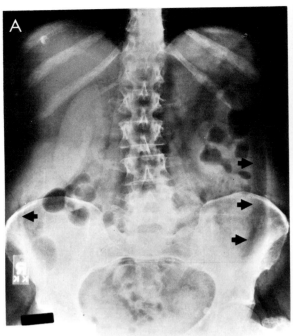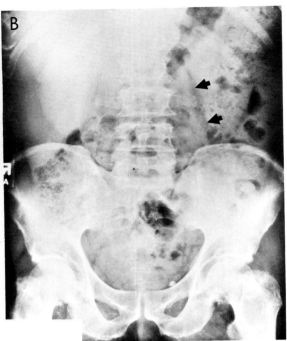

FIG 5–7.
Normal anatomy: flank stripes and psoas shadows. **A,** same patient as Figure 5–3. The left flank stripe is very wide *(arrows),* and the right is very narrow. This is a normal variation. The thin white shadow *(single arrow)* between the narrow flank stripe and the cecal gas is the right lateral gutter. This is a potential space. This white shadow widens if there is free blood in the peritoneal cavity. **B,** normal abdominal film of a different patient, showing narrow flank stripes on both sides. Note that the left psoas margin is more clearly shown than the right in this patient.

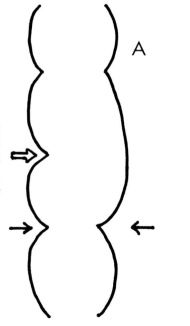

FIG 5–8.
A, haustrations are deep indentations that may be eccentric *(open arrow)* or matched across lumen *(closed arrows).* **B,** valvulae conniventes are small indentations that are matched across the lumen. The transverse mucosal folds sometimes have the appearance of stripes or a stack of coins.

tics: (1). *General location.* The small-bowel mesentery is attached centrally; therefore, loops of bowel in the central abdomen are more likely to be small bowel. (2). *Valvulae conniventes.* Small bowel is characterized by tiny indentations that always line up across the lumen. These sometimes extend completely across the lumen, giving the appearance of a stack of coins (Fig 5–8,B). In distended jejunum, you will always see valvulae conniventes. They are not effaced by distention. In the ileum, the valvulae conniventes are less well developed and are often not visible in distended loops. (3). *The "bent-finger sign."* A loop that looks like a bent finger is characteristic of small bowel (see Fig 5–12). This most useful small-bowel characteristic has not been emphasized in the literature.

Gas outside the bowel is always significant. It may take one of several forms: a crescent beneath the diaphragm (Fig 5–10), a "gull-wing" configuration in the biliary tract (see Fig 5–54), a speckled appearance in pockets (see Fig 5–139), streaky and bubbly collections in the retroperitoneum (see Fig 5–41). Other examples are included in the case material to follow.

Abdominal masses, even when large, may be very difficult to detect on abdominal radiographs because the radiographic density of the mass may be the same as that of the surrounding soft tissues (see Figs 5–30 and 5–31). When the mass displaces bowel loops, contains calcium, is adjacent to a fat interface, or is of a density different from that of the surrounding tissue, it is more readily detected. Detection of masses requires systematic film viewing.

The Acute Abdomen

Film Routine

Radiographic examination of the abdomen is often productive in the evaluation of a patient with abdominal pain. This section will present step by step criteria for film interpretation.

For initial evaluation of any type of acute abdominal pain, a supine abdominal film is inadequate. A minimum series for the acute abdomen includes a supine film centered at the iliac crest, an upright film centered at the crest, and an *upright* chest film. The chest film should be a conventional 6-foot PA film if the patient's condition permits him to stand. This view is essential to abdominal evaluation because it provides the best visualization of free air in the peritoneal cavity. Additionally, pneumonia, atelectasis, or pleural fluid may be concomitants or a manifestation of acute abdominal disease. The supine abdominal film is essential for detecting fluid or blood in the peritoneal cavity and for identifying gas in bowel loops. An upright or decubitus film of the abdomen is necessary for detecting air-fluid levels. The decubitus view of the abdomen is useful when the patient is unable to stand. However, one should realize that, unless special wall-mounted Bucky equipment is available, technically excellent decubitus films are virtually impossible to obtain because of limitations imposed by the grid cassette. We prefer an upright view when obtainable, as it contains more diagnostic information and is of better technical quality.

A special technique is extremely helpful in obtaining upright abdominal and chest films in patients unable to stand unassisted. Upright films may be obtained on debilitated patients by using compression binders, provided the patient is neither hypotensive nor a victim of multiple trauma. A compression binder is placed over the patient's knees. A second compression binder is placed over the patient's chest, between the breasts and the armpits. The compression binder at the knees keeps the patient from falling by preventing the knees from buckling. The compression binder across the chest helps to immobilize the patient on the table. If a compression binder is not available, tape is a good substitute. Extend the tape across the patient and attach it to both edges of the table. Use a small towel or gauze to prevent the tape from adhering to the patient's skin.

The technologist then establishes the factors to be used for an upright abdominal film and an upright Bucky chest film before actual filming is begun. A cassette is placed in the Bucky tray and the patient is positioned for a supine abdominal film. After this film has been obtained, the cassette is replaced, the table is tilted upright, the tube is positioned, and an upright abdominal film is obtained immediately. With the table still upright, the cassette is quickly changed and the x-ray tube is positioned for an upright Bucky chest film. As soon as the technologist exposes this film, the table is immediately returned to the horizontal position. With this method, both an upright abdominal and an upright Bucky chest view can be obtained with the patient in the upright position for less than 1 minute. This technique is useful for patients on whom upright films would not otherwise be obtainable, but should not be used on patients in shock. Also, it may not be feasible for some patients with fractures.

The alternative to the upright abdominal film when the patient is unable to stand is a left lateral decubitus view. This is made with the patient's *left side down,* using a grid cassette with the cassette and the x-ray tube centered to include the upper right edge of the abdomen on the film. Free air is localized between the liver and the peritoneum.

A right lateral decubitus film of the abdomen *(right side down)* is of limited or no value in detecting free

Expected

677-0010

Mark Seabolts

peritoneal air because distended bowel loops in contact with the peritoneum of the upright left side of the abdomen cannot, in most instances, be distinguished from free air.

In some institutions, the filming routine consists of supine and upright films with the upright film centered high to include the diaphragm. We have encountered several problems in using this technique. The technologist, not being certain of the level of the diaphragm in many patients, tends to center too high and thus fails to obtain some crucial information in the lower abdomen. Using a technique satisfactory for abdominal penetration tends to burn out details of the lung and diaphragm margins. The film is therefore of limited value for lungs and for evaluation of the margin of the diaphragm for free air.

It is a mistake to expect an accurate visualization of free air under the diaphragm on erect films of the abdomen. Patients are often quite ill. A slight movement of the diaphragm will obscure small amounts of air. Chest films or left lateral decubitus views are infinitely more reliable, the former because of shorter exposure times and the latter because the air is not in contact with the diaphragm.

Additional views may occasionally be useful in selected patients. These consist of two supine films made 15 minutes apart for evaluating changes in the distribution of small-bowel loops in patients with suspected obstruction. A lateral view (horizontal beam lateral) of the anterior abdomen made with the patient supine on the x-ray table may at times be useful in evaluating air-fluid levels in obese patients.

Film quality is often a problem in the emergency setting because of the inability of the patient fully to cooperate, inability to obtain standard views, the necessity for grid cassettes, and the stress under which the staff must work.

Bowel Obstruction

Terminology

Bowel obstructions fall into two categories. Mechanical obstruction occurs when the lumen is blocked because of adhesions, twisting, or an intraluminal mass. Paralytic obstruction results from inhibited peristalsis.

Mechanical obstruction may be strangulating, in which there is interference with blood supply, or simple, which includes all nonstrangulating obstructions. Mechanical obstruction may occur in the small intestine or the colon.

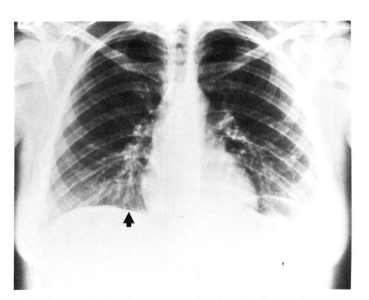

closed arrow). Fecal content of colon is shown by *open diamonds*. A small-bowel loop with stripes incident to valvulae conniventes is shown by the *open arrow*.

FIG 5–9 (left).
Normal bowel anatomy. Haustrations are shown by *closed arrows*. Note that in some instances these may be matched across the lumen of the bowel (*opposing closed arrows*), but in others they are not (*single vertical closed arrows*, but in others they are not (*single vertical

FIG 5–10 (right).
Upright chest. *Arrow* indicates free air under right hemidiaphragm. Also note bowel gas within the splenic flexure of the colon under left hemidiaphragm.

Adynamic ileus, paralytic ileus, reflex ileus, neurogenic ileus, nonobstructing ileus, nonobstructing distention, adynamic distention, and aerophagia are all different names for the same entity. Opinion varies as to the principal mechanism by which gas accumulates in bowel that is not mechanically obstructed. In this text, the term "adynamic ileus" is preferred because it is the one most commonly used and understood in clinical practice. Localized or generalized bowel atony best explains the radiographic findings, which may consist of a single atonic loop (sentinel loop), gaseous distention of the entire small bowel and colon, or any degree of distention between the two.

This section outlines the diagnostic criteria for various types of obstruction.

The Nonspecific Abdomen

Most bowel gas is swallowed air. Gas that has passed through the pylorus into the small intestine is rapidly absorbed or transported. It clears the small intestine in less than 20 minutes. A slack abdominal wall, labored respiration, or prolonged supine position may contribute to some retention of gas in the small bowel. Retention of gas is therefore common in aged or bedridden patients. A variable amount of small-bowel gas is normal in children. In the ambulatory adult patient, there is ordinarily little or no small-bowel gas detectable on routine abdominal films.

The significance of gas within small-bowel loops may be difficult to interpret. We use the following guidelines for interpreting small-bowel gas patterns.

Distended small-bowel loops are always abnormal. We consider 3 cm to be the upper limit of normal for the diameter of the small bowel. Distended small-bowel loops with air-fluid levels are always abnormal and are more significant than distention alone.

Air-fluid levels in nondistended small bowel are more difficult to interpret. They should be looked upon as abnormal but nonspecific in nature. We routinely recommend follow-up examinations in such cases since this sign may represent the earliest findings of significant abdominal disease.

Scattered air in nondistended small-bowel loops falls into the gray zone between normal and abnormal. We tend to minimize the significance of this finding, which is often seen in normal patients (Fig 5–11). This pattern is seen in older or bedridden patients and is associated with air swallowing from sipping drinks or meals through straws. This also explains why extensive small-bowel gas is normal in many infants and neonates, who may swallow more air than liquid when feeding.

Although some small-bowel gas may be present in some individuals in the absence of any disease process, the possibility of significant intra-abdominal disease should always be considered when small bowel gas is observed.

In patients with acute abdominal pain, the most frequently encountered radiographic finding is an isolated loop of gas-containing small bowel in the upper left quadrant or central abdomen. Any distended (3 cm) gas-containing small-bowel loop encountered under these circumstances may be considered a "sentinel loop." It usually represents a localized adynamic loop secondary to some acute disease process. Although sentinel loop has long been recognized as a feature of acute pancreatitis, it may also occur in a large variety of intra-abdominal conditions such as acute cholecystitis, acute appendicitis, blunt abdominal trauma, back trauma, peritonitis, bowel obstruction, myocardial infarction, acute gastroenteritis, mesenteric adenitis, and other acute processes.

Although nonspecific, the sentinel loop may be a hallmark of an acute intra-abdominal process. Identification is extremely important because it serves as a clue to the presence of acute intra-abdominal disease, but it will provide no specific information as to the nature of the process. The sentinel loop is most often seen in the upper abdomen, but may be identified anywhere; its location is not necessarily related to the location of the disease process. For example, acute appendicitis, a right lower quadrant inflammatory process, may produce a left upper quadrant sentinel loop.

Gas and fluid that have passed the ileocecal valve remain in the colon for varying periods and may be readily detectable on abdominal films. The colon absorbs substantial fluid, but it is not unusual to find colon air-fluid levels in normal patients. Additionally, air-fluid levels may be noted in the colon in patients incident to enemas given at home prior to presenting at the emergency department. Therefore, fluid in the colon must be considered within normal limits at any time.

An 18-year-old girl came to the emergency department complaining of abdominal pain and tenderness. Supine and upright films of the abdomen were obtained (Fig 5–12). In evaluating the films systematically, a number of interesting features can be identified. Bone structure is intact. The lumbar spine is scoliotic with the patient standing, but straight on the supine film. The lung bases and costophrenic angles are clear. No calcifications or concretions are identified. Several tiny artifacts are noted, including one over the left greater trochanter. The liver edge varies substantially in prominence on comparison of the su-

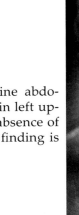

FIG 5–11.
The nonspecific bowel gas pattern in the supine abdomen. Note the isolated loop of small-bowel gas in left upper quadrant with valvulae conniventes. In the absence of distention or air-fluid level, as in this case, the finding is nonspecific and may be normal.

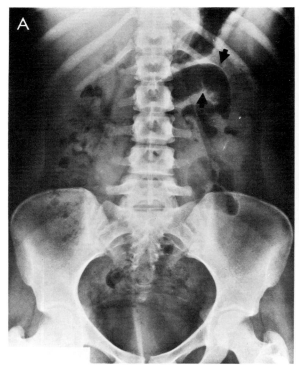

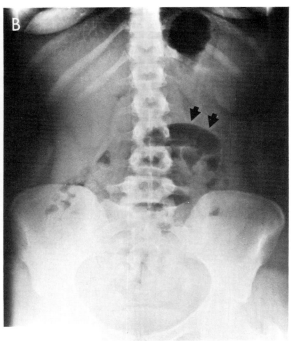

FIG 5–12.
The bent-finger sign. Supine **(A)** and upright **(B)** films of the same patient. *Arrows* point to a small-bowel loop, which resembles a bent finger. In this case the bowel loop is distended and therefore represents a sentinel loop.

pine and upright films. The spleen is readily identified and is moderately enlarged. The kidneys are rather poorly delineated. Both psoas shadows are normal. The flank stripes are very well demonstrated bilaterally. The urinary bladder and paravesical fat (over the dome of the bladder) are well shown. Fecal content is identified in the colon in a picture-frame distribution. Haustrations are not prominent. Stomach gas is visible in the left upper quadrant medial to the spleen. Just below this on both the supine and upright films is a beautiful example of a bent-finger, unequivocally incident to gas in an isolated loop of small bowel (sentinel loop) in the left upper quadrant. Valvulae conniventes are rather poorly defined. Gas is not identified outside the bowel.

On examination in the emergency department, this patient was found to have a small mass in the left inguinal region and was admitted to the surgical service with a tentative diagnosis of incarcerated hernia. When seen by a surgeon, the mass was thought to be a lymph node. A heterophil antibody test was strongly positive. The diagnosis was acute infectious mononucleosis presenting as an acute abdomen. This finding also explains the enlarged spleen.

Summary

An isolated gas-containing loop of small bowel is a nonspecific finding often seen in several types of acute intra-abdominal disease. The sentinel loop may be seen in any of a large variety of acute conditions, including early mechanical obstruction. When a distended small-bowel loop is identified, the patient requires careful clinical observation and evaluation. Appreciation of the nonspecific abdomen is an important concept for first-encounter physicians. It is the most frequently encountered radiographic finding in patients presenting with abdominal pain and serves as an indication that the patient has some type of acute disease.

Mechanical Obstruction

In adults, gas is normally recognized in the stomach and colon. In upright patients, stomach gas accumulates in the fundus of the stomach beneath the left hemidiaphragm, forming an air-fluid level with the liquid gastric content. Gas and fecal material are normally scattered through the colon. Air-fluid levels may also at times be noted in the normal colon.

Because the small bowel does not ordinarily contain gas, air-fluid levels there usually indicate disease. Like gas in the normal small intestine, fluid is rap-

idly transported from the pylorus to the colon. When the small intestine becomes completely mechanically obstructed for any reason, intestinal content (gas and fluid) cannot be propelled by peristalsis beyond the point of obstruction. The bowel loops proximal to the obstruction become distended with gas and fluid. When the small bowel is obstructed, fluid absorption is decreased. Distention of bowel loops leads to changed circulatory dynamics. Gas is not formed in an obstructed loop, but obstruction decreases absorption. The presence of small-intestine air-fluid levels on an upright abdominal film should always raise the issue of mechanical obstruction. When correlated with clinical findings, a significant error will rarely be made. One should be aware that fluid may be due to laxatives, narcotics, prolonged adynamic ileus, or acute gastroenteritis (see Fig 5–26).

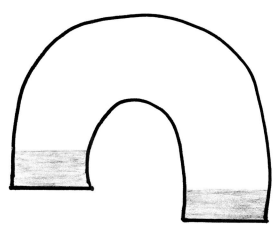

FIG 5–13.
Diagram of a dynamic loop. Fluid is shown in a single loop of small bowel at two different levels. The *shaded area* is fluid; the *clear area* is gas.

Distended small bowel loops layer out one on the other on the supine film. In the upright film, the air-fluid levels form a stepladder pattern. Active peristalsis causes some of the air-fluid levels to be at different levels in the same loop. These "dynamic loops" are the result of peristalsis attempting to propel fluid against an obstruction. Dynamic loops are virtually diagnostic of mechanical obstruction (Fig 5–13).

When obstruction is prolonged, the bowel wall may become edematous, causing the loops to appear separated. Fat in the mesentery, however, may also separate bowel loops.

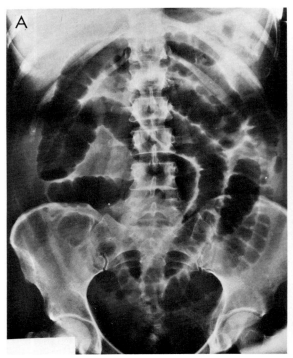

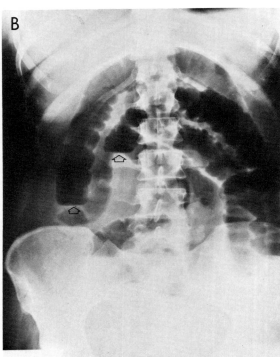

FIG 5–14.
Mechanical small-intestinal obstruction. **A,** supine film. There are multiple gas-filled loops of small bowel arranged in a cluster in the central abdomen. Note the valvulae conniventes and multiple bent fingers. The colon is almost devoid of gas. A rectal bubble can be identified. **B,** upright film. Multiple air-fluid levels are identified *(arrows).* Several of these appear to be at different levels in the same loop. These are dynamic loops with active peristalsis attempting to propel bowel content past a point of complete obstruction.

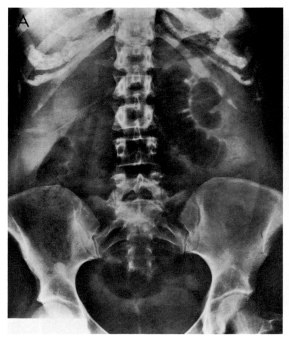

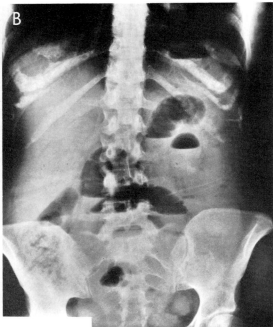

FIG 5–15.
Mechanical small-intestinal obstruction. **A,** the supine film shows distended small bowel. **B,** the upright film shows dynamic air-fluid levels.

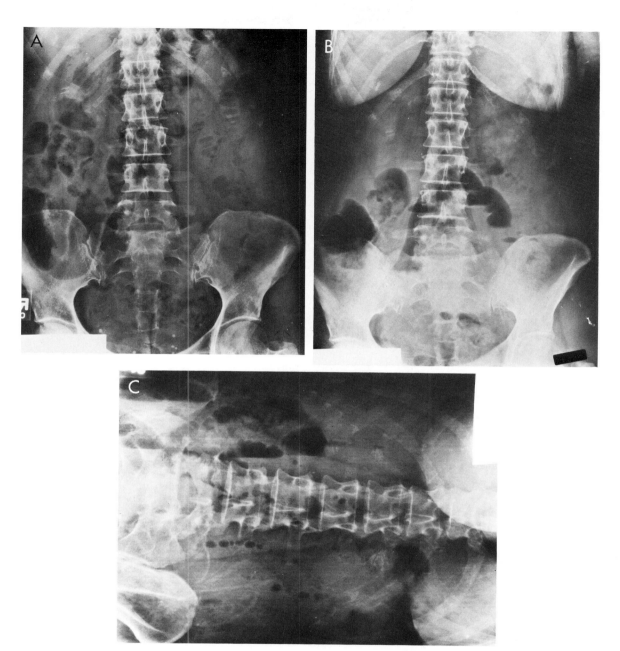

FIG 5–16.
Mechanical small-intestinal obstruction. **A,** supine film. Note the paucity of findings. **B,** upright film. Note dynamic air-fluid levels. **C,** decubitus view. Note that dynamic air-fluid levels are less well shown than on the upright film.

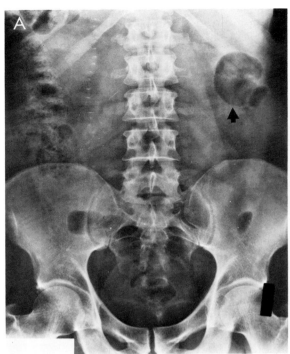

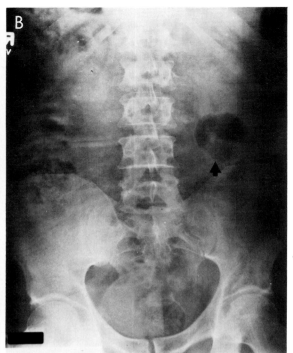

FIG 5–17.
Sentinel loop. **A,** supine view. Note the small-bowel loop with the appearance of a bent finger in the left upper quadrant.

Since the bent finger is distended, it represents a sentinel loop. **B,** same patient, upright view. Although often seen as part of the sentinel loop, no air-fluid level is present in this case.

FIG 5–18.
Progression of the bent finger to full-blown adynamic ileus in same patient as Figure 5–17. **A,** supine film shows gaseous distention of large and small bowel. **B,** upright film

shows an air-fluid level in the colon in the right upper abdomen. There is an air-fluid level projected over the sacrum, which could be large or small bowel.

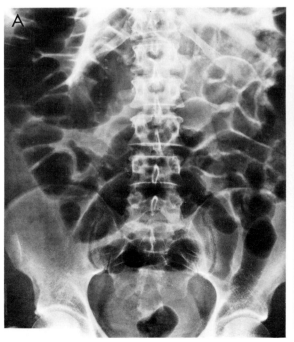

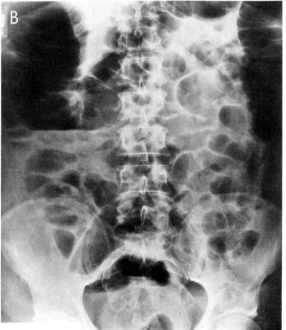

In complete mechanical small intestinal obstruction, the colon may or may not contain gas and fluid. This depends in part on how long the obstruction persists. Early on, gas and fluid that were present in the colon prior to the obstruction may remain indefinitely. The rectal bubble is simply colon gas and has no special significance. In some patients, the colon contents will be evacuated. If the obstruction is complete, the colon may contain little gas, fluid, or fecal material. It should be remembered, however, that air-fluid levels in the colon are normal at any time.

Summary

Classic plain film findings in mechanical small intestinal obstruction are multiple gas-filled loops of small bowel and (in the upright view) dynamic air-fluid levels (Figs 5–14 to 5–16).

Adynamic Ileus—The Mechanism of Gas Accumulation

Swallowed air may remain in the stomach for varying periods, depending on the activity and position of the patient. After it has passed through the pylorus, it is normally transported rapidly through the small intestine or absorbed by the intestinal mucosa. Gas that passes through the ileocecal valve may remain in the colon for relatively long intervals before it is absorbed or expelled.

When circulation in mesenteric vessels decreases, gas absorption is lowered. Complex neurogenic and circulatory mechanisms work directly and indirectly to affect peristalsis and absorption of gas and fluids from the intestine. Derangement of these mechanisms occurs in a variety of situations, including shock, cardiac decompensation, peritonitis, pneumonia, spinal injuries, postoperative infectious disease, uremia, severe blunt trauma, collagen diseases, medication reactions, acute pancreatitis, acute cholecystitis, pelvic inflammatory disease, pelvic peritonitis, acute disk or back injury, colic from biliary stone, urinary stone, and others. Restriction of excursion of the diaphragm also lowers absorption. Patients with chronic obstructive lung disease swallow more than the normal amount of air, which tends to increase intestinal gas.

A common feature of early adynamic ileus of any etiology is that virtually no fluid is found in the small bowel.

Fluid may accumulate in adynamic loops distended for several hours because the prolonged distention interferes with circulatory dynamics, decreasing fluid absorption. These fluid levels, however, are different from the fluid levels seen in mechanical obstruction, which are more likely to be dynamic loops. Moreover, when multiple adynamic loops containing fluid levels are observed, the presence of even one dynamic loop indicates an underlying mechanical obstruction.

The sentinel loop is the beginning stage of adynamic ileus. One should realize that radiographic examination of a patient presenting with an acute abdomen may demonstrate any degree of gaseous distention, from a single sentinel loop through pronounced gaseous distention of multiple loops, depending on the duration and severity of the disease process.

A 40-year-old female presented at the emergency department with abdominal pain and was admitted to the surgical service. The most significant finding on her films was a sentinel loop in the left upper quadrant (Fig 5–17). The following morning, repeat abdominal films (Fig 5–18) showed a large amount of gas scattered through multiple loops of large and small bowel. An air-fluid level in the right abdomen was definitely in the colon and, therefore, of no significance. The patient was examined by a surgeon, who diagnosed acute appendicitis and operated. At surgery, acute gangrenous appendicitis was found. The films show progression of the sentinel loop into a full-blown adynamic ileus.

An elderly man presented in the emergency department with abdominal pain and distention. A suprapubic cystostomy tube was present. After examination, the tentative diagnosis was adynamic ileus secondary to urinary tract infection. However, when films were obtained, a consolidating left lower-lobe pneumonia was noted. The pneumonia in this patient was completely unsuspected until the chest film was obtained, an occurrence that emphasizes the importance of obtaining such films in every patient who presents with acute abdominal findings. The radiologic and clinical diagnosis was adynamic ileus secondary to pneumonia (Fig 5–19).

The child who presents with clinical findings of acute abdomen should be particularly suspect. Not infrequently, a child who has not had a chest film has been operated on for acute appendicitis. Surgery reveals a normal appendix, and follow-up chest examination shows pneumonia as the etiology of the acute abdominal symptoms.

Distal Colon Obstruction Versus Adynamic Ileus

Twenty to twenty-five percent of all cases of intestinal obstruction involve the colon. Malignant neoplasm is by far the most common cause, accounting for 80% of cases of acute colon obstruction. Other

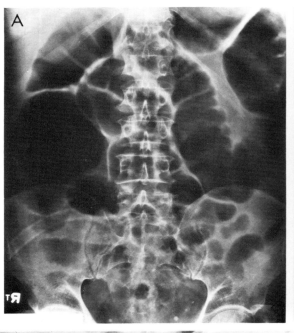

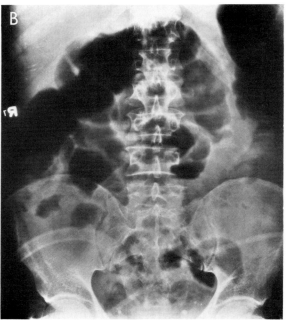

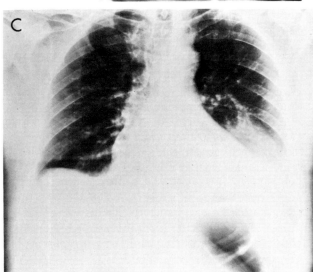

FIG 5–19.
Adynamic ileus secondary to pneumonia. **A,** the supine film shows distended large and small bowel. Note suprapubic tube. **B,** the upright film shows distended large and small bowel. An air-fluid level is present in the central abdomen. **C,** the chest x-ray shows left lower-lobe pneumonia.

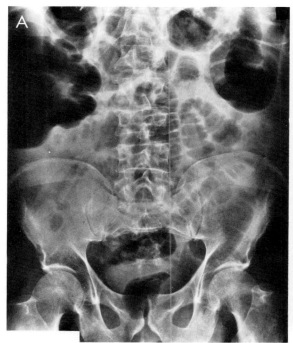

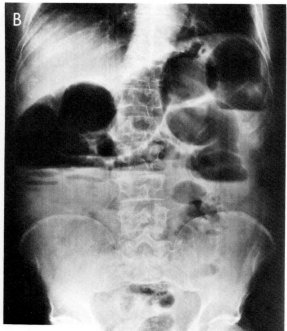

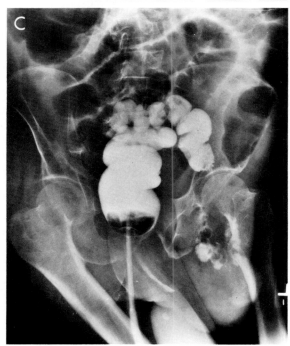

FIG 5–20.
Distal colon obstruction. **A,** supine film shows large-bowel gas in a picture-frame distribution. Small-bowel gas is central. There is a bent finger in the left central abdomen. Valvulae conniventes can be identified. **B,** upright film shows multiple air-fluid levels in large and small bowel. **C,** water-soluble contrast enema shows a distal colon obstruction from incarcerated inguinal hernia.

causes are incarcerated inguinal hernia, acute diverticulitis, fecal impaction, and, rarely, extrinsic malignancy. In the small bowel, adhesions are the most common cause of obstruction.

Mechanical distal colon obstruction has plain-film radiographic findings virtually identical to those of end-stage adynamic ileus (small- and large-bowel distention).

Fecal impaction can be a problem in the elderly. Feces may become impacted proximal to an obstructing lesion but, in the elderly, impaction usually results from chronic constipation. Impactions are also seen in patients with mental retardation, spinal neurologic disorders, and myxedema. A distended colon in a child suggests the possibility of Hirschsprung's disease.

In patients with large amounts of both large- and small-bowel gas, the principal entities in the differential diagnosis in the emergency setting are adynamic ileus of any cause or distal mechanical colon obstruction.

Contrast enema is useful in identifying or ruling out colon obstruction when the clinical picture is not clear.

A 65-year-old man presented at the emergency department with a distended abdomen and acute abdominal pain. The supine film showed multiple distended loops of small bowel in the central abdomen and substantial gas throughout the colon as well. The upright film showed multiple air-fluid levels. Some of these were definitely in the colon, but some of them appeared to be in the small bowel. The presence of small-bowel fluid in this patient was consistent with mechanical or adynamic obstruction of any cause. Contrast enema was performed to confirm that an incarcerated hernia was the cause of the obstruction (Fig 5–20). If the clinical diagnosis is not clear, as in the patients shown in Figures 5–18 and 5–19, contrast enema is useful.

Summary

Adynamic ileus may be identified in any one of several stages, from an isolated single loop of distended small bowel to full-blown gaseous distention of both large and small bowel. The distended small bowel is usually, but not always, devoid of air-fluid levels. When air-fluid levels are present, they are not of the dynamic type.

Summary of Basic Concepts for Recognition of Simple, Classic Obstructions

1. A sentinel loop is a reliable nonspecific indicator of some acute intra-abdominal problem.
2. "Classic" mechanical small-intestinal obstruction is characterized by distended small intestine with dynamic air-fluid levels.
3. Adynamic ileus may produce varying degrees of large- and small-bowel distention, usually without small-bowel air-fluid levels and always without dynamic air-fluid levels.
4. Fluid levels in the colon and stomach are normal.
5. Distal colon obstruction produces radiographic findings identical to those of adynamic ileus. A contrast enema provides differentiation.

Barium Versus Water-Soluble Contrast

Barium sulfate is an insoluble particulate substance which is combined with various suspending agents. It is the standard substance for gastrointestinal examination and is not absorbed by the intestinal tract. It has a moderately high viscosity, which varies with manufacturers' specifications and dilutions. In the mid-1950s, water-soluble agents (Gastrografin, oral Hypaque) were introduced for gastrointestinal examination as well. There are significant differences in the two types of contrast. An understanding, therefore, of the uses and limitations of each is essential to optimal patient care.

Water-soluble contrast has a low viscosity. When administered orally, it rapidly traverses the small intestine and generally enters the colon within 2 hours. It has a significant laxative effect.

Water-soluble contrast is not absorbed from the intact intestinal tract in 95% of normal adult patients. Because of low viscosity, however, it will readily penetrate points of intestinal perforation, and is therefore useful in evaluating for obscure or suspected intestinal perforation. Water-soluble contrast will penetrate perforated intestinal mucosa, gain access to the circulation, be excreted by the kidneys, and become visible in the urinary bladder in 2 to 4 hours. This occurs whether the perforation is at the esophageal, gastric, small-intestinal, or colonic level. Visualization of orally administered water-soluble contrast in the urinary bladder 2 to 4 hours after administration is a reliable indicator of intestinal perforation in adults. There are about 5% false positive results.

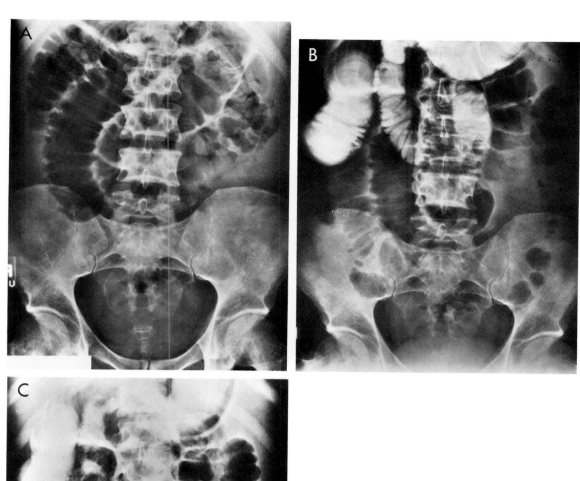

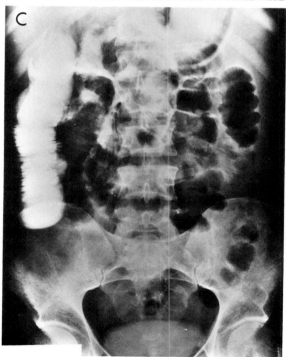

FIG 5–21.
Intestinal perforation. **A,** supine film. Note the distended small bowel in the upper abdomen. **B,** supine film 2 hours after oral water-soluble contrast. The stomach and jejunum are opacified. Contrast can be seen in the urinary bladder as well. **C,** supine film 4 hours after oral contrast. There has been an increase in density of the urinary bladder.

There are some limits on the use of water-soluble contrast. Because it is hygroscopic and draws substantial amounts of fluid into the bowel lumen, it alters water balance and is therefore of particular concern in children. In addition, although not absorbed from the intact intestinal tract in most adults, it is readily absorbed from the normal intestinal tract in 50% of children. The absorbed contrast is excreted by the kidneys and becomes visible in the urinary bladder, causing a false positive diagnosis of intestinal perforation in children. Neonates and infants are especially vulnerable to the osmotic side effects of these agents. For these reasons, water soluble contrast is not recommended as an oral contrast agent in children. Currently, newer water-soluble contrast agents, such as metrizamide, are being developed. These newer agents can be used at isotonic or near-isotonic concentrations. Originally used exclusively in myelography, these agents are finding new, widespread applications, but are currently quite expensive.

In the abdomen water-soluble contrast is of substantially lower radiographic density than barium. Because low viscosity permits it to pass by points of partial obstruction and because of the relatively low radiographic density, oral water soluble contrast is of limited value in detecting intestinal obstruction. For these reasons, oral administration of water-soluble contrast should be limited to patients in whom intestinal perforation is suspected.

Because barium has a higher radiographic density and greater viscosity, it is of substantial value in detecting mechanical small-intestinal obstruction. It is more reliable for this purpose than oral water-soluble contrast and is the agent of choice when oral contrast is indicated to evaluate obstruction.

Surgeons sometimes object to the oral administration of barium for intestinal obstruction because the presence of barium in the lumen may make intestinal anastomosis more difficult, should this be necessary. This problem should be kept in mind if surgical intervention is planned.

Barium should not be given orally when both large and small bowel are distended because of the possibility of a low colon obstruction. The barium will impact in the colon and further complicate the obstruction. In this situation, a contrast enema is the procedure of choice.

When an emergency contrast enema is indicated for a patient who has not had prior colon preparation, water-soluble contrast rather than barium is the agent of choice. Because of its low viscosity, it will flow through an unprepared colon more readily than barium. If the colon is partially obstructed to retrograde flow, the aqueous contrast is more likely to get by the lesion and help establish its nature (see Fig 5–20). If the colon is perforated from acute diverticulitis or colon carcinoma, aqueous contrast is less hazardous to the patient, since it is absorbed and excreted by the kidneys. If barium comes in contact with the peritoneum, it may cause granulomas and adhesions.

A 44-year-old female presented at the emergency department with severe abdominal pain and distention. She was receiving vincristine for Hodgkin's disease. A nasogastric tube was introduced. The patient was too ill for an upright or decubitus film. A supine film (Fig 5–21,A) showed extreme gaseous distention of multiple loops of small bowel in the upper central abdomen. There was some slight separation of bowel loops, suggesting exudate or bowel-wall edema. Clinical findings favored peritonitis. For further evaluation of the possibility of intestinal perforation, 50 cc of oral water-soluble contrast was introduced into the nasogastric tube. A film after 2 hours (Fig 5–21,B) showed that the contrast had not progressed beyond the midjejunum. Some opacification of the urinary bladder was noted. After 4 hours (Fig 5–21,C), there had not been significant progression of contrast beyond the midjejunum. There had been an increase in the intensity of opacification of the urinary bladder.

The findings indicated mechanical small-intestinal obstruction and intestinal perforation. At autopsy, the patient was found to have multiple small-bowel perforations from vincristine therapy, with diffuse peritonitis and mechanical small-bowel obstruction.

Summary

Water-soluble contrast
1. Traverses bowel rapidly, has low viscosity, pulls fluid into the bowel lumen.
2. Is favored for oral administration in suspected bowel perforation.
3. Should not be administered orally to children, particularly infants.
4. Is favored for the contrast enema on an unprepared colon.

Barium
1. Has better radiographic density.
2. Is more reliable for oral use in evaluating small-intestinal obstructions.
3. Is favored as an oral contrast agent unless intestinal perforation or colon obstruction is suspected.

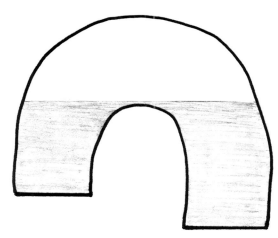

FIG 5–22.
Diagram of the "tortoise shell" sign. As fluid increases in an obstructed loop, the air-fluid level appears round on the top and flat or notched on the bottom. The *shaded area* is fluid, the *clear area* is gas. Compare with Figure 5–13.

FIG 5–23.
Strangulation obstruction. **A,** upright AP view. Multiple small-bowel loops (distended bent fingers) containing dynamic air-fluid levels are indicative of mechanical obstruction. **B,** upright lateral view. Several loops are present which are flat on the bottom and curved on the top—the tortoise shell sign *(arrows).* At surgery, the patient was found to have strangulation obstruction from incarcerated strangulated inguinal hernia.

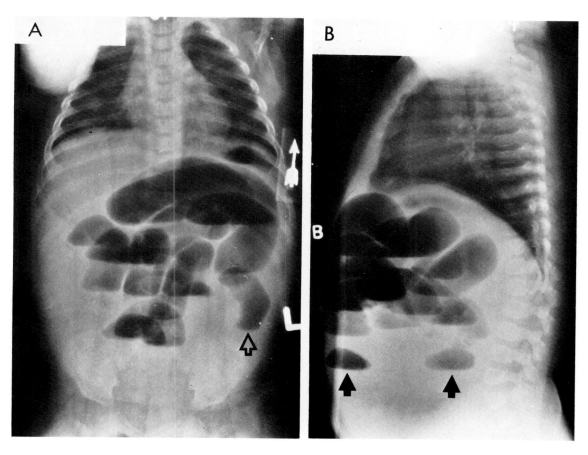

FIG 5–24.

Strangulation obstruction. **A**, supine view. In the left upper quadrant there is a tiny collection of small-bowel gas *(arrow)*. Close inspection shows some parallel stripes across it incident to valvulae conniventes. The finding is minimal. **B**, upright view. The film shows two tortoise shell signs *(arrows)*. One of these precisely corresponds to the small gas-filled loop on the supine film. The patient was operated on and found to have a strangulation obstruction from adhesions incident to an old appendiceal abscess. The films demonstrate that upright views are mandatory for full evaluation of abdominal pain or possible bowel obstruction.

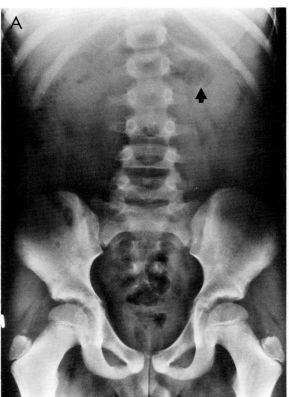

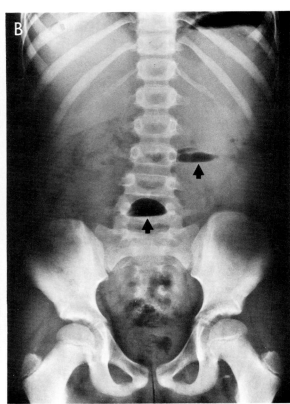

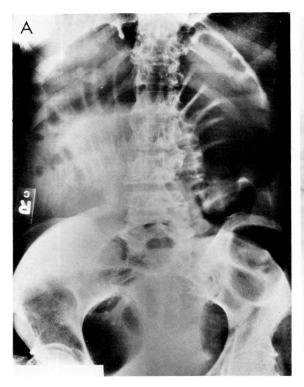

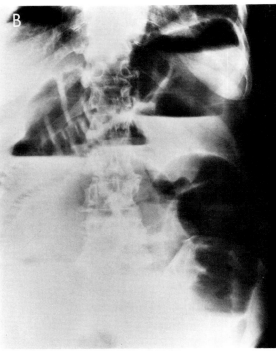

FIG 5–25.

Obstructing carcinoma of the colon, producing massive distention of the colon and small intestine. **A**, supine film. In colon obstruction, the degree of small-intestinal distention depends on the relative competence of the ileocecal valve. In this patient an incompetent valve has resulted in massive distention of the small bowel. **B**, upright film. Note that the small bowel contains a very large amount of fluid, suggesting strangulation. Note the "string of beads" in the right abdomen. The strangulation pattern of the small bowel is secondary to impaired circulation from prolonged distention.

Strangulation Obstruction

Strangulation obstruction implies impaired vascular supply to obstructed bowel. It is most often due to adhesions, twisted loop, or incarcerated hernia, which constrict the bowel lumen sufficiently to obstruct both the lumen and the blood supply. The altered circulatory dynamics interfere with the normal absorption of gas and fluid and, in fact, cause a large amount of fluid to accumulate in the bowel lumen. This feature is characteristic of strangulation.

If the bowel contains gas and fluid, an air-fluid level may be noted on upright abdominal films. If the bowel contains only fluid, however, the air-fluid level may not be visible radiographically, and the loop may therefore not be readily detectable by plain film examination. Multiple fluid-filled small-bowel loops may simulate a mass if they are completely closed.

Tiny collections of gas, which have the appearance of a string of beads or pearls, represent gas trapped within the recesses of the valvulae conniventes of dilated, fluid-filled small-bowel loops.

As a large amount of fluid accumulates in the bowel lumen, the air-fluid levels assume a characteristic appearance, round on the top and flat on the bottom. This "tortoise shell sign" simply indicates that there is a large amount of fluid in the bowel (Fig 5–22). A large amount of fluid in the small bowel is characteristic, but not diagnostic, of strangulation obstruction.

Large amounts of intraluminal fluid in the small bowel may result from any obstruction in which prolonged distention of the mucosa compromises blood supply. This is, in effect, strangulation, since the blood supply is diffusely compromised. Although not as acute, its consequence is the same as a localized strangulation as may be seen with adhesions, incarcerated hernia, or twisted loop. The possibility of strangulation should be suspected in any patient in whom a large amount of small-bowel fluid accumulates.

If a closed loop is bent on itself, it assumes the shape of a coffee bean, with the doubled width of the opposed walls resembling the cleft of the bean. This is called the "coffee bean sign" of strangulation obstruction and may be seen in closed loop obstruction of the small bowel or colon. It is much more readily recognized in the colon. In volvulus of the colon, this finding is also called the horse collar sign. In discussing volvulus of the colon, we prefer the term "horse collar sign" because it is more descriptive of the large distended loop. In evaluating the small intestine, we have found the tortoise shell sign far more valuable in recognizing strangulation. It is seen with great frequency. The coffee bean sign is seen infrequently.

Because of the changed circulatory dynamics, strangulation is a crucial diagnostic problem. Clinically, it is characterized by sudden onset of pain, or constant pain, with leukocytosis and abnormal tenderness to palpation.

True strangulation obstruction may be easily overlooked on plain film examination. One third of all serious obstructions caused by adhesions and bands have scanty or no radiographic findings. If there is severe pain, clinical evidence of obstruction, and negative plain film findings, suspect strangulation.

Oral barium is recommended in all doubtful cases. The risk of barium use is negligible, while the risk of not making the diagnosis is large. After barium ingestion, the patient must lie right side down for 30 minutes. This is important because, if the patient remains supine, the barium may pool in the gastric fundus and not leave the stomach. With the patient on the right side, the barium should reach the obstruction within 1 hour.

The patient in Figure 5–23 demonstrates that evaluation of the abdomen is more difficult in children than in adults. Fascial and fat planes are much less well developed in the child making the identification of normal anatomical structures such as kidneys, flank stripes, psoas shadows, urinary bladder, and perivesical fat more difficult. Further, the haustrations and valvulae conniventes are less well developed in a child, making differentiation between large and small bowel less marked. Children may normally have large amounts of gas in both large and small bowel. Children up to 2 years of age usually have large amounts of small-bowel gas. Between 2 and 5 years of age there are varying amounts of small-bowel gas; above 5 years of age, gas may be present in a child who has been crying for long periods before or during filming. Air-fluid levels are, however, always significant (Figs 5–24 to 5–26).

Summary of Basic Concepts for Recognition of Strangulation and Less Common Obstructing Small-Intestinal Lesions

1. Substantial fluid in the small bowel suggests strangulation. The tortoise shell sign indicates a large amount of small-bowel fluid. Therefore, although the sign is not specific for strangulation, the possibility should be considered.

2. In strangulation obstruction or high simple obstruction, there may be little or no gas in the small bowel.

3. Fluid-filled, small-bowel loops may simulate a mass on plain films.

4. Unless bowel perforation is suspected, oral barium is useful in the diagnosis of obscure strangulation obstruction, high simple obstruction, and masses.

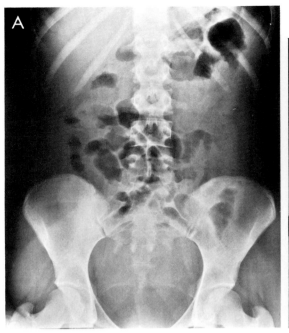

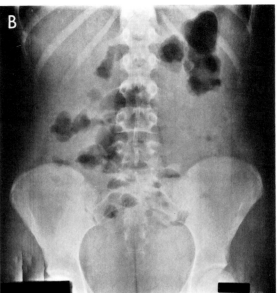

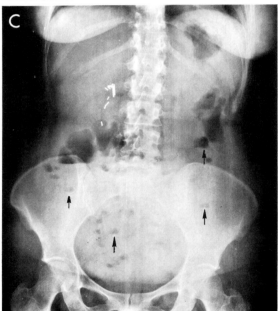

FIG 5–26.
Acute gastroenteritis. **A,** supine view. There are several nondistended small-bowel loops in the central abdomen. **B,** same patient, upright view. Note the fluid levels in the nondistended small bowel. **C,** different patient, upright view. There is a large amount of fluid in multiple nondistended small-bowel loops *(arrows).* Surgical clips are from prior cholecystectomy. These two patients are quite different from patients with strangulation obstruction. Although the small bowel contains fluid (a large amount in the patient shown in **C**), the loops are not distended. Note differences from Figures 5–23, 5–24, and 5–25.

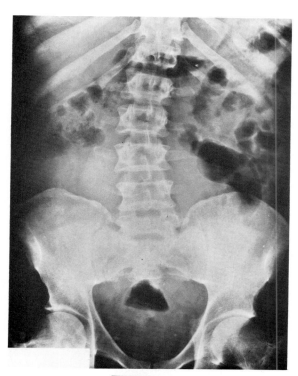

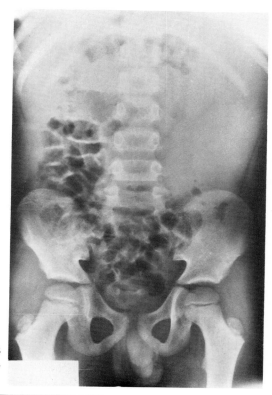

FIG 5–27 (top left).
Very large lower abdominal mass. Note the soft tissue density in the central abdomen with the curved upper margin displacing bowel gas. Margins of the bladder are faintly visible adjacent to the rectal bubble.

FIG 5–28 (top right).
Enlarged spleen displaces bowel gas out of left upper quadrant of abdomen.

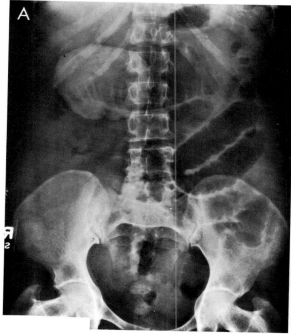

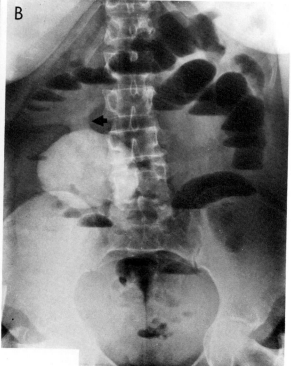

FIG 5–29.
Large abdominal mass external to patient. **A,** supine film. Note the mass in the right upper abdomen and multiple distended small-bowel loops. **B,** upright film. Note that the mass is attached to a pedicle *(arrow)*. Multiple dynamic air fluid levels indicate mechanical obstruction of the small bowel. Also note several tortoise shell signs, indicating a large amount of fluid in the small bowel. The mass is unrelated. On examination in the emergency department, a large pedunculated soft tissue mass was noted on the patient's back.

Abdominal Masses

Masses inside the abdomen (Figs 5–27 and 5–28), even when large, may be difficult to detect because the radiographic density of the mass is the same as the radiographic density of the surrounding soft tissues. Masses that efface or displace bowel loops are more readily recognized. Fluid-filled bowel loops, such as those which occur with strangulation obstruction or intussusception, may produce a subtle abdominal mass. Most clinicians have had the experience of palpating a relatively large abdominal mass only to be surprised at not being able to see it on plain abdominal films. Intra-abdominal masses may be notoriously difficult to see on plain films unless contrast is used to delineate displaced bowel loops.

Masses outside the abdomen (Fig 5–29) are generally much more readily recognized on plain abdominal films because there is a sharp interface between the surrounding air and the soft tissue density of the mass. Colostomy openings, for example, although small in size, ordinarily produce a soft tissue mass density because of this air–soft tissue interface.

Abdominal masses of all types are much more readily depicted on computed tomography than on plain films. The entire bowel must be opacified with contrast in order that fluid-filled bowel loops cannot be mistaken for a mass. Intravenous contrast is also useful in most instances because vascular enhancement is helpful in recognizing masses in the major organs (liver, spleen, pancreas, kidneys) and in evaluating aneurysms.

Intussusception

The diagnosis of ileocolic intussusception in a small child is usually suspected on the basis of cramping abdominal pain and blood in the stool. Plain films of the abdomen are often normal. A soft tissue mass incident to the intussusception of the ileum into the colon may at times be recognized in the upper central or right upper abdomen on plain film examination. A mass can often be palpated on careful clinical examination. Contrast enema is useful for confirmation of diagnosis. The intussusception may be reduced during the procedure.

Two patients came to the emergency department at different times with cramping abdominal pain and bloody stools. In both instances, a vague mass could be identified above the right iliac crest incident to the intussusception (Fig 5–30). The diagnosis in both patients was confirmed with barium enema. Both cases demonstrated how difficult it is to see even large abdominal masses on plain films. In most patients with intussusception, plain films will be negative. The initial suspicion must rest on clinical grounds.

High small-intestinal obstruction may not be characterized by the classic radiographic findings of intestinal obstruction (Fig 5–31). In many patients with high small-intestinal obstruction, abdominal films are entirely normal. The diagnosis should be suspected in any patient with abdominal pain and persistent vomiting. Contrast ingestion with follow-up filming 30 minutes later will almost always confirm the diagnosis. A 30-minute film should be obtained even though patients usually vomit the contrast. They invariably retain enough to permit the diagnosis to be made. After the contrast has been introduced into the stomach, positioning the patient with the right side down is essential to prevent the contrast from pooling in the gastric fundus, as it does if the patient is supine (Fig 5–32).

Internal hernias constitute a complex problem that generally will not be readily recognized in the first patient encounter.

Hernias may occur through defects in the mesentery, omentum, broad ligaments, into the lesser sac through the foramen of Winslow; or they may be retroperitoneal, in the paraduodenal, pericecal, or intrasigmoid area.

Clinically, internal hernias generally present with chronic or recurring abdominal pain. Barium work-up is required for diagnosis.

Pyloric stenosis (Fig 5–33) is usually suspected clinically in infants with projectile vomiting. In most patients with pyloric stenosis, the plain films will be normal because the patient has vomited. Rarely, radiographic findings of gastric outlet obstruction may be observed. Careful examination of the patient often reveals a small palpable mass in the region of the pylorus. Oral barium study is useful for further evaluation when the diagnosis is suspected. In some cases, the "olive" (hypertrophic pyloric valve) may be demonstrated by real-time ultrasonography.

Free Air in the Peritoneum— Intestinal Perforation

Intestinal perforation in a large percentage of patients involves the stomach, proximal duodenum, or large bowel. All normally contain large amounts of gas. For this reason, perforation of any of these structures allows large amounts of gas to enter the peritoneal cavity. The gas is readily detectable beneath the right hemidiaphragm on an upright film, or between the liver and the peritoneum on a left lateral decubitus abdominal film.

In the upright position, free air in the peritoneal cavity will invariably be seen under the right hemidia-

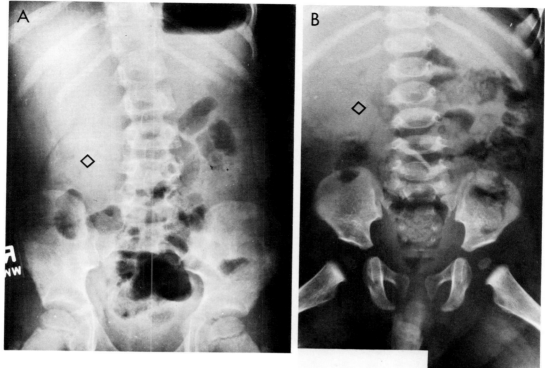

FIG 5–30.
Ileocolic intussusception. **A,** supine film. Note a vague soft tissue mass between the liver edge and the right sacroiliac joint *(diamond)*. **B,** supine film, different patient. Again, there is a poorly defined soft tissue mass in the right abdomen *(diamond)*.

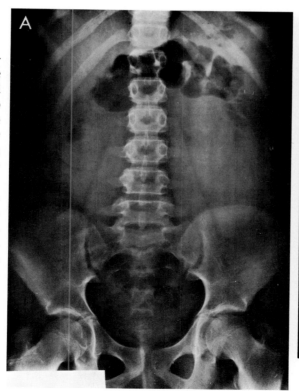 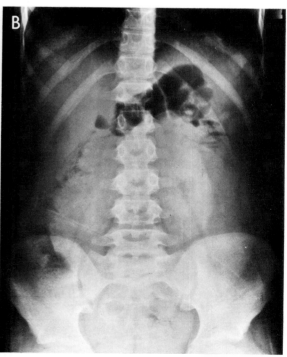

FIG 5–31.
Proximal small-intestinal obstruction. A 12-year-old female with severe acute abdominal pain. **A,** supine film. There is no small-bowel gas and very little stomach gas. A large, vaguely outlined central abdominal mass is present. **B,** upright film. Very little change from supine film. There are no small-bowel air-fluid levels. On the basis of clinical findings, the patient was operated on and found to have jejunal ileal intussusception. The vaguely defined abdominal mass is fluid-filled small bowel. This is an example of strangulation obstruction with fluid but no gas in the small bowel.

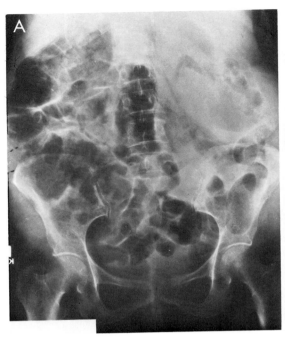

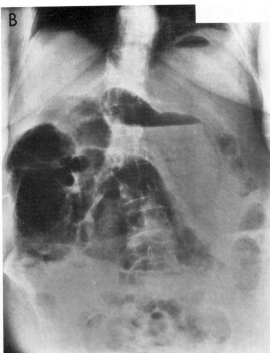

FIG 5–32.
Fluid-filled stomach simulating a left upper quadrant mass. **A,** supine film. Mass in left upper quadrant with superimposed bowel gas. **B,** upright film. The mass remains. Note the air-fluid levels in the gastric antrum indicating that the mass is fluid-filled stomach. There is considerable gas in the bowel as well. The patient was operated on and found to have a partial jejunal obstruction from adhesions. This is an example of high small intestinal obstruction in which the patient has not vomited.

FIG 5–33.
Two patients with pyloric stenosis. **A,** supine film. There is a large amount of gas overdistending the stomach. Bowel beyond the stomach is almost devoid of gas. **B,** different patient, upright film. There is a large amount of fluid overdistending the stomach. There is an air-fluid level and a small amount of gas scattered through the colon.

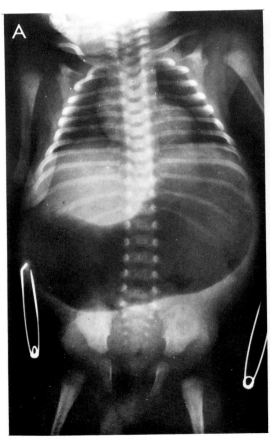

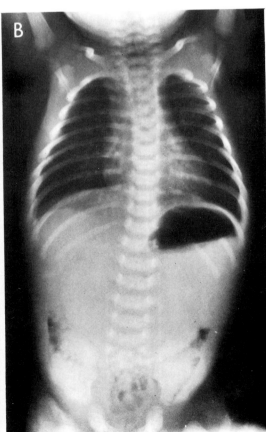

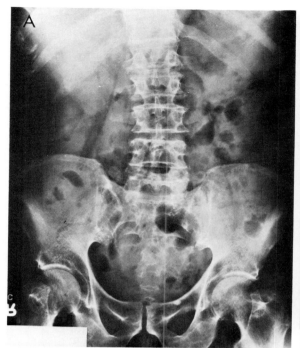

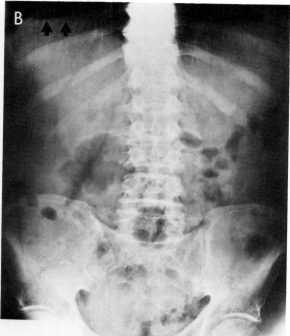

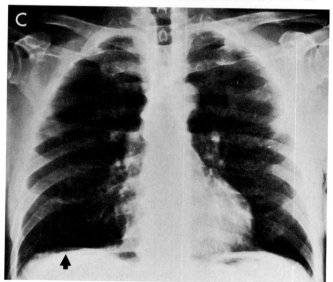

FIG 5–34.
Free air in the peritoneum. The patient presented with excruciating epigastric pain. Electrocardiogram and serum amylase levels were normal. **A,** supine film. There is minimum intraluminal small-bowel gas in the central abdomen. **B,** upright abdominal film. Note a small amount of free air beneath the right hemidiaphragm *(arrows)*. It is quite difficult to see because of exposure factors and position of the diaphragm. **C,** upright chest film. The free air is more readily visible *(arrow)*. Free air is generally more easily seen on upright chest film.

phragm, but may or may not be seen under the left hemidiaphragm because the gas has free access to the right hemidiaphragm through the right gutter. There is limited access of air to the left hemidiaphragm in some patients because of the phrenicocolic ligament in the left upper quadrant. This ligament interferes with free flow through the left gutter to the left hemidiaphragm.

A lesser sac abscess from intestinal perforation is virtually the only situation in which an air-fluid level beneath the left hemidiaphragm may be anticipated without accompanying free air on the right. This situation occurs from perforation of the posterior wall of the stomach. When it may be clinically necessary to determine whether the air-fluid level on the left represents a lesser sac abscess or normal air in the stomach, a water-soluble contrast swallow will make the distinction. If the fluid is in the stomach, the contrast will mix with it immediately. If the air-fluid level is in a lesser sac abscess, the contrast will mix with it slowly. Fluoroscopy or upright abdominal films, including a standing lateral view, made immediately after the ingestion should make the difference readily apparent.

A large amount of free air is most often due to a perforated duodenal ulcer or a perforated colon carcinoma. A perforated appendix usually does not produce a large amount of intraperitoneal gas. Benign pneumatosis intestinalis may produce pneumoperitoneum. Perforation of a colon diverticulum usually leads to a localized abscess rather than pneumoperitoneum. Perforation of the rectum may produce free intraperitoneal gas or retroperitoneal gas. Gas lateral to the rectum suggests extraperitoneal perforation of the rectum or a low colon diverticulum. Intraperitoneal or retroperitoneal gas is generally readily recognizable on abdominal computed tomography.

The small intestine is normally almost devoid of gas; therefore, perforation beyond the level of the duodenum would be expected to produce only minimal intraperitoneal air. It has been shown that an amount of intraperitoneal air as small as 2 cc can be identified if the patient is maintained in an upright position for 20 minutes prior to filming. However, this is rarely feasible because patients with intestinal perforation are often quite ill. An alternative procedure is to send the patient to the x-ray department lying left side down on the cart. The time prior to filming can therefore be effectively used. With the patient in this position, the air will accumulate over the surface of the liver, between it and the peritoneum of the right abdominal wall. When an upright or lateral decubitus film is obtained, small amounts of air will be detectable.

Supine films alone are not adequate to diagnose free air. On supine views, free air in the peritoneal cavity may be difficult or impossible to recognize, even in large amounts. A series of eight normal patients each had 1,000 cc of free air introduced into the peritoneal cavity by pelvic pneumography. In only three patients could the air be identified with certainty on supine abdominal films.

Normally, one sees only the inside of any bowel loop delineated by air. In the presence of large amounts of free air in the peritoneal cavity, both sides of the bowel wall may be visualized (Rigler's sign). Examples are shown in Figures 5–34 to 5–37. Occasionally, free air may be identified along the liver edge or in other locations in the abdomen on a supine film, but diagnosis may be uncertain because omental fat may simulate free air. In rare cases, free intraperitoneal gas may be detected with the patient supine because of gas trapped in pockets that do not conform to contours of bowel, or by delineating the peritoneal ligamentous attachments to the anterior abdominal wall, such as the falciform ligament of the liver, the urachus, and the remnants of the omphalomesenteric vessels. The latter extend superiorly in the form of an inverted "V" to the umbilicus. A tilted or cross-table lateral view may show air anterior to the liver above the falciform ligament.

Summary

1. Perforated small bowel usually produces little or no free air.

2. Large amounts of free peritoneal air may be difficult or impossible to recognize on supine abdominal films.

3. Upright films can be obtained in most patients by using compression binders.

4. Free air, if in large amounts, can always be identified in the upright position beneath the right hemidiaphragm.

5. An isolated air-fluid level beneath the left hemidiaphragm may be seen with perforation of the posterior wall of the stomach.

6. Free air in the peritoneal cavity and/or the retroperitoneal space are generally readily visible on abdominal computed tomography.

Interposition

Interposition of the colon between the liver and the right hemidiaphragm (Fig 5–38) is a normal variant (Chilaiditi's syndrome). Patients are invariably asymptomatic. Interposition should not therefore be confused with conditions it may simulate, such as ret-

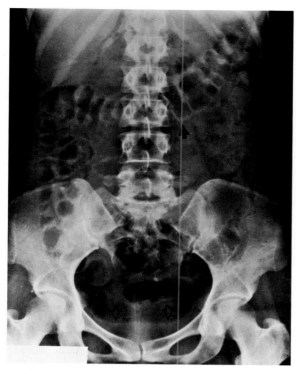

FIG 5–35.
Free air in peritoneal cavity. Note that air outlines pelvic recesses *(open arrows)*, providing a good demonstration of their anatomy. Blood accumulating in the pelvic recesses is the basis for the "dog ear" sign. In this patient, the *open arrows* are in the middle of the dog's ears, which are of gas density rather than fluid density here. *Closed arrows* indicate free air, which sharply defines the outer wall of the colon.

FIG 5–36 (bottom left).
Free air in peritoneal cavity. The air forms a sharp interface with the margins of the urinary bladder, making it appear unusually dense. Also, air sharply defines inner and outer walls of the cecum and greater curvature of stomach.

FIG 5–37 (bottom right).
Intestinal perforation. Note air on both sides of bowel wall *(arrow)*.

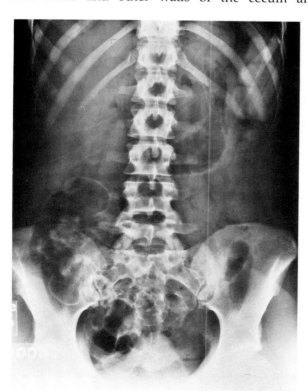

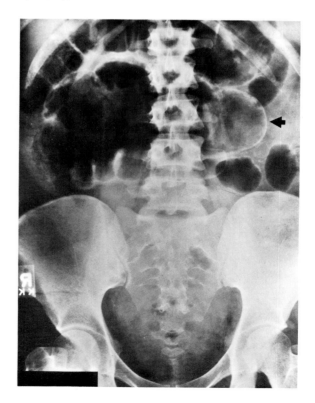

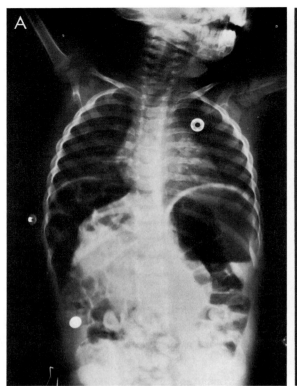 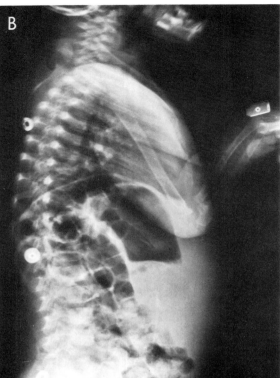

FIG 5–38.

Interposition of the colon between the liver and right hemidiaphragm. A 2-year-old male was brought to the emergency department because mother said she thought he had swallowed a foreign body. The child was extremely frightened and cried continuously through the x-ray procedure. **A,** upright AP film. There is a large amount of swallowed gas in bowel. The stomach is distended with gas and contains fluid.

There is a large amount of gas beneath the right hemidiaphragm. **B,** upright lateral film. Bowel gas extends superiorly behind the liver to interpose between the liver and the right hemidiaphragm. A vague density on the lateral view suggests a low-density ingested foreign body obscured by gastric fluid. Note the gown snaps and safety pin on the films. These represent poor x-ray technique. All surface opaque material should be removed from the patient before filming.

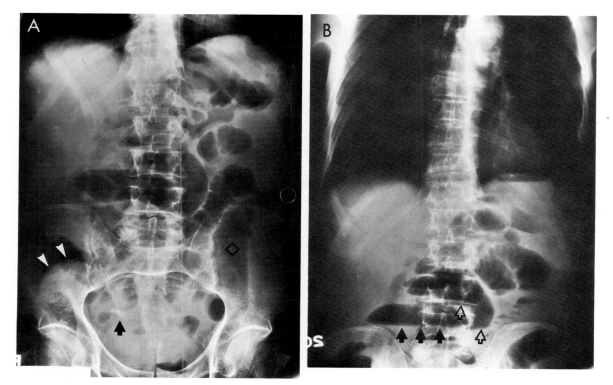

FIG 5–39.
Coprolith, appendiceal abscess. **A,** supine abdominal film. There is an oval calcification projected along the right margin of the sacrum *(black arrow).* Also note multiple bent fingers in the central abdomen. Gas in the descending colon in the left lower abdomen *(diamond)* has a typical sausage-like configuration. A soft tissue mass projects into the cecal gas in the right lower quadrant *(white arrows).* **B,** upright abdominal film. Note gas in multiple loops of small bowel in the central abdomen. The air-fluid level beneath the left hemidiaphragm is due to gas and fluid in the stomach. The loop projected over the lower lumbar spine *(open arrows)* shows fluid at two different levels in the same loop (dynamic loop), indicating mechanical obstruction *(open arrows).* Lower and to the right, a flat fluid level extends across a loop of bowel *(closed arrows).* This is the tortoise shell sign indicative of substantial intraluminal fluid accumulation. The presence of one dynamic loop strongly suggests mechanical obstruction. At surgery, the patient was found to have a large appendiceal abscess secondary to perforated gangrenous appendicitis, with associated small intestinal obstruction secondary to the appendiceal abscess.

FIG 5–40 (right).
Coprolith *(arrow),* appendiceal abscess. Supine film. A soft tissue mass is suggested by absence of gas in the area.

FIG 5–41 (below).
Retroperitoneal perforation of appendix. **A,** upright abdominal film. Note numerous tiny gas bubbles projected to the right of the spine. These represent gas within the right retroperitoneal tissues, dissecting superiorly to the right hemidiaphragm. Also note mild scoliosis and absence of right psoas shadow. **B,** upright chest film shows extraperitoneal gas beneath right hemidiaphragm *(arrows).* The appearance differs from free air, which is in a single space while extraperitoneal gas is dispersed through interstices of retroperitoneal fat. Differentiation from interposition of the colon (see Fig 5–38) should not be a problem. Patients with retroperitoneal perforation of the appendix are clinically ill; patients with interposition are not.

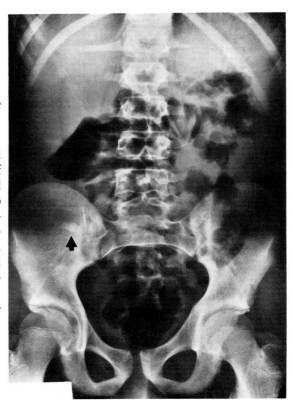

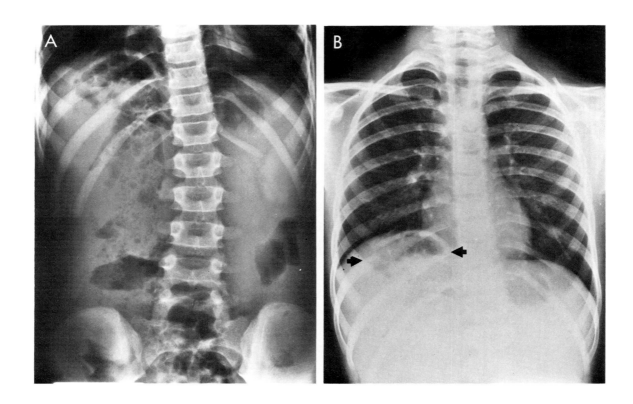

roperitoneal air or subphrenic air. Interposition is more common at the extremes of age. It may be recurrent, but patients are rarely aware of any change in symptoms, whether interposition is present or not. It occurs in patients with a lax attachment of the liver. The interposed bowel may intervene between the dome of the liver and the diaphragm, either anteriorly or posteriorly.

Appendicitis, Coproliths, Appendiceal Abscess, Perforation

Acute appendicitis is one of the most frequent diseases seen in the emergency department. It should be recognized that most patients with acute appendicitis have completely normal plain films when they first present. For this reason, appendicitis may be one of the most difficult diagnoses to make with certainty. Abdominal films early in the disease may be negative, but a "sentinel loop" may be identified with substantial frequency as an indication that some acute process is present. In patients in whom the first encounter is delayed, the condition may have progressed to a full-blown adynamic ileus.

In some patients, a soft tissue mass representing an appendiceal abscess may be present (Fig 5–39,A). Obliteration of the flank stripe or some extra-alimentary gas within the appendiceal abscess may be identified.

Rarely, the appendix may perforate intraperitoneally, releasing free air into the cavity, or may perforate retroperitoneally, producing retroperitoneal dissection of gas. Free air is most readily detected in the upright or left lateral decubitus abdominal film. Retroperitoneal perforation with retroperitoneal dissection of gas has a characteristic appearance. Plain film findings include multiple small gas bubbles extending from the right midabdomen superiorly to the diaphragm, obliteration of the right psoas shadow, and lumbar scoliosis. The radiographic findings in retroperitoneal perforation of the appendix are essentially identical to those found in traumatic retroperitoneal rupture of the duodenum.

At times, gas may be identified within the appendiceal lumen. At one time, the presence of gas was considered a sign of gangrenous appendicitis, but subsequent studies indicate that it is usually a normal finding. Gas appears with greater frequency in an uninflamed retrocecal appendix because its anatomical position facilitates the entrance of gas in the erect position.

Barium enema has been advocated by some as an effective means of diagnosing doubtful cases. If the appendix fills with barium on retrograde barium enema, acute appendicitis is virtually excluded, but if the appendix does not fill, which is the case in a substantial number of normal patients, the diagnosis remains in doubt. Barium enema to diagnose acute appendicitis is performed with some risk because the increased intraluminal pressure in the colon could perforate the devitalized appendix.

An inspissated, calcified mass impacted in the lumen of the appendix is called an appendiceal coprolith, appendicolith, or calcified fecolith. Appendiceal coproliths may be round or oval and frequently show concentric lamination with a lucent center, but usually they conform to the appendiceal lumen. Coproliths occur in 25% of resected appendices, but only 10% contain sufficient calcium to be radiographically visible.

Appendiceal gangrene and perforation are reported more frequently in the presence of a coprolith. Possibly, the coprolith renders the inflamed appendix more susceptible to these complications. When a coprolith is identified on plain films of the abdomen in a patient who presents with acute abdominal findings, there is a high correlation (90%) with acute appendicitis; 50% will be gangrenous or perforated. A coprolith is an "Aunt Minnie" that can generally be readily recognized (Figs 5–39,A and 5–40). In some patients, it may be necessary to rule out urinary tract calculus. Calcified mesenteric lymph nodes can usually be distinguished radiographically from coproliths because they are dense with irregular margins, do not show concentric laminations, and are not ring shaped. Ureteral calculi have a wide variety of shapes, but they are usually round or oval. They may have concentric laminations but rarely have lucent centers. Phleboliths have a round or oval shape, usually with a lucent center. They are round principally in the perirectal venous plexus. They are usually multiple and generally occur below the level of the ischial spines. A single right-sided phlebolith could mimic an appendiceal coprolith.

After perforation, coproliths may lodge elsewhere in the peritoneal cavity and may be associated with an abscess (Figs 5–39 to 5–41).

Summary

Abdominal films are usually negative in patients with acute appendicitis. Specific signs of right lower quadrant inflammation can sometimes be identified. In the acute abdomen, the presence of a coprolith has a high association with gangrenous appendicitis.

Acute Pancreatitis and Cholecystitis

Acute pancreatitis and cholecystitis occur relatively frequently and, in the acute phase, the clinical find-

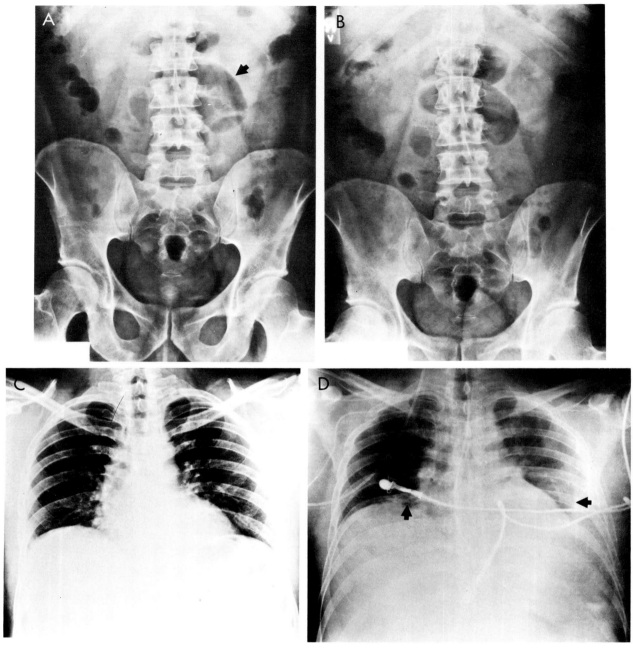

FIG 5–42.
Acute pancreatitis. **A,** supine film. Note sentinel loop, upper central abdomen *(arrow).* **B,** upright film. Sentinel loop is unchanged. There is no air-fluid level. **C,**

upright chest film is normal. **D,** portable chest film the following morning. Note high position of both leaves of the diaphragm. There is left pleural fluid *(arrow)* and right basilar atelectasis *(arrow).*

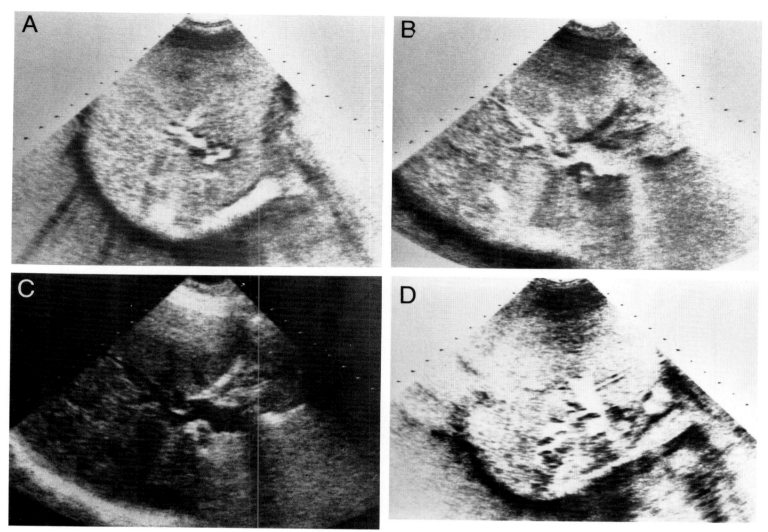

FIG 5–43.
Typical sonographic appearance of dilated intrahepatic bile ducts. Ultrasound is preferable to CT and nuclear studies for evaluation of biliary duct size. **A** and **B,** light background format. **C,** dark background format, same image as **B. D,** different patient, same diagnosis.

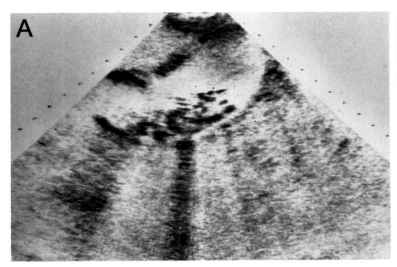

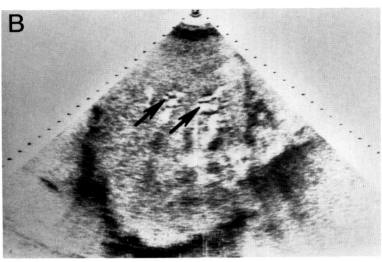

FIG 5–44.
A 68-year-old female with acute cholecystitis. **A,** sonogram images of the gallbladder show multiple shadowing densities which represent stones. **B,** sonogram of the liver shows dilated tubular structures in the portal region consistent with dilated bile ducts and implies the presence of an obstructing stone in the common duct.

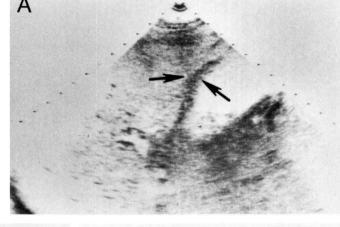

FIG 5–45.
Acute cholecystitis with cystic duct obstruction in an 88-year-old man. The sonogram (**A**) shows thickening of the gallbladder wall as a dark echogenic stripe (*arrows*). Low level echogenicity is present in the dependent portion of the gallbladder. The nuclear scan (hepatobiliary study, [**B**] early, [**C**] late) fails to visualize the gallbladder, but rather demonstrates normal visualization of the liver, common bile duct, and proximal small bowel including duodenum. This combination of imaging findings may be present in acalculus cholecystitis or in acute cholecystitis with obstruction of the cystic duct.

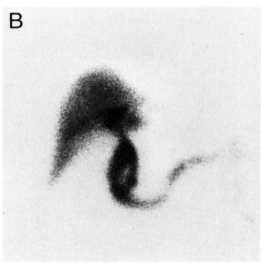

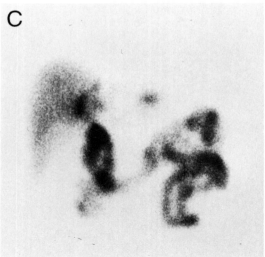

ings are dramatic.

The plain film findings may be normal, especially early in the disease. The sentinel loop, although not specific, may be a useful clue (Fig 5–42, A and B).

The effects of acute pancreatitis on adjacent structures may be extensive. These include lesser sac peritonitis and fluid, exudate over the dome of the liver and down the right gutter, gastrointestinal bleeding, left and right pleural effusion, pneumonia, and atelectasis (Fig 5–42, D). Lesser sac abscess in acute pancreatitis is characterized by elevation of the left hemidiaphragm, left pleural effusion, and a lesser sac fluid collection. Computed tomography and ultrasound are both useful for evaluation of possible acute pancreatitis.

The ileus may have a specific pattern characterized by a cutoff sign (ileus to the splenic flexure due to extension of pancreatic inflammatory process into the mesentery).

Acute cholecystitis may be characterized by calculi, sentinel loop, enlarged gallbladder, focal ileus, and, rarely, gas accumulation in the gallbladder (emphysematous cholecystitis).

Plain roentgenograms will often be nonspecific in the differential diagnosis of pancreatitis versus cholecystitis. Emergency ultrasound may be useful and confirmatory. An enlarged edematous pancreas has a characteristic ultrasound appearance. Pseudocysts are often discovered in pancreatitis patients with acute, severe pain. Dilated biliary ducts are easily recognized (Figs 5–43 and 5–44). A normal ultrasound of the gallbladder may be reassuring, but acalculous cholecystitis may be missed and, therefore, we prefer the hepatobiliary scan, which may be useful in differentiating acute cholecystitis from acute pancreatitis (Figs 5–42 and 5–45). Obstruction of the cystic duct is a feature of acute cholecystitis. Therefore, nondelineation of the gallbladder after an appropriate interval favors acute cholecystitis. Accumulation of the hepatobiliary agent in the gallbladder rules against acute cholecystitis.

If gas-producing organisms infect the edematous, distended gallbladder, both gas and pus may develop. Ulceration and necrosis of the mucosa allows gas to enter the submucosa and possibly the gallbladder as well.

Pelvic Inflammatory Disease, Pelvic Mass, and Ectopic Pregnancy

Abdominal films in pelvic inflammatory disease, like acute appendicitis, may be negative. Localized adynamic ileus (the nonspecific abdomen) is often present. A mass may be appreciated on plain films by indentation of the bladder or displacement of bowel loops. A fluid-filled sigmoid colon may simulate a pelvic mass.

An ectopic pregnancy resulting from tubal rupture may present with blood in the peritoneal cavity (lateral gutters and pelvic recesses).

Pelvic sonography is the method of choice for evaluating a pelvic mass of any type, including ectopic pregnancy (Figs 4–46 to 4–53).

The timing of ultrasonography should be correlated with the HCG (human chorionic gonadotropin) test. Refinements in radioimmunoassay of the beta subunit of human chorionic gonadotropin have enabled the diagnosis of ectopic pregnancy as early as 10 days after conception (3.5 weeks menstrual age). The serum beta-HCG is more sensitive and specific than the urine pregnancy test.

If the serum pregnancy test is negative, ectopic pregnancy can be excluded. If the serum HCG is positive, the principal role of ultrasound is to demonstrate the presence or absence of a viable intrauterine pregnancy. The presence of a well-formed gestational sac and fetal pole within the uterus virtually excludes ectopic pregnancy.

Failure to demonstrate a viable intrauterine pregnancy in a patient with positive pregnancy test does not necessarily indicate ectopic pregnancy. Other possibilities include a pregnancy of less than 5 to 6 weeks, incomplete abortion, or nonviable intrauterine pregnancy.

The demonstration of fluid in the cul-de-sac and an adnexal mass is strong evidence of ectopic pregnancy. However, an adnexal mass is not seen in a significant number of ectopic pregnancies. Therefore, if the pregnancy test is positive and the uterus is empty, ectopic pregnancy must be considered possible until proven otherwise.

A quantitative HCG is extremely helpful in this circumstance. If the serum HCG is 6,500 mIU/ml or greater, a well-defined gestational sac should be visible in the uterus. The absence of a well-defined gestational sac and serum HCG above 6,500 mIU/ml would be strong evidence against a viable intrauterine pregnancy. Ectopic pregnancy is therefore likely.

If the serum HCG is less than 6,500 mIU/ml and no well-defined gestational sac is demonstrated, the possibility of an early intrauterine pregnancy (less than 6 weeks menstrual age), incomplete abortion, or ectopic pregnancy must be considered. In these cases, it is appropriate to perform serial quantitative HCGs and follow-up ultrasound examinations. In early normal intrauterine pregnancy, the HCG will double in value every 2 days. If the serum HCG fails to rise normally and follow-up scans do not show an intrauterine

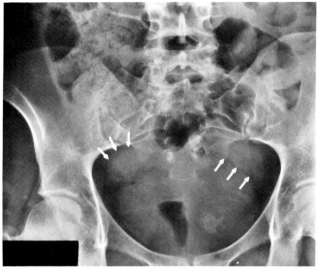

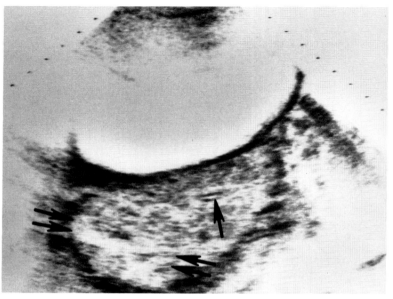

FIG 5–46 (left).
Ruptured tube from ectopic pregnancy. Supine view. Note blood in the pelvic recesses resembling dog ears *(arrows)*.

FIG 5–47 (right).
The 22-year-old female had a positive pregnancy test and complained of abdominal pain. Representative transverse sonogram shows the uterus empty (note endometrial canal *(single arrow)* and a right solid adnexal mass *(double arrows)*. Ectopic pregnancy was confirmed at surgery.

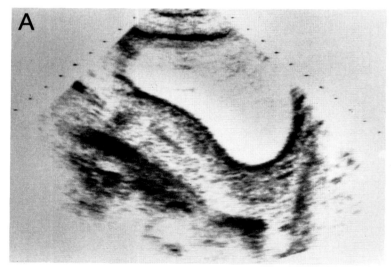

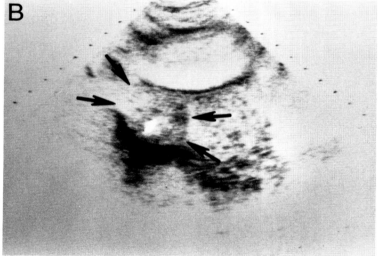

FIG 5–48.
Another example of ectopic pregnancy. **A,** the longitudinal scan shows empty uterus and prominent endometrial canal. **B,** the transverse scan shows a right adnexal mass *(arrows)*. At surgery, an unruptured cornual pregnancy was found.

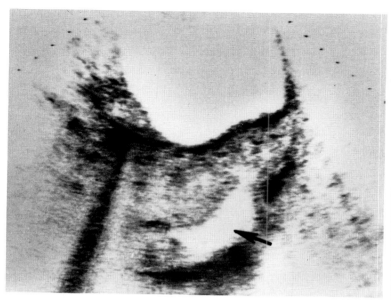

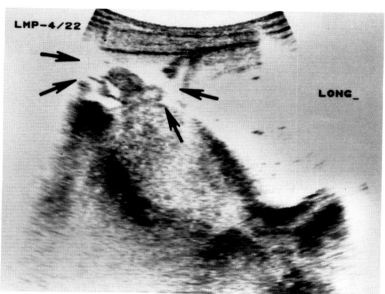

FIG 5–49 (top left).
Transverse sonogram reveals typical appearance of free fluid in the cul-de-sac *(arrow)*. Sexually active female with a negative pregnancy test. The finding is common in inflammatory conditions. Appearance is similar in ruptured ectopic pregnancy.

FIG 5–50 (top right).
The pregnant 18-year-old battered wife presented to the emergency department in a hypotensive state. Pelvic sonography showed a viable 12- to 13-week intrauterine pregnancy (not included). In addition, there was free intraperitoneal fluid (blood) cephalad to the bladder. Note echogenic bowel loops "floating" *(arrows)* in sonolucent fluid (blood) cephalad to the bladder. Ruptured spleen was diagnosed at surgery.

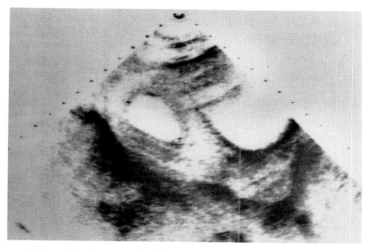

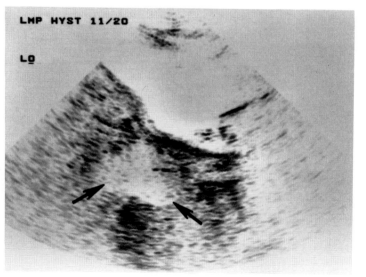

FIG 5–51 (bottom left).
Longitudinal sonogram in a 20-year-old female. Blighted ovum is the most likely diagnosis. No fetal pole or evidence of a viable pregnancy other than an empty sac in the uterus is seen. Occasionally a hydatidiform mole in the early stages may have a similar presentation.

FIG 5–52 (bottom right).
The patient presented to the emergency department 2 weeks posthysterectomy with a fever of 103°F. Longitudinal sonogram of the pelvis shows absence of the uterus. The bladder is echo-free. Posterior to the bladder a hypoechoic area seen *(arrows)* proved to be an abscess. Purulent material was aspirated from the lesion.

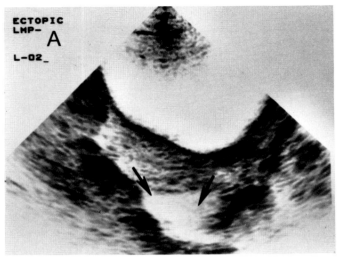
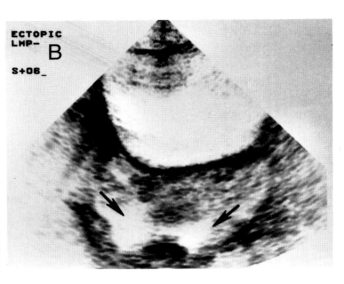

FIG 5–53.
Ectopic pregnancy. **A,** longitudinal pelvic sonogram shows free fluid posterior to the uterus consistent with blood in the cul-de-sac. **B,** transverse sonogram (*arrows* indicate the same fluid collection).

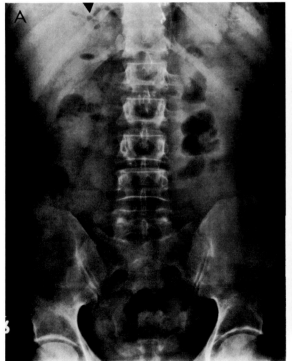
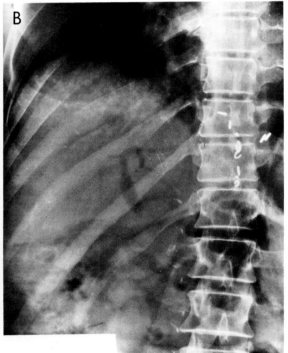

FIG 5–54.
Air in biliary tree. **A,** upright abdominal film. Note "gull wing" configuration of air in right and left hepatic ducts *(arrow).* A small air bubble at the liver margin is most likely in the duodenal bulb. **B,** supine film (enlarged) of same patient. Gas fills common and left hepatic ducts. Note the surgical clips. The gas in the biliary tree in this instance is due to prior biliary intestinal anastomosis.

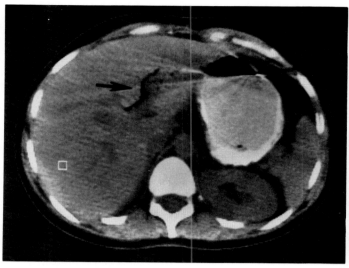

FIG 5–55 (top left).
Gas in the biliary tree, as shown in this patient, can be an ominous finding such as may be seen in gas-producing infections. This patient had undergone a prior choledochojejunostomy. The air-filled duct is seen in the left lobe of the liver as an S-shaped gaseous lucency *(arrow)*.

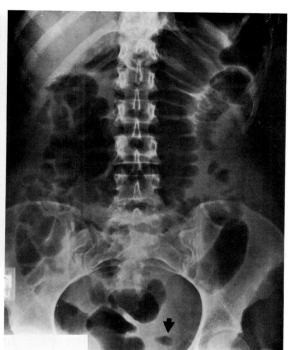

FIG 5–56 (top right).
Acute diverticulitis. Supine film. Substantial gas is scattered through the colon. There is minimal gas in multiple loops of small bowel. Superimposed on the left side of the urinary bladder is a small gas collection *(arrow)*, which is a small amount of gas in a pelvic abscess secondary to acute diverticulitis with perforation. The margins of the abscess are not seen. Diagnosis was confirmed with water-soluble contrast enema.

FIG 5–57 (bottom right).
Longitudinal midline sonogram of the pelvis in a female with diverticular disease of the colon. The uterus was removed 5 years earlier. A fluid collection is shown posterior to the bladder. This proved to be a diverticular abscess at surgery.

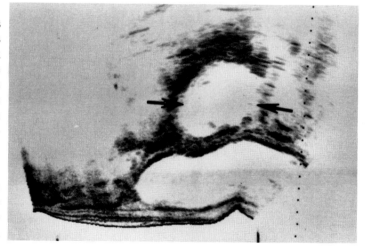

pregnancy, an endometrial curettage would be helpful in differentiating incomplete abortion and ectopic pregnancy. If HCG does increase to expected levels, follow-up scans can be performed until a normal viable intrauterine pregnancy can be demonstrated.

The combined use of ultrasound and serum HCG measurements should result in detection of most cases of ectopic pregnancies.

Gallstone Ileus

Gallstone ileus, perforation of a gallstone into the duodenum, is a relatively rare cause of intestinal obstruction. If the gallstone is sufficiently large, it may cause mechanical small-intestinal obstruction, in which case the radiographic findings are typical of mechanical obstruction. If the gallstone is of sufficient density, it may be possible to identify it on abdominal films as the cause of obstruction. The diagnostic triad for gallstone ileus consists of a large, solitary gallstone in the midabdomen, dilated loops of small bowel proximal to the stone and, possibly, air in the biliary tree.

Gallstone ileus is a disease of the elderly. An inflammatory fistula forms between the gallbladder and the duodenum. This duodenal biliary fistula may allow intestinal gas to pass into the biliary radicals in the liver. The calcific density of the stones may be small on plain film x-ray. A calcified nidus may be surrounded by a thick uncalcified coating. A gallstone that obstructs the small bowel may be much larger than it looks on plain film, if it is detectable at all.

Eighty percent of patients with gallstone ileus develop air in the gallbladder or bile ducts. In some patients (20%), spontaneous closure of the fistula after stone passage or a pre-existing cystic duct occlusion prevents air from entering the biliary tree.

Air in the biliary tree (Figs 5–54 and 5–55) is not pathognomonic of cholecystoenteric fistula due to gallstone erosion. Surgical fistulization (cholecystoenterostomy and choledochoenterostomy) is the most common cause. A less common cause is duodenal ulcer perforation.

Acute Diverticulitis

Patients with acute diverticulitis (Fig 5–56) generally present with the rather typical clinical findings of left lower quadrant pain and tenderness. Plain film diagnosis of colon perforation in acute diverticulitis is unusual, inasmuch as the perforation is generally extraperitoneal and localized. Occasionally, one will see evidence of a left lower quadrant or a left pelvic mass, gas in a pelvic abscess, or free air in the peritoneal cavity. The diagnosis is most often a clinical one and, where indicated, may be confirmed with water-soluble contrast enema. This procedure, however, involves some risk of perforation.

When retroperitoneal perforation of a sigmoid diverticular abscess occurs, it may lead to the development of a sinus tract in the skin of the abdominal wall, the flank, or the left thigh. Infection follows the fascial planes of the retroperitoneum into the subcutaneous tissues. The breakdown of overlying skin is followed by the formation of a draining sinus. Occasionally, the draining sinus first calls attention to a pre-existing diverticulitis.

An inflammatory mass surrounding a perforated sigmoid diverticulum may entrap an adjacent small-bowel loop, causing small-intestinal obstruction. Abdominal distention, crampy abdominal pain, and vomiting may ensue (Fig 5–57).

Peritonitis

Acute peritonitis produces intraperitoneal fluid. The intestinal gas pattern is that of adynamic ileus. In some circumstances, it may be difficult to distinguish peritonitis from mechanical intestinal obstruction. In fact, a combination of the two may be present because the infection causes fluid to collect in pockets and adhesions to form. The peritoneal inflammation may cause separation of gas-filled bowel loops by fluid. The inflammation may obliterate the flank stripes. For this reason, detection of fluid in the lateral gutters may be difficult or impossible. The infection readily crosses the diaphragm, and basilar pleural fluid and atelectasis may therefore be noted.

If oral contrast is clinically indicated for differentiating adynamic ileus from mechanical obstruction, water-soluble contrast is the agent of choice because of the risk of peritonitis secondary to obscure intestinal perforation.

Intra-abdominal abscess may result from bowel perforation at any level. The most common origins are appendix, colonic diverticulum, or gastric or duodenal ulcer. Any of these may perforate intra- or retroperitoneally. Intraperitoneal perforation usually results in pericecal, lateral gutter, subhepatic, subphrenic, or pelvic gutter localization. Retroperitoneal abscess may also originate from kidney, pancreas, or spine. Perforation of the posterior wall of the stomach will result in lesser sac abscess. Abscesses in any location may be quite large and may contain localized gas. Ultrasound and computed tomography are the methods of choice in the search for suspected fluid collections and abscesses (Figs 5–57 to 5–59).

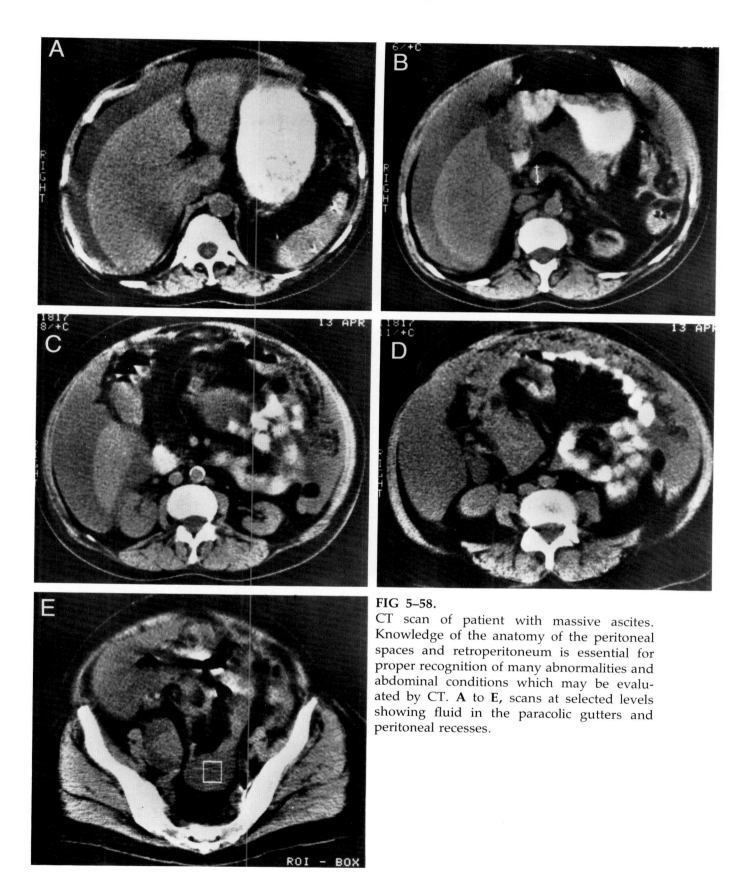

FIG 5–58.
CT scan of patient with massive ascites. Knowledge of the anatomy of the peritoneal spaces and retroperitoneum is essential for proper recognition of many abnormalities and abdominal conditions which may be evaluated by CT. **A** to **E,** scans at selected levels showing fluid in the paracolic gutters and peritoneal recesses.

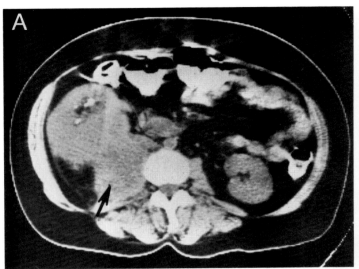

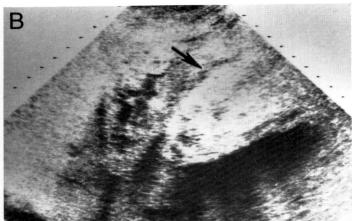

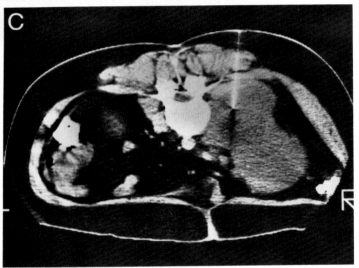

FIG 5–59.
CT and ultrasound demonstration of psoas abscess. The patient was an insulin-dependent diabetic with night sweats. **A,** CT scan shows large psoas abscess on the right *(arrow)*, displacing the right kidney anteriorly. **B,** sonogram in the longitudinal plane shows large "hypoechoic" mass lesion posterior to the kidney *(arrow)*. The lesion was aspirated with CT guidance. **C,** the needle tip is shown in the lesion with the patient in the prone position. Frank purulent material was obtained.

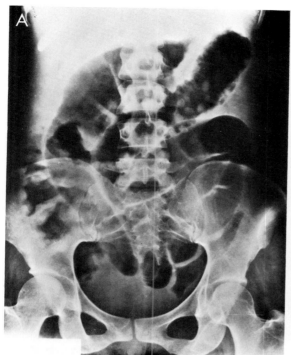 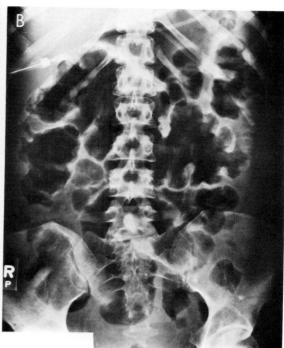

FIG 5–60.

Toxic megacolon. **A,** supine view of patient with ulcerative colitis. Note gaseous distention of colon and multiple nodular mucosal masses in transverse colon. **B,** supine film of another patient with ulcerative colitis. Note the massive distention of the colon. The mucosal nodularity is less prominent, and there is less small-bowel gas. Massive distention in toxic megacolon signifies impending perforation. Clinical findings should clearly differentiate toxic megacolon and volvulus.

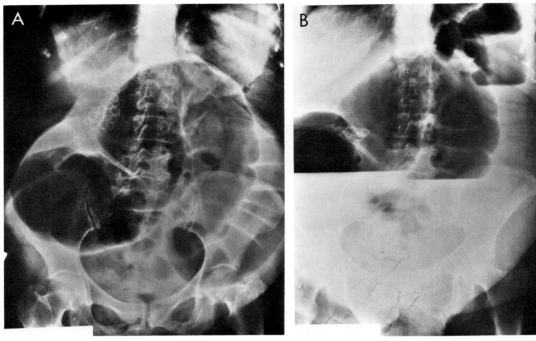

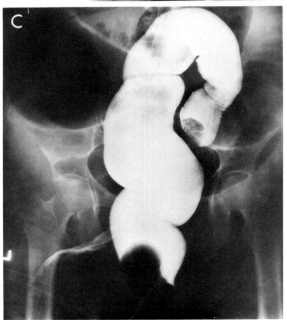

FIG 5–61.
Obstructive colon carcinoma, producing massive distention of colon simulating volvulus. **A,** supine film. Massive gaseous distention of colon. Also note the cluster of gallstones in right upper quadrant. **B,** upright film. Large amount of fluid in distended colon. Fluid levels in hepatic flexure, transverse colon, and splenic flexure. **C,** contrast enema shows obstruction of left colon.

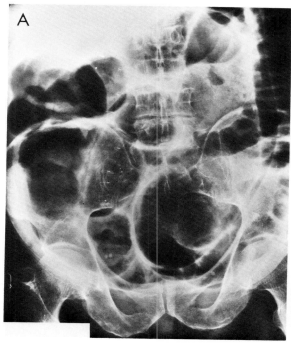

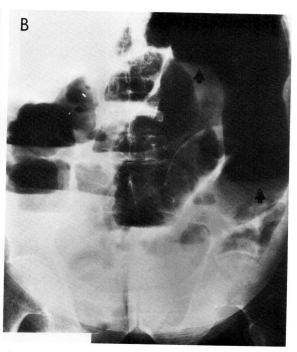

FIG 5–62.
Sigmoid volvulus. **A,** supine film. Note massive distention of virtually the entire colon. The closed loop cannot be specifically identified. **B,** upright film. Note

large amount of fluid in large and small bowel. The twisted loop can be identified in the left upper quadrant. Fluid in the loop is at two different levels (*arrows*).

FIG 5–63.
Volvulus of colon. **A,** supine film with typical horse collar configuration of sigmoid volvulus. The twisted

loop has also been called the coffee bean sign. **B,** upright film shows air-fluid levels.

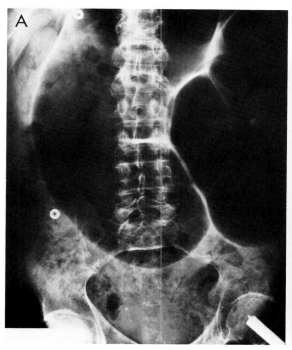

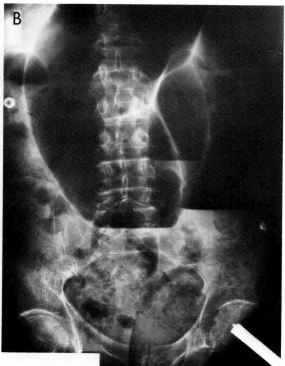

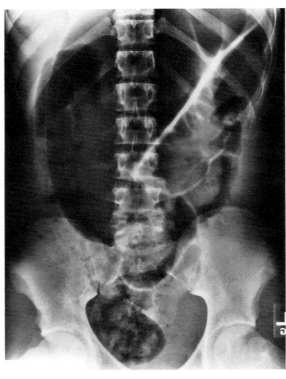

FIG 5–64.
Supine film showing typical horse collar sign of sigmoid volvulus.

FIG 5–65.
Cecal volvulus. **A,** supine film. Note oval configuration of the obstructed cecum in right abdomen and distended small bowel loops in the left central abdomen. The stomach is distended in left upper quadrant. **B,** upright film shows air-fluid levels in cecum, small intestine, and stomach. The tortoise shell configuration of the air above the fluid indicates a large amount of fluid in the loops.

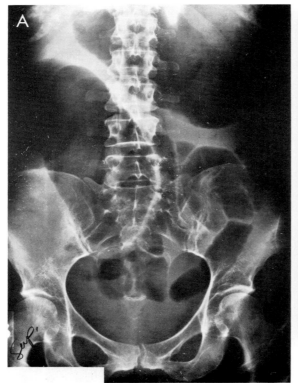

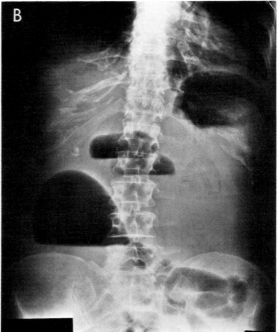

Summary of Basic Concepts for Recognizing Inflammatory Lesions

1. Radiographic findings in acute appendicitis are usually negative. Sentinel loop may be a clue.

2. A coprolith is highly reliable evidence of acute appendicitis in patients with clinically acute abdomen.

3. A sentinel loop is often present in acute pancreatitis and acute cholecystitis. Hepatobiliary scan is useful in distinguishing the two. Ultrasound may confirm gallstones, dilated bile ducts, enlargement of the pancreas, and pseudocysts.

4. Patients with gallstone ileus may have air in the biliary tree; however, air is most often due to prior biliary intestinal anastomosis.

5. Acute diverticulitis usually presents with typical clinical signs.

6. Ultrasound and computed tomography are the methods of choice for diagnosing intra-abdominal fluid and abscesses.

7. Pelvic inflammatory disease, pelvic masses, and ectopic pregnancy are best evaluated with pelvic sonography.

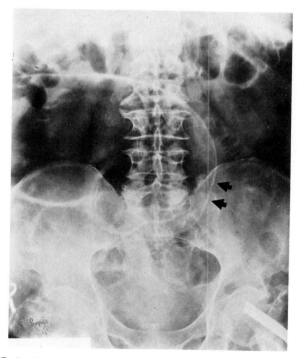

FIG 5–66.
Cecal volvulus. Colon perforation from strangulation. Supine film. Note that bowel wall *(arrows)* is clearly delineated, indicating free air in the peritoneal cavity, outlining the massively dilated cecum.

Volvulus

Volvulus of the colon is generally associated with an unusually long mesentery. The redundant loop may twist 180 to 360 degrees and usually involves either the sigmoid colon or the cecum. The striking radiographic feature in each is the presence of massively distended colon.

When a patient presents with acute abdominal pain and films show a massively distended colon, one must suspect the possibility of volvulus. Massively distended colon may be incident to other things, but none is particularly common or especially difficult to distinguish.

Acute mesenteric thrombosis may, in rare instances, present plain film findings similar to those of volvulus. A contrast enema will readily make the distinction. On introduction of contrast, the colon is obstructed in patients with volvulus but not in those with mesenteric thrombosis.

Substantial gaseous distention of the colon may occasionally be seen in patients with toxic megacolon (Fig 5–60), but clinical features and visible mucosal ulcerations in the colon will usually make the diagnosis.

Low colon obstruction from carcinoma (Fig 5–61) may, in some instances, produce a massively distended colon. The distinction can be made after a water-soluble contrast enema because the obstruction incident to volvulus is often characterized by a "bird's beak" configuration, whereas obstruction from colon carcinoma is more typically characterized by an "apple core" configuration.

Volvulus most frequently involves the cecum or sigmoid portion of the colon. Less frequently, it may involve the transverse colon, stomach, or small intestine. For the first-encounter physician, determining the type of volvulus is not of high priority. Typically, sigmoid volvulus (Fig 5–62) forms an inverted U (Figs 5–63 and 5–64), cecal volvulus an oval loop (Figs 5–65 and 5–66). Either loop may be found anywhere in the abdomen.

Summary

1. Volvulus is characterized by massive distention of the colon.

2. It is generally easy to distinguish from other causes of massive distention.

3. Diagnosis is urgent because strangulation will lead to perforation.

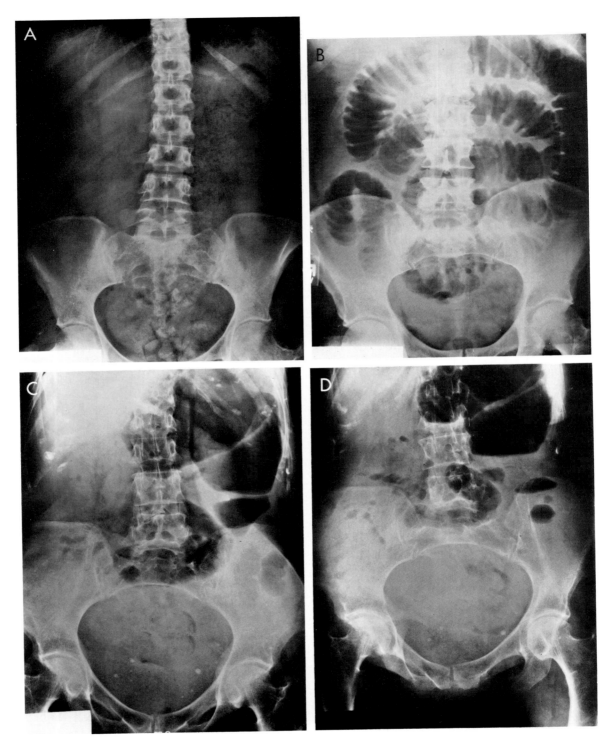

FIG 5–67.
Three patients with acute mesenteric ischemia. **A,** the gasless abdomen. **B,** classic x-ray picture of mechanical small-intestinal obstruction. **C,** atypical presentation. Gas and fluid in small intestine; isolated distention of splenic flexure with gas and fluid. **D,** same patient as **C,** upright film. Note air-fluid levels in loop in left upper quadrant and small-bowel air-fluid levels. X-ray findings are indistinguishable from volvulus. An angiogram may be indicated for diagnosis, depending on clinical findings.

Mesenteric Ischemia

The diagnosis of mesenteric ischemia is always difficult. Clinically, this entity may be characterized by sudden onset of severe pain or by an insidious onset of moderate pain. Most patients present with an acute abdomen or with GI bleeding. Twenty percent vomit blood. Blood in the stool or diarrhea is frequent.

There are various forms of mesenteric ischemia, including arterial thrombosis or embolism, venous thrombosis, and nonocclusive mesenteric ischemia. Ischemic colitis may result when any of these entities interferes with the colonic vascular supply. Infarction of small or large bowel may occur, depending on the degree of severity. Nonocclusive mesenteric ischemia is most often seen in older patients and is associated with digitalis use. Atherosclerotic disease of the mesenteric circulation may present as abdominal angina. Not all cases of mesenteric ischemic disease represent mesenteric vascular catastrophe. The conditions interfering with blood supply run an entire spectrum. Likewise, the gas pattern may run the spectrum from normal through sentinel loop, full-blown paralytic ileus, or full-blown mechanical obstruction. The classic radiologic picture is that of mechanical small-intestinal obstruction with gaseous distention of the colon to the splenic flexure. Fluid and gas may collect rapidly in the devitalized small bowel. Clinically, there is usually early hyperperistalsis with later secondary ileus.

In many instances, only minimal fluid may accumulate early in the small-bowel loops. For this reason, the plain film findings may make it impossible to distinguish mesenteric ischemia from adynamic ileus secondary to acute gallbladder, pancreatitis, appendicitis, etc.

Contrast enema with water-soluble contrast medium is useful in ruling out a colon obstruction when distention of small and large bowel occurs. Water-soluble contrast may be given by mouth to differentiate mechanical obstruction and ileus. Barium should not be used because of the possibility of bowel perforation.

The gasless abdomen has been described in the radiologic literature on mesenteric thrombosis. Bowel ischemia, particularly with venous mesenteric occlusion, may produce huge quantities of intraluminal fluid in the small intestine. This process gives rise to the gasless abdomen, a suggestive but not pathognomic sign of ischemia. Absence of bowel gas may also be the result of vomiting, high small-intestinal obstruction, or strangulation obstruction, or it may be normal. Clinical correlation is essential in evaluating the gasless abdomen.

Specific plain film findings occasionally seen are edema of the bowel wall with increased thickness and change in contour. Edema or intraperitoneal fluid may cause thickening of the bowel wall and, consequently, separation of bowel loops. If the separation of loops is localized, suspect thickened bowel wall. Bowel-wall thickening is more typical of venous thrombosis, which may produce some narrowing of the bowel lumen.

Bowel supplied by the superior mesenteric artery is most frequently involved. Inferior mesenteric arterial occlusion occurs with some frequency in patients with atherosclerosis, but collateral blood from the superior mesenteric artery will often replace the inferior mesenteric artery distribution.

Venous thrombosis is seen with congestive heart failure, producing venous stasis. Mesenteric thrombosis is more common in middle-aged and elderly patients with cardiovascular, renal, and respiratory abnormalities. Arterial occlusion may be embolic or atherosclerotic. Mesenteric angiography may be useful in the diagnosis and should be performed as soon as possible if bowel ischemia is suspected. Angiography should be performed before barium studies.

Impaired vascularity and inadequate collateral circulation ultimately cause bowel-wall necrosis. Intestinal gas enters the bowel wall and ascends through the mesenteric veins to reach the intrahepatic branches of the portal vein. Through-and-through necrosis leads to bowel-wall perforation and pneumoperitoneum. The radiographic findings of bowel-wall gas, portal vein gas, or gas entering the peritoneum indicate a grave prognosis.

Acute mesenteric ischemia may have a variety of radiographic presentations. Unless infarction is massive, plain films are likely to be negative. When less than 50% of the small bowel is infarcted, a minority of patients show evidence of distention. Distention is more characteristic of venous infarction or extensive arterial infarction. Figure 5–67,A shows the abdomen almost devoid of gas. A stomach bubble can be identified. There is fecal material mixed with a small amount of gas to the left of the spine and in the pelvic area. This appearance has been described as the "gasless" abdomen. Figure 5–67,B shows pronounced gaseous distention of multiple loops of small intestine, typical of acute mechanical small-intestinal obstruction. The colon in this patient is devoid of gas, except for a rectal bubble. Figures 5–67,C and D show localized gaseous distention of the splenic flexure associated with some small-bowel gas in the central abdomen. The upright view shows multiple small-bowel air-fluid levels.

The diagnosis of acute mesenteric ischemia could not be made from the films alone in any of these three patients. Figure 5–66,A is consistent with the normal; Figures 5–66,C and D are consistent with volvulus and mesenteric ischemia. The colon would be completely obstructed to the retrograde flow of contrast in volvulus, but would be unobstructed in ischemia.

In the healing phase of ischemic bowel disease, the affected bowel may become stenotic as a result of scarring of the bowel wall (Fig 5–68).

Summary

Nonspecific radiographic findings in mesenteric ischemia are:

1. Very little intestinal gas in the early stage of infarction. (This must be associated with clinical signs of infarction, inasmuch as a paucity of intestinal gas may be normal.)

2. Distention of the small intestine and the colon to the splenic flexure.

3. Fluid levels caused by mechanical small-intestinal obstruction.

4. Rapid increase in bowel distention.

Clinical suspicion should lead to early angiography.

The Decision Tree (The Acute Abdomen)

Minimum routine includes supine and upright abdominal and *upright* chest films.

A negative plain film examination does not rule out significant abnormality. Diagnosis depends on clinical evaluation.

Sentinel loop indicates a high probability of significant intra-abdominal pathology. Further clinical evaluation and observation are indicated.

Distended large and small bowel with no small-bowel air-fluid levels could be incident to low colon obstruction or adynamic ileus of any cause (end stage of the sentinel loop).

Multiple, dynamic, small-bowel air-fluid levels probably represent mechanical small-intestinal obstruction. Clinical evaluation is required to exclude other causes of small-intestinal fluid.

A large amount of fluid in the small bowel (tortoise shell sign) suggests strangulation. This sign is also seen in vascular impairment incident to prolonged bowel distention.

Massively distended colon is most commonly due to volvulus.

Flank Pain (Ureteral Colic)

Ureteral colic is a frequently encountered problem in most emergency departments. Clinical and urographic diagnoses are generally straightforward and uncomplicated. Plain-film diagnosis may be straightforward if a clearly visible ureteral calculus correlates with the patient's clinical findings. More often, however, plain films of the abdomen are negative or show one or more small calcific densities projected along the margin of the bladder, any one of which might be a ureteral calculus or phlebolith. If the calcification is round and has a central lucent hole or is projected below the iliac spine, it is more likely to be a phlebolith. If it is irregular in shape, it is more likely to be a ureteral calculus. Often, however, excretory urography is necessary for the differentiation. Whenever the diagnosis is in doubt, a urogram usually resolves the question.

Unilateral urographic nonfunction associated with ureteral colic suggests acute ureteral obstruction from calculus. It is suggested that delayed films at intervals of ½, 1, 2, 4, and 8 hours be obtained in this situation. Acute ureteral obstruction may cause a transient absence of contrast accumulation in the collecting system, but with delayed films the ureter can often be delineated to the level of the obstruction.

In patients in whom stone obstruction has been present over a prolonged interval, the excretory urogram shows a slightly delayed pyelogram, with delineation of a slightly dilated collecting system to the level of the ureteral obstruction. Stones usually lodge at one of three levels of the ureter: the ureteral pelvic junction, the point at which the ureter crosses the iliac vessels, or at the ureteral vesical junction. The most common stones are calcium oxalate and calcium phosphate. Uric acid calculi are less frequent. Cystine and xanthine stones are rare. Only uric acid, xanthine, and pure mucoprotein matrix calculi are radiolucent.

"Renal calculus" is a term referring to stones in the kidney which may be in different locations. "Nephrolithiasis" refers to calculi within the pyelocalyceal system. "Nephrocalcinosis" signifies numerous small stone calcifications, either medullary or cortical in location.

Nephrocalcinosis usually has a recognizable cause and often signals hypercalcemic, hypercalciuric, or hyperoxaluric states, or an underlying renal structural change (glomerular or tubular). Nephrolithiasis frequently has no underlying recognizable cause. It is usually not accompanied by nephrocalcinosis.

Perirenal inflammation is characterized by flank pain with tenderness to direct percussion of the flank.

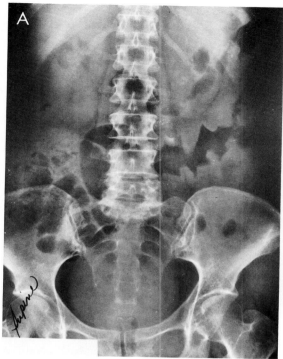

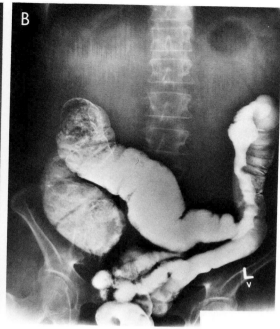

FIG 5–68.
Ischemic bowel disease of long standing, with stenosis of the distal transverse colon. The patient is a 53-year-old woman with a 20-pound weight loss over several months. She had some rectal bleeding during this period, although not marked. **A,** supine film. The "thumbprinting" configuration of the colon, due to edema of the bowel wall, is typical of chronic localized ischemic disease. **B,** contrast enema confirms the stenotic segment of the colon with thumbprinting.

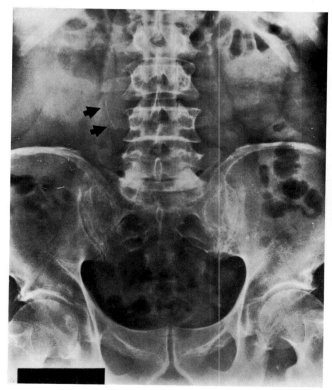

FIG 5–69.
Dissecting abdominal aortic aneurysm *(arrows)*. The patient presented with right-flank pain typical of right ureteral colic.

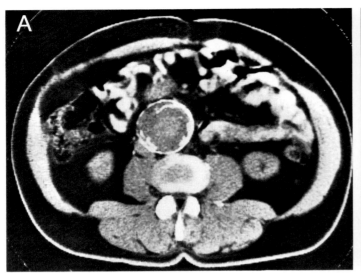

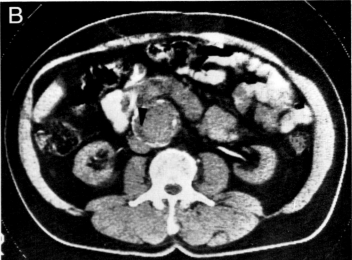

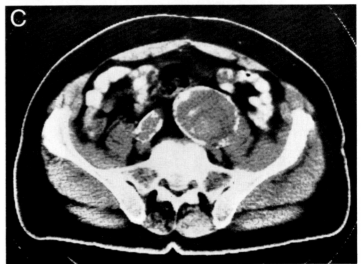

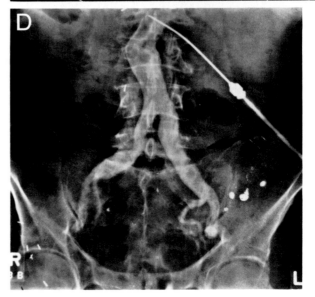

FIG 5–70.
Extensive abdominal aortic aneurysm. In this case, the aneurysm extends to above the level of the renal arteries and beyond the aortic bifurcation to the left iliac artery. This is important information for the surgeon who is faced with the prospect of cross-clamping the aorta above the renal arteries. **A** and **B,** the distal abdominal aorta is calcified. *Arrowhead* depicts interface between contrast enhanced flowing blood and lower density thrombus. At the time of presentation this patient was in renal failure with evidence of lamellar thrombus occluding the renal artery origins. **C,** shows the involvement of the left iliac artery. **D,** translumbar aortogram performed 6 years prior. This technique is contraindicated in the presence of aneurysm. The angiogram injection by whatever technique defines the lumen of the vessel, while CT or ultrasound give broader information on total caliber, including thrombus. *Arrow* depicts calcific margin of left iliac artery aneurysm.

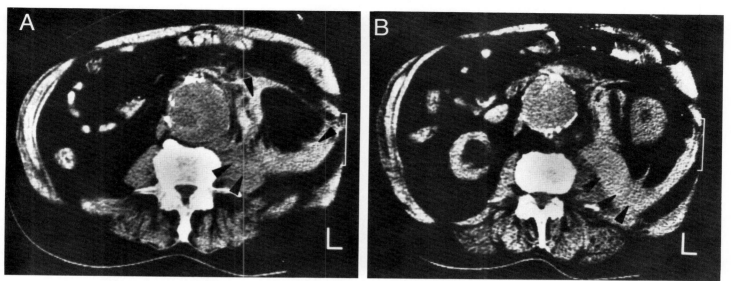

FIG 5–71.
Leaking abdominal aortic aneurysm. Note extension to the left flank and psoas region (*arrowheads*).

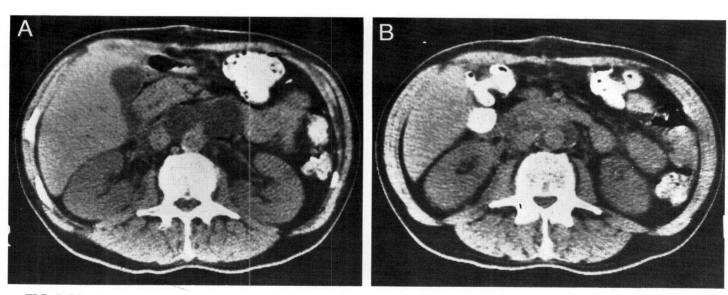

FIG 5–72.
This 59-year-old man presented to the emergency department with abdominal pain and a falling hematocrit. He had previously undergone repair of an abdominal aortic aneurysm. **A** and **B,** CT scan shows a large, relatively low-density hematoma surrounding the abdominal aorta. A bleeding site at the margin of the prior aortic repair was found at surgery. The patient survived.

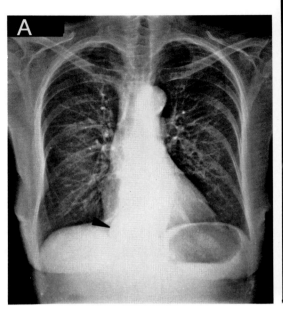

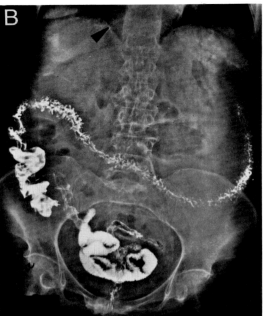

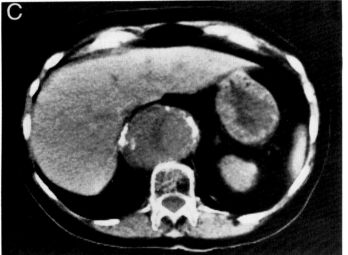

FIG 5–73.
Uncommon presentation of abdominal aortic aneurysm in a 78-year-old woman. The aneurysm extended from the esophageal hiatus to the celiac axis and is visualized on the chest radiograph (**A**) and abdomen film (**B**) obtained during a barium enema. Computed tomography scans (**C, D, E**) show the elliptical shape of the aneurysm, the eccentric mural thrombus, and the aortic lumen which is opacified by contrast injection.

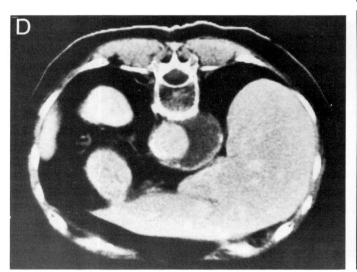

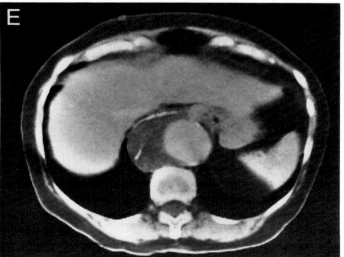

Radiographic findings consist of scoliosis with concavity toward the side of inflammation, loss of delineation of psoas margin on the affected side, and gas accumulation in the intestine from adynamic ileus. Computed tomography is useful in suspected perirenal inflammation.

Occasionally, an unusual problem is encountered in patients with renal colic. The patient in Figure 5–69 was admitted through the emergency department with a diagnosis of right ureteral colic. The film shown, obtained before intended excretory urography, shows a calcific shell projecting to the right of the spine. The patient, while on the x-ray table waiting for contrast injection, suddenly complained of excruciating abdominal pain and went into shock. He died within minutes of a ruptured dissecting abdominal aortic aneurysm.

Either ultrasound or contrast enhanced abdominal computed tomography may be useful for evaluation of suspected abdominal aorta aneurysm (Figs 5–70 to 5–74).

Figure 5–75 shows a film taken before an excretory urogram for left ureteral colic. The film is completely normal.

Intravenously injected contrast extravasated around the upper left ureter. This finding is diagnostic of ureteral rupture from stone obstruction and requires no specific treatment.

A more typical first-encounter situation in a patient presenting with ureteral colic is shown in Figure 5–76. There are two tiny opaque densities projected along the left margin of the urinary bladder, either of which could be a ureteral calculus. Excretory urography resolved the issue.

Delayed films are useful in definitely establishing that diminished function of one kidney associated with acute ureteral colic is due to stone obstruction. In Figure 5–77,B, contrast in the dilated ureter to the level of the stone is shown after 40 minutes. In Figure 5–77,C, the left ureter is very faintly opacified to the level of the stone after 1 hour. In spite of markedly compromised excretion of contrast, the diagnosis of stone obstruction is confirmed.

Testicular Torsion

Testicular torsion may present as flank or groin pain. Close examination often localizes the symptoms specifically to the scrotum. Radioisotope studies are valuable in differentiating torsion from acute epididymo-orchitis. Dynamic and static images of the scrotum will generally show evidence of decreased blood flow to the affected side relative to the normal side

(Fig 5–78) when torsion is present. Conversely, increased flow or activity may be seen in inflammatory conditions. This test can therefore be a useful aid in determining the need for immediate surgical exploration.

Summary

1. Intravenous urography is often necessary to differentiate ureteral calculi and phleboliths.

2. Unilateral flank pain associated with ipsilateral diminished or absent renal function usually indicates obstructing ureteral calculus. Uncommon causes, e.g., obstructing neoplasm, renal artery thrombosis, or dissecting aneurysm, must also be considered.

The Pregnant Patient—Radiation Exposure During Pregnancy

Whether a radiographic examination should be performed when pregnancy is known is a matter of medical judgment. Because of possible fetal injury from radiation, knowledge of specific guidelines is essential to an informed decision in any specific situation. In addition, when a plain film examination is performed prior to knowledge of pregnancy, guidelines are necessary in patient management.

If the pregnancy is past the first trimester, the fetal parts are completely formed. Therefore, there is no possibility of x-ray exposure producing a fetal anomaly. However, there are reports in the literature of a slightly higher incidence of leukemia late in life in patients who were exposed to radiation in utero during the second and third trimester of pregnancy. For this reason, limiting x-ray exposure during the second and third trimester of pregnancy is prudent.

Our policy in second- and third-trimester pregnancy is to perform radiographic examination as necessary to handle an acute medical problem in any patient. The number of exposures, however, is limited to the minimum necessary to obtain the information. Where possible, the examination is deferred.

It is possible that radiation exposure during the first trimester of pregnancy will produce fetal anomalies. How much exposure may be given to the patient and under what circumstances? The review by Brent and Goarsen is a particularly good summary of the effects of radiation exposure during pregnancy. They point out that, with age, the fetus becomes progressively less sensitive to the effects of radiation.

Every effort must be made to avoid irradiating patients early in pregnancy. This principle is the basis for the "10-day rule," which states that the abdominal

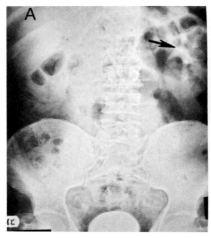

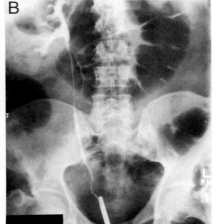

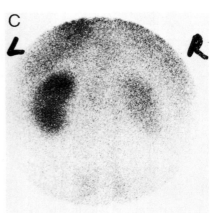

FIG 5–74.

A 52-year-old man presented to the emergency room with acute flank pain. Several imaging studies followed. **A,** excretory urogram, 15-minute film. *Arrow* points to normal finding of contrast in left-sided collecting system. There is poor nephrogram visualization on the right, with delay in calyceal visualization. There was speculation as to the presence of a nonopaque calculus. **B,** right retrograde pyelogram shows no evidence of a calculus in the normal anatomy of this collecting system. **C,** renal scan. Glucoheptonate static scan 2 minutes postintravenous injection shows poor visualization of the right kidney. The flow study also showed decreased blood flow to the right kidney. **D,** angiogram films (1-early and 2-late arterial phase) showed distortion of the right kidney and stretching of the capsular vessels *(arrowheads),* suggesting subcapsular hematoma. **E,** right renal venogram (subtraction film). The renal vein and its branches are widely patent without evidence of renal vein thrombosis. **F,** CT scan shows hyperdense right nephrogram. Subcapsular hematoma surrounds right renal parenchyma. There is also "thickening" of the tissue planes of the retroperitoneum consistent with bleeding. *Performance of the CT scan earlier in the sequence might have obviated the need for several of the correlating studies performed.*

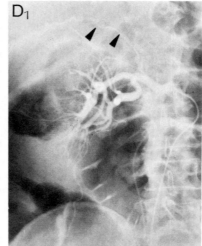

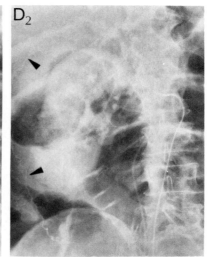

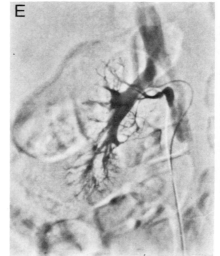

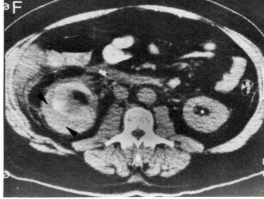

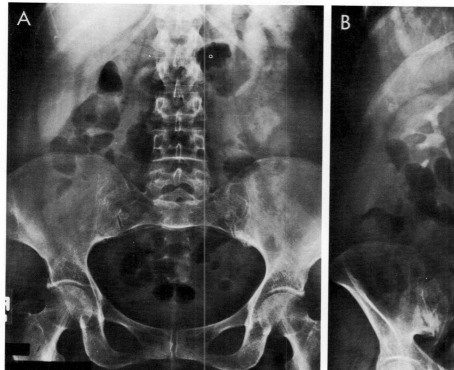

FIG 5–75.
Ureteral rupture from stone obstruction. **A,** patient with left ureteral colic. Normal film preliminary to excretory urogram.

B, same patient; normal right urogram. Note extravasation of contrast outside left ureter *(arrow)*, indicating ureteral rupture from stone obstruction. The nonopaque stone is not seen.

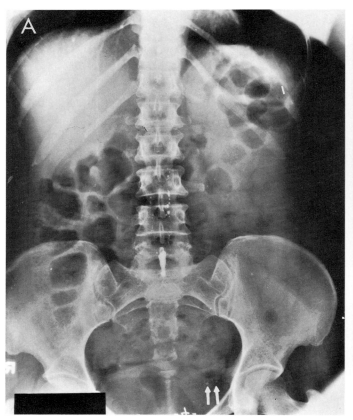

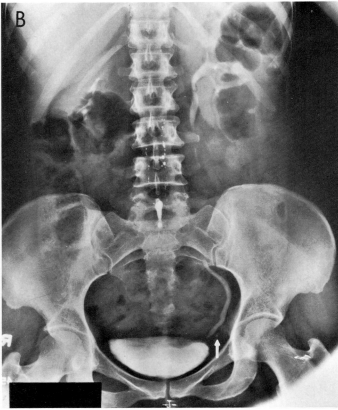

FIG 5–76.
Patient with left ureteral colic. **A,** supine film. Note retained contrast in spinal canal from prior myelogram. Two tiny concretions *(white arrows)* in the left pelvis are quite difficult to see. **B,** same patient; normal right urogram. Note partial obstruction of distal left ureter. The more medial of the two concretions precisely corresponds to the location of the distal left ureter. It is obscured by this contrast. The more lateral of the two concretions is a phlebolith outside the ureter *(arrow).*

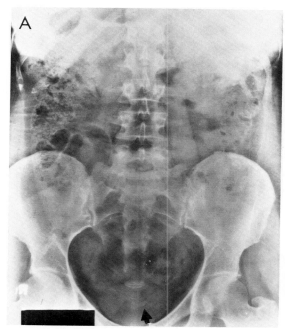

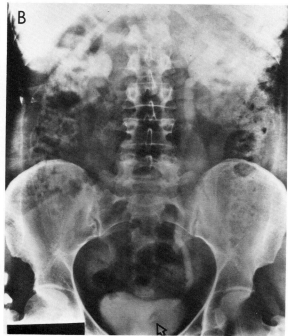

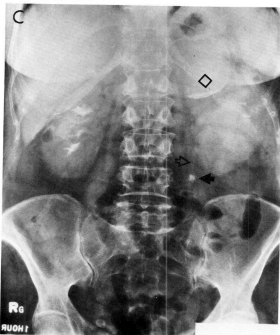

FIG 5–77.
Value of delayed films. **A,** patient with left ureteral colic. There is a large, oval, very low-density concretion projected along the left edge of the coccyx *(arrow)*. **B,** IVP of same patient. On the initial films, there was poor excretion of contrast by the right kidney. After 40 minutes, a dilated left ureter to the level of the obstructing calculus is shown *(arrow)*. Note halo around the calculus. At cystoscopy, the calculus was found to be in a ureterocele. **C,** IVP of a different patient; one-hour delayed film. Normal right urogram. Obstructing calculus in the mid-left ureter. Note very faint contrast in the ureter to the level of the obstructing stone *(open arrow)*. The patient also has a calcified pseudocyst of the pancreas *(diamond)*.

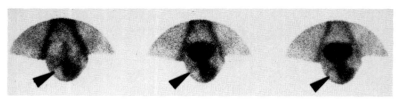

FIG 5–78.
Testicular torsion. Images of the scrotum at 2, 7 and 10 minutes post-injection of blood pool tracer. Nuclear scan shows absence of perfusion of the right testicle (*arrowhead*). The left testicle is normal. Note progressive increase in bladder activity over time.

3. Shielding the abdomen with a lead apron during these exposures further reduces fetal exposure by a factor of eight.

4. One fluoroscopic procedure—such as a barium enema or upper GI series—yields 5 rad.

These "rule-of-thumb" radiation dose estimates are high (therefore on the conservative side) for most modern x-ray equipment. The actual dose in both radiography and fluoroscopy varies greatly among institutions, depending on a variety of factors. Whenever a more precise determination of fetal exposure is necessary, the radiologic physicist should be consulted immediately.

If a review of the examination techniques (i.e., type of exam, kilovolt peak, etc.) determines that the fetal dose may have exceeded 1 rad, a more complete dosimetric evaluation should be carried out. With

area of a female of reproducing capacity should not be irradiated outside the first 10 days of her menstrual cycle. This ensures that no zygote or embryo is exposed to x-rays. If any radiographic examination of the abdominal area in such a patient is not urgent, it should be deferred. The "rule of 10" has recently been revised to the "rule of 14," allowing radiation exposure during the first 14 days of the menstrual cycle.

After several months of pregnancy, the risk of radiating an unknown embryo becomes small, because the patient is generally aware of her condition. With current rapid pregnancy testing and routine questioning of patients about possible pregnancy in most emergency departments, the pregnancy is often known (or can be determined) before x-ray examination is considered.

The door of each x-ray room in many hospitals bears a sign: "Women of childbearing age, if there is any possibility that you might be pregnant, tell the technologist before the x-rays are taken."

During the first trimester of pregnancy, under many circumstances, radiologic examination should not be conducted. However, if a pregnant patient escapes detection and is irradiated, what is the subsequent responsibility to the patient and what should be done?

The first step is to estimate the fetal radiation dose. Some simple rules of thumb are useful:

1. One film in which the maternal pelvis is included in the direct beam yields 1 rad. Such examinations include the abdomen, lumbar spine, sacrum and coccyx, pelvis and hips.

2. One film in which the maternal pelvis is not included in the direct beam—such as skull, chest, extremities—yields 0.1 rad.

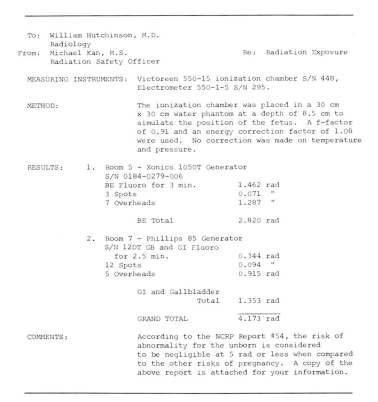

```
To:   William Hutchinson, M.D.
      Radiology
From: Michael Kan, M.S.                    Re:  Radiation Exposure
      Radiation Safety Officer

MEASURING INSTRUMENTS:  Victoreen 550-15 ionization chamber S/N 448,
                        Electrometer 550-1-5 S/N 295.

METHOD:                 The ionization chamber was placed in a 30 cm
                        x 30 cm water phantom at a depth of 8.5 cm to
                        simulate the position of the fetus. A f-factor
                        of 0.91 and an energy correction factor of 1.08
                        were used. No correction was made on temperature
                        and pressure.

RESULTS:    1.  Room 5 - Xonics 1050T Generator
                S/N 0184-0279-006
                BE Fluoro for 3 min.          1.462 rad
                3 Spots                       0.071  "
                7 Overheads                   1.287  "

                     BE Total                 2.820 rad

            2.  Room 7 - Phillips 85 Generator
                S/N 12DT GB and GI Fluoro
                    for 2.5 min.              0.344 rad
                12 Spots                      0.094  "
                5 Overheads                   0.915 rad

                GI and Gallbladder
                          Total              1.353 rad

                GRAND TOTAL                  4.173 rad

COMMENTS:               According to the NCRP Report #54, the risk of
                        abnormality for the unborn is considered
                        to be negligible at 5 rad or less when compared
                        to the other risks of pregnancy. A copy of the
                        above report is attached for your information.
```

FIG 5–79.
Typical calculation of radiation dose to fetus.

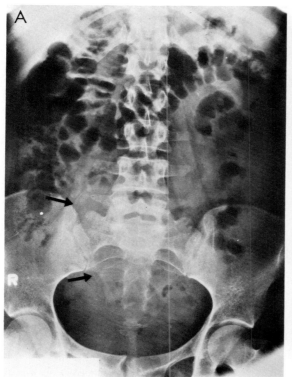
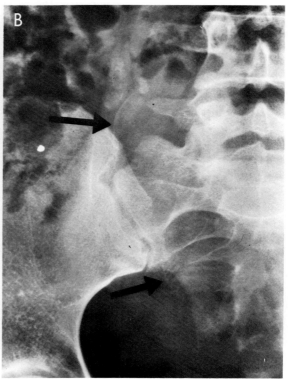

FIG 5–80.
Early pregnancy. A 22-year-old female presented in the emergency department with symptoms suggesting urinary tract infection. On questioning, the patient denied the possibility of pregnancy. An excretory urogram was requested. **A,** supine film of abdomen before urography. There is a vertical curvilinear shadow *(upper arrow)* to the right of the top of the fifth lumbar transverse process. A cluster of parallel curvilinear shadows *(lower arrow)* can be identified along the right margin of the sacrum. The upper shadow is a fetal skull; the lower shadow, fetal ribs. **B,** same patient, magnified view. This is an early pregnancy (16–18 weeks). Although the patient had denied pregnancy, the x-ray evidence is unequivocal. The excretory urogram was deferred. At term, the patient delivered a normal infant.

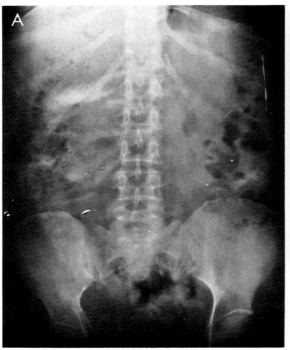

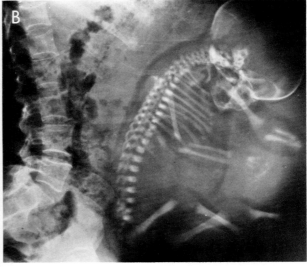

FIG 5–81.
Motion unsharpness. A 23-year-old patient presented at the emergency department with the statement, "Doctor, I am 9 months pregnant and I am in labor." **A,** supine film of the abdomen, blurred image. **B,** lateral view clearly shows a fully mature fetus in breech presentation. On the supine film, the fetal skull can be identified in the right upper quadrant and fetal back along the right margin of the uterus. The fetus was moving when the supine film was obtained, obscuring fetal detail. A structure as large as a 9-month fetus may be obscured if it happens to be in motion when a film is obtained. The lesson in this patient is also clearly applicable to other radiographic examinations. For example, in abdominal films made with mobile equipment on patients in distress, motion unsharpness is often a problem, and the limitations imposed on diagnostic accuracy should be clearly recognized.

FIG 5–82.
Septic abortion. Gas bacillus infection of uterus. A 37-year-old woman brought to the emergency department in septic shock. She was too sick to be sent to x-ray for an abdominal film. A film made with mobile apparatus was therefore obtained. The uterus is enlarged. The wall is thick *(open arrows).* The outer wall can be identified by indentation of gas in the cecum. The inner wall is outlined by gas filling the uterine cavity. Note the large pear-shaped collection of gas projected over the sacrum and lower lumber spine. The vague densities projected in the region of both hip joints *(black arrows)* are calcifications in the soft tissues of the buttocks due to gluteal fat necrosis (injection granuloma) attributed to prior penicillin shots. The diagnosis was gas-producing infection of the uterus. An emergency hysterectomy was performed. The patient survived.

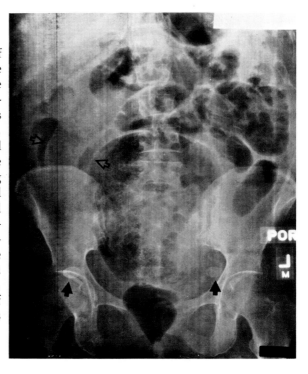

knowledge of the types of examinations performed and the techniques and apparatus employed, the physicist can accurately measure the fetal dose. Phantoms and dosimetry materials are available to ensure that this determination is accurate (Fig 5–79).

Once the fetal dose is known, the referring physician and radiologist should determine the gestational age at which x-ray exposure occurred. With this information, there are two alternatives: allow the pregnancy to continue or terminate it.

There are very few authoritative recommendations regarding whether or not abortion is indicated.

1. In man, diminished body growth, head size, and mental development have been observed in children of mothers who received 50 rad during the early months of gestation, and some disturbances of growth may occur after as little as 25 rad.

2. There is no stage of gestation during which an exposure of 50 rad is not associated with a significant probability of an observable pathologic effect on the embryo. From a clinical point of view, an absorbed fetal dose of 10 rad at any time during the first trimester of gestation can be considered a practical threshold for the induction of congenital defects. With doses of less than 10 rad, the probability of adverse effects becomes negligible.

3. Fetal doses below about 1 rad do not indicate induction of abortion. Fetal doses between 1 rad and about 10 rad indicate therapeutic abortion only in the presence of other complications. Fetal doses above about 10 rad presumably always indicate abortion.

4. Risk associated with fetal doses in excess of 20 rad may be unacceptably high, but a dose below 10 rad would never, in itself, justify a recommendation for abortion.

In view of the available evidence, Bushong has developed a 10-to-25-rad rule. Below 10 rad, a therapeutic abortion is not indicated unless there are additional mitigating circumstances. Between 10 and 25 rad, one must carefully consider the precise time of irradiation, emotional state of the patient, the effect an additional child would have on the family, and other social and economic factors.

In Bushong's experience, fetal doses have been consistently low. His experience covers at least 50 questionable cases in the past 10 years. Fetal doses usually ranged from 1 to 3 rad; none has exceeded 10 rad.

Occasionally, a patient may not be aware that she is pregnant, and it is important that the pregnancy may be detected on the initial scout film before urography or gastrointestinal examination is carried out (Fig 5–80). This determination is at times complicated by fetal movement, which may obscure a rather late pregnancy (Fig 5–81). Complications of pregnancy, such as septic abortion or the need for pelvimetry may necessitate radiation exposure. The cost-benefit ratio here is considered acceptable (Fig 5–82).

References

Because current information on radiation exposure in pregnancy is not generally included in textbooks readily available in emergency departments, and because of its timely nature, a short reference list is included here.

The reference list has been updated for the second edition of this book, and the reader is specifically directed to the more recent references for current information. No reason has emerged from the current literature for altering recommendations of the first edition.

Brent RL, Gorson RO: Radiation exposure in pregnancy. *Curr Top Radiol* 1972; 2:3–48.

Bushong SC: Pregnancy in diagnostic radiology: Radiation control procedures. *Appl Radiol* 1976; July-August: 63–68.

Bushong SC: Radiation exposure in our daily lives. *Physics Teacher* 1977; 15:135–144.

Hale J, Thomas JW: Radiation risks for patients having x-rays. *Nurse Practitioner,* December, 1985.

Hammer-Jacobson E: Therapeutic abortion on account of x-ray examination during pregnancy. *Dan Med Bull* 1959, pp 113–122.

NCRP Report 54, *Medical Radiation Exposure of Pregnant and Potentially Pregnant Women.* Washington DC, National Council on Radiation Protection, 1977.

NCRP Report 53, *Review of NCRP Radiation Dose Limits for Embryo and Fetus in Occupationally Exposed Women.* Washington DC, National Council on Radiation Protection, 1977.

Neumeister K, Wasser S: Clinical data for radiation embryology 1984 Report. *Radiation and Environmental Biophysics,* New York, Springer-Verlag, 1985.

Proposed Rules Procedures to Minimize Medical X-ray Exposure of the Human Embryo and Fetus. Recommendations for Medical Radiation Exposure of Women of Childbearing Potential. *Federal Register* vol 44, no 225, November 20, 1979.

Ritenour ER: Health effects of low-level radiation: Carcinogenesis, teratogenesis, and mutagenesis. *Seminars in Nuclear Medicine,* vol XVI. 1986; 2(April):106–117.

Sternberg J: Radiation and pregnancy. *Can Med Assoc J* 1973; 109:51–57.

Taylor L: Problems of radiation double standards: The exposure of potentially pregnant persons. *Health Physics* vol 49. 1985; 6(Dec):1043–1052.

Wagner LK, Lester RG, Saldana LR: *Exposure of the Pregnant Patient to Diagnostic Radiations (A Guide to Medical Management).* Philadelphia, JB Lippincott Co, 1985.

Blunt Abdominal Trauma

Blunt trauma to the abdomen may be especially difficult to diagnose because serious intra-abdominal injuries can be masked by more obvious, but less lethal ones. Intra-abdominal injuries that are ultimately fatal

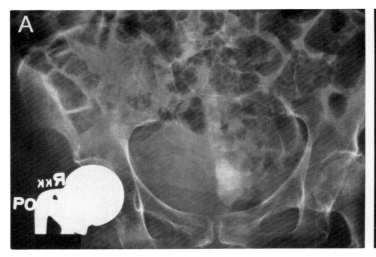

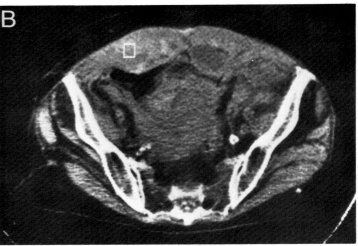

FIG 5–83.
Rectus sheath hematomas. **A,** plain film of the pelvis shows a density displacing the contrast filled bladder. **B,** CT scan shows bilateral rectus sheath hematomas.

The patient was on anticoagulant therapy. Compare the thickness of the rectus muscles *(white box)* to the thicknesses shown in other scans in this chapter, such as Figures 5–70, C and 5–90, E.

FIG 5–84.
Computed tomography scan shows a low-density area in the posterior right lobe of the liver representing a massive intrahepatic hematoma. Note rim of fluid (blood) at anterior liver margin *(arrowheads)*. Gas in abdominal wall is related to chest tube placement.

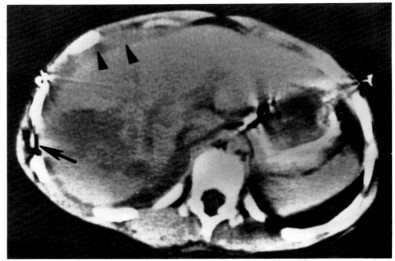

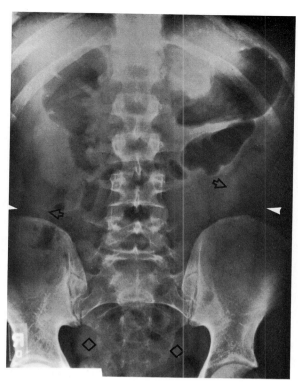

FIG 5–85.

Free blood in peritoneal cavity. A 23-year-old unconscious male brought to the emergency department by the rescue squad, in shock, with head injury and multiple extremity fractures. A supine film of the abdomen shows a large amount of blood in both lateral gutters between the peritoneal fat line *(white arrow)* and cecum on the right *(open arrow),* and between the peritoneal fat line *(white arrow)* and descending colon on the left *(open arrow).* In addition, there is blood in the pelvic gutter *(diamonds,* dog ear sign). A large amount of free blood in the peritoneal cavity was readily apparent on plain film in this particular patient. Substantial intraperitoneal blood (more than 250 cc) is necessary before it is detectable on plain films.

FIG 5–86.

Fluid in the descending colon simulating free blood in peritoneal cavity. Note that there is no colon gas medial to the fluid *(diamond)* along the left flank stripe. The fluid is in the descending colon, not the lateral gutter. There is a slight separation of gas in the cecum from the flank stripe on the right *(circle).* This is the upper range of normal for the width of the potential space of the lateral gutter. The inferior hepatic angle is clearly shown. There is no fluid between the liver and the flank stripe *(arrowhead).* Fluid in the sigmoid colon simulates pelvic mass *(square).*

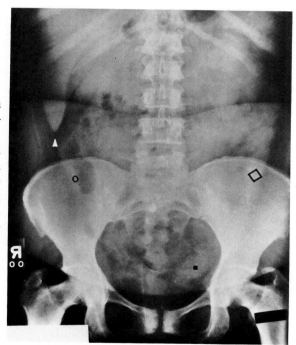

may seem nonexistent for several hours after the injury. It is important to be knowledgeable about these conditions, which may be overlooked during the initial evaluation.

The role of radiology in the diagnosis and management of abdominal trauma has steadily increased in importance. Abdominal plain film examination is valuable in the initial detection of hemorrhage, extraluminal air, or hematomas. Hematomas may present either as a localized mass or organ enlargement (Figs 5–83 and 5–84). Radiographic examination is essential for the diagnosis of rupture of the diaphragm, duodenum, or urinary bladder, and for detection of major visceral vascular occlusion or injury.

Radiographic Technique

As a general rule, mobile-unit films of the abdomen should not be attempted when conventional ones can be obtained. Because of the necessity for a stationary grid and because of the short tube-film distance, mobile-unit films are not of the same diagnostic quality that is obtained with the patient on an x-ray table. Motion unsharpness is a major problem in mobile-unit abdominal films because of the long exposure times required. Any patient motion diminishes the quality of the image obtained. Mobile-unit abdominal films may be required in certain circumstances, but they should be avoided whenever conventional films can be obtained without endangering the patient (see Fig 5–81).

Supine abdominal and chest films should be the first steps in roentgenographic evaluation of the patient with blunt abdominal trauma. These studies may provide all the information that is necessary and are often all that can be performed.

If the patient is unconscious or a victim of multiple trauma, the examination may be limited to the supine position, necessitating the use of both perpendicular and horizontal-beam techniques. These techniques are particularly applicable to the abdomen and vertebral column.

When possible, an upright or left lateral decubitus view should be obtained because free air is more readily detectable in these projections.

Additional information may, at times, be gained from two supine films taken 5 minutes apart. A change in gas pattern or fluid distribution may make free blood, free air, or obscure fracture more readily detectable when the films are compared. Computed tomography, ultrasound, nuclear medicine, and angiography are all useful in evaluating various aspects of blunt abdominal trauma including intra-abdominal or retroperitoneal hemorrhage, organ injury, or intra-peritoneal or retroperitoneal gas. The method of choice would depend on available expertise and technology and on specific clinical circumstances.

Intraperitoneal or retroperitoneal gas is less readily seen by ultrasound than by computed tomography.

Nuclear medicine is most useful for organ injury.

Angiography is indicated for evaluation of organ injury or bleeding and may be useful for treatment of hemorrhage by means of vascular embolization.

Contrast material should not be given orally or rectally if abdominal angiography is being considered.

Blood in the Peritoneal Cavity

Intraperitoneal bleeding follows injury to the spleen, liver, mesentery, intestinal tract, and omentum. Occasionally, it results from bladder trauma and, rarely, from injury to the pancreas. In hemoperitoneum, blood accumulates in the paracolic gutter, between the lateral wall of the colon and the parietal peritoneum. On the plain supine radiograph of the abdomen, the blood within the paracolic gutter appears as a homogeneous soft tissue density, interposed between colon and the radiolucent flank stripe, which displaces the colon medially. In evaluating this condition, it is important to identify the colon by its content, since small-bowel gas may normally be separated from the flank stripe. Unless the colon is identified, fluid-filled small bowel may give rise to a false positive interpretation. Additionally, fluid in the descending colon may simulate fluid in the lateral gutter. Always keep in mind that the lateral gutter lies between the colon and the flank stripe on both right and left. When the hemoperitoneum is secondary to hepatic rupture, the normally visible inferior angle of the liver is obliterated by the density of the adjacent free blood (Figs 5–85 and 5–86).

Intraperitoneal fluid that accumulates in the most dependent portion of the peritoneal cavity, that is, in the pouch of Douglas, produces two globular soft tissue densities in the pelvis above the pubic rami. This blood within the pelvic recess displaces the gas-filled loops of small bowel up out of their normal position within the pelvis. The density of the blood in the pouch of Douglas is usually separated from the density of the urinary bladder by a thin radiolucent stripe caused by the extraperitoneal fat between the dome of the bladder and the pelvic peritoneum. This complex of roentgenographic changes has been described as the dog ear sign (see Figs 5–46 and 5–85).

Fluid or blood within the pelvic peritoneal space is distinguished from extraperitoneal blood or urine by the fact that the intraperitoneal fluid collections are sharply demarcated laterally. The soft tissues of the obturator internus muscle and the urinary bladder remain radiographically visible, while the same soft tissue shadows are completely obliterated by extraperitoneal fluid collections (see Figs 5–93 and 5–94).

Ultrasound is the method of choice for confirmation of fluid in the pelvic recess. Peritoneal lavage is a useful form of paracentesis when single-needle or four-quadrant needle aspiration does not produce diagnostic material. The chief problem with this technique is that both false positive and false negative results occur. Another problem is that of slightly bloody fluid return in patients with blunt abdominal trauma. Two to three milliliters of blood in the 500-ml lavage will cause a slightly bloody appearance, but should not make surgery mandatory. Negative needle aspiration or lavage paracentesis with normal fluid return does not rule out significant abdominal damage. Neither of these procedures will detect subcapsular or intraparenchymal bleeding. Retroperitoneal bleeding will also be missed. Needle aspiration is more reliable in detecting liver injury rather than splenic or retroperitoneal bleeding.

Retroperitoneal hemorrhage obliterates the psoas and renal shadows. In the pelvis, it displaces the bladder and the rectum. A large accumulation between the parietal peritoneum and the flank stripe obliterates the lucency of the flank stripe and displaces the parietal peritoneum medially.

For confirmation of retroperitoneal hemorrhage or hematoma, computed tomography is the modality of choice. Radionuclide scanning of various organs has been remarkably successful in demonstrating relatively symptomless injury, as well as in accurately delineating the extent of severe trauma. The noninvasive character of isotope scanning techniques is obviously attractive, particularly in patients with multiple and complicating coexistent injuries.

Spleen

Rupture of the spleen is the most common intraabdominal injury. Fracture of the left lower ribs is associated in about 50% of adults, but associated rib fracture in children is rare. Conversely, about 5% of patients with rib fractures have spleen injury.

Ruptured spleen may be of three types: (1) extensive laceration with immediate massive intraperitoneal hemorrhage; (2) small capsular tear; or (3) intracapsular hemorrhage, either subcapsular or intrasplenic.

Most patients with immediate massive intraperitoneal hemorrhage from ruptured spleen die. A significant number of patients with ruptured spleen present with obscure clinical and radiographic findings.

With a high index of suspicion, splenic injury should not be missed because of the availability of simple confirmatory methods such as isotopic scanning, ultrasound, and computerized tomography.

Clinically, left shoulder pain suggests the diagnosis of splenic rupture (Kehr's sign). Blood may be identified in the flanks and pelvis. Plain-film findings in splenic rupture include splenic enlargement, distention of the stomach with thickened rugal folds along the greater curvature, medial displacement of the stomach, or inferior displacement of the colon.

The most valuable clinical sign of splenic rupture is the presence of a mass in the left upper quadrant (Fig 5–87). If there is suspicion of a ruptured spleen, the patient should be carefully examined radiographically for possible mass. A splenic mass displaces the stomach and transverse colon. A right posterior oblique film of the abdomen, if available, may show the splenic mass. The presence of such a mass should be strong presumptive evidence of possible splenic rupture. Visualization of what appears to be a slightly enlarged splenic outline is consistent with subcapsular hemorrhage, while the presence of mass is a valuable sign. However, the absence of a mass on initial plain film examination does not rule out splenic rupture.

Certain signs may be contributory, especially if several coexist.

1. Obscuration of splenic shadow by adjacent blood (here, the splenic outline may not be clearly visible, but the presence of a left upper quadrant mass may be inferred by displacement of adjacent organs).

2. Elevation and restriction of the left hemidiaphragm.

3. Atelectasis and pleural effusion.

4. Prominent gastric mucosal folds.

5. Irregularity of the gastric curvature of the stomach, which may be serrated or indented.

6. Haziness or obliteration of the left renal or psoas shadow.

7. Displacement of stomach (gastric air bubble), splenic flexure, or kidney.

8. Gastric dilatation.

9. Rib fracture.

10. Separation of bowel loops by fluid.

11. Adynamic ileus from blood leaking into the peritoneal cavity.

Splenic disease (infectious mononucleosis, malaria, blood dyscrasia) increases the likelihood of rupture. Rupture may occur without obvious trauma or with minimal trauma if the spleen is diseased.

If the spleen is ruptured or lacerated, blood may be confined to the left upper quadrant by the phrenicocolic ligament or because the hemorrhage is subcapsular. For this reason, negative peritoneal lavage does not rule out splenic rupture.

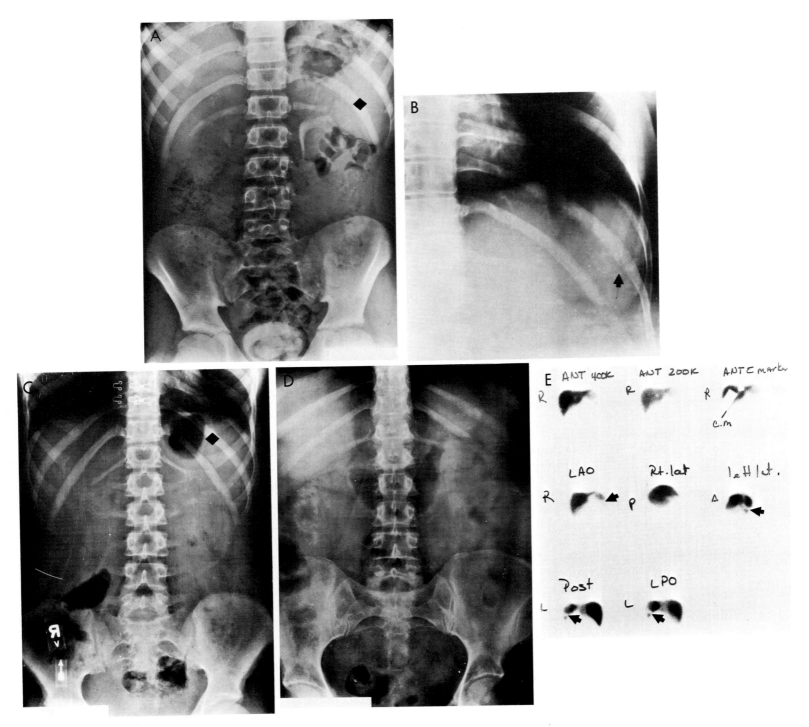

FIG 5–87.

Ruptured spleen. **A,** there is a left upper quadrant mass *(diamond).* In addition, the mucosal pattern of the gastric fundus is accentuated. This is an indirect sign that may be associated with splenic rupture. **B,** there is a fracture of the left eleventh rib. The margins of the splenic mass can be seen just below the base of the *black arrow.* The left upper quadrant is totally devoid of gas. **C,** there is a straight lateral margin of the gastric fundus resulting from compression from a mass *(diamond).* **D,** there are no detectable margins to a mass, but the left upper quadrant is devoid of gas, and gas in the stomach is medially displaced, indicating a mass. **E,** spleen scan, multiple views. *Arrows* point to splenic disruption.

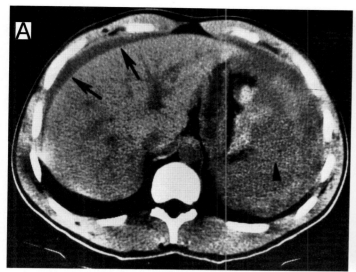

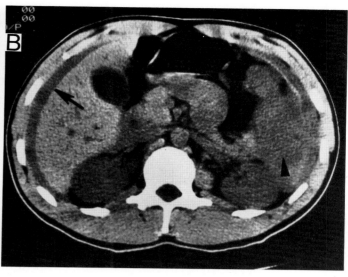

FIG 5–88.

Computed tomography scan without IV or oral contrast in auto accident victim. Note distortion of spleen with poorly defined areas of low density *(arrowheads)*. The ruptured spleen was removed at surgery. Note also a low-density crescentic rim at the liver margin indicating free intraperitoneal blood *(arrows)*. **A,** scan through midliver, stomach and spleen. **B,** same patient, slightly lower level.

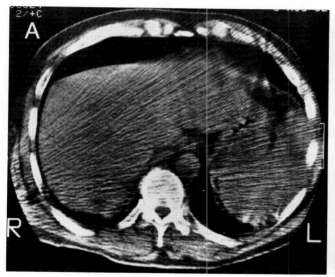

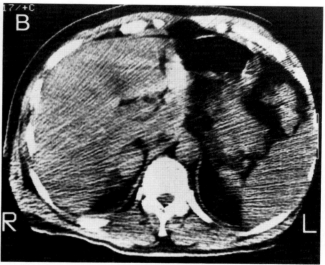

FIG 5–89.

Suboptimal CT scan. Angiography (not shown) yielded the appropriate diagnosis of severe splenic contusion and subcapsular hematoma. **(A** and **B),** the CT which had been performed first was inconclusive due to streak artifact. This often happens when patients cannot cooperate with respiratory maneuvers or when the extremities must be included in the scan field. At surgery a ruptured spleen was removed.

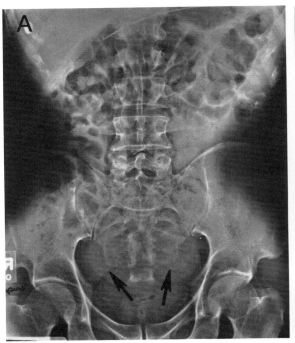

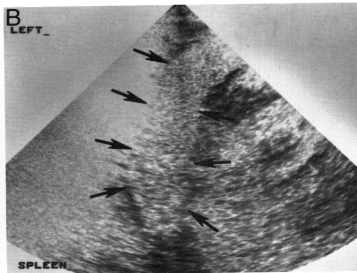

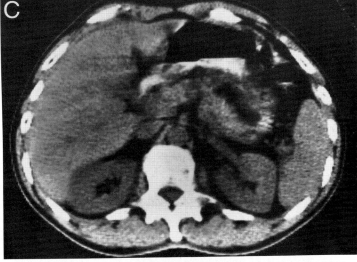

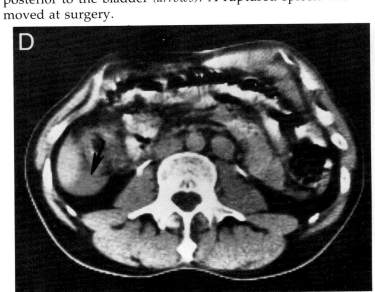

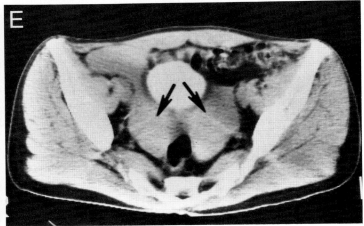

FIG 5–90.
A 41-year-old accident victim. **A,** plain film of the abdomen shows a vague density above the bladder suggesting the possibility of free fluid *(arrows).* Because of this finding, additional studies were performed. **B,** sonogram with rib-shadowing artifact shows normal sonographic texture and appearance of the spleen *(arrows).* **C,** CT scan of the upper abdomen shows normal appearance of the liver, spleen, pancreas, and kidneys. **D,** CT image at the inferior edge of the right lobe of the liver shows minimal fluid (blood) adjacent to the liver margin. **E,** CT image of the midpelvis shows massive fluid accumulation (blood) in the peritoneal recesses posterior to the bladder *(arrows).* A ruptured spleen was removed at surgery.

Severity of the clinical situation may preclude roentgen examination. Only when leakage of blood is slow or ceases temporarily is a radiographic examination performed.

When time permits, ultrasound, isotopic scanning (Fig 5–87), or rapid-sequence computed tomographic scanning are reliable methods of evaluating splenic trauma (Figs 5–87 to 5–90). Angiography is useful in cases where other studies have proved unsatisfactory or as a part of another angiographic evaluation. However, since newer angiographic techniques permit transcatheter embolization and occlusion of bleeding splenic arteries and other visceral blood vessels, surgical intervention may be eliminated or deferred in some cases. When this expertise is available, angiography may be the method of choice for evaluation as well.

Viscus Perforation

Perforation of a hollow viscus rarely results from blunt trauma. When it does occur, however, it may produce intraperitoneal, retroperitoneal, or mediastinal accumulation of gas. Perforation of the esophagus is especially difficult to detect early.

By virtue of its direct continuity with the stomach, the esophagus may be injured by trauma below the diaphragm. The chest film is the most valuable single diagnostic aid when rupture of the esophagus is suspected. Pneumothorax, pleural fluid, mediastinal emphysema, and soft tissue emphysema of the chest wall and neck may be identified. Oral water-soluble contrast is useful for confirmation if clinically indicated.

Perforation of the stomach, the first part of the duodenum, or the colon will produce ample free gas in the peritoneal cavity. Gas from extraperitoneal perforation of the colon may extend up both sides of the retroperitoneal space and outline the psoas and renal areas. This gas tends to change little with change in the patient's position, while intraperitoneal gas, of course, shifts markedly.

The oral or rectal use of water-soluble contrast media, such as Gastrografin or oral Hypaque solution, is helpful for diagnosis of perforated viscus, since the contrast usually extravasates into the peritoneal cavity. The extravasation, however, may be difficult or impossible to recognize because of the low contrast density of water-soluble medium. Unless the patient is in shock, the contrast will concentrate in the urinary bladder within 2 to 4 hours in sufficient density for radiographic definition (see Fig 5–21).

Perforation of the small intestine following blunt trauma to the abdomen is rare. Additionally, because of the paucity of air normally present in the small intestine, free air in the peritoneal cavity may be minimal or absent. If small-intestinal perforation from blunt trauma is suspected, and free air is not demonstrated, oral water-soluble contrast might be considered for its usefulness in detecting obscure intestinal perforation at any level. In children, however, its use is limited by normal absorption from the intestinal tract.

Jejunal and ileal perforation occur with seatbelt injuries. Fifty percent of the injuries in a collected series were transverse fractures of the vertebral body and/or separations of the articular facets. The seatbelt sign (lower abdominal abrasions, contusion, ecchymosis) may be a tip-off. Less than half of the radiographs in patients with these injuries show free air.

Duodenal Injury

The duodenum's fixed retroperitoneal position directly over the upper lumbar spine makes it the most commonly injured segment of the intestinal tract. The most common site of duodenal rupture is the second or third portion. A direct blow to the upper midabdomen compresses and shears the duodenal wall against the vertebral body. Concomitant contusion of the pancreatic head frequently occurs.

Duodenal injuries are classified as follows:
   I. Hematoma (intramural).
   II. Perforation (retroperitoneal, intraperitoneal)
   III. Perforation and minor pancreatic injury
   IV. Perforation and major pancreatic injury

Intramural hematoma and retroperitoneal perforation occur with approximately equal frequency. Intraperitoneal perforation is rare. Clinically, there is a history of trauma. The patient usually has signs of peritoneal insult with abdominal rigidity and pain on palpation. Pain often radiates to the back. There may be massive emesis. The patient may be unconscious or in shock. Clinical confirmation may be obtained by aspiration of blood through a nasogastric tube.

Retroperitoneal perforation of the duodenum is demonstrated by extraluminal gas that tends to conform to the anatomical spaces outlined by fascial planes. The air may surround the right kidney or consist of dispersed bubbles (see Fig 5–41). The plain film findings in retroperitoneal perforation of the appendix or the duodenum are identical.

Approximately half of the patients with retroperitoneal duodenal laceration show retroperitoneal air. Duodenal injury results in the escape of blood, duodenal enzymes, and fluid into the retroperitoneal tissues. Without retroperitoneal air, the diagnosis becomes more difficult and rests on progressive obscur-

FIG 5–91.
Ruptured left hemidiaphragm. The lower half of the left chest is opaque. The appearance suggests marked elevation of the left hemidiaphragm, with compression of lung or large left pleural fluid collection. The chest x-ray is typical of diaphragmatic rupture. A chest x-ray suggesting abnormal position of the diaphragm following blunt trauma to the abdomen should cause a high index of suspicion for rupture. Diagnosis is readily confirmed by introducing water-soluble contrast into the stomach through a nasogastric tube.

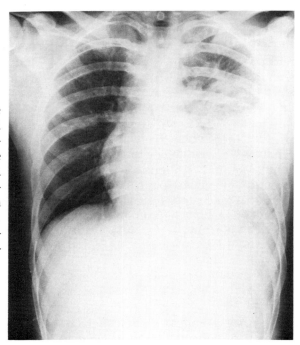

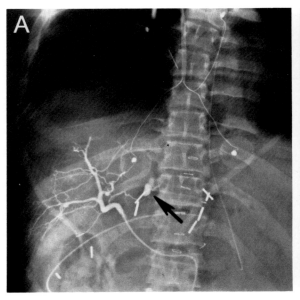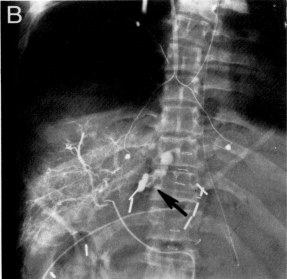

FIG 5–92.
This multiple trauma victim was rushed to surgery from the emergency department. A small bowel perforation was repaired. Small surface lacerations of the liver were present, but a bleeding site could not be seen. Postoperatively the patient continued to hemorrhage. After transfusion of 15 units of blood products, an angiographic search for active bleeding was performed including pelvic and visceral angiography. A selective right hepatic angiogram showed hemorrhage to the peritoneal space. After angiographic embolization, the patient stabilized. **A,** early arterial phase; *arrow* marks the bleeding site. **B,** late arterial phase; contrast accumulation indicates significant active hemorrhage.

ing of adjacent structures by the inflammatory process.

If not diagnosed and treated, retroperitoneal sepsis is rapidly fatal (mortality 70%–90%). The mortality rate increases in direct proportion to the length of time between injury and definitive treatment. The symptoms may have a delayed onset. Within 12 to 24 hours after injury, signs of sepsis, including leukocytosis and fever, develop. Increasing continuous pain in the right flank and back is common. With these symptoms, and in the absence of retroperitoneal air, an oral water-soluble contrast study is indicated to evaluate the integrity of the duodenum. The contrast is administered and the patient placed in the right lateral decubitus position for 5 to 10 minutes. Delayed films may show Gastrografin outside the perforated bowel lumen.

If contrast is not seen outside the bowel lumen, a 2- or 4-hour delayed film of the urinary bladder should be obtained. Water-soluble contrast may be too low in density to be seen as it leaks from a bowel perforation, but will be detected in the bladder in 2 to 4 hours if the bowel lumen is perforated (see Fig 5–21).

Approximately 50% of retroperitoneal ruptures of the duodenum is associated with trauma to the pancreas. With simple contusion of the pancreas, radiographic findings will be negative, but serum amylase levels may be elevated.

With laceration of the pancreas, the clinical and plain film findings are those of acute pancreatitis. These include severe deep epigastric pain, elevated left or right hemidiaphragm, basilar atelectasis, pleural fluid, scoliosis, adynamic ileus, loss of radiographic visualization of normal structures and fascial planes, possible viscus displacement from a mass, and elevated serum amylase levels.

Intramural duodenal hematoma occurs in children, usually following a fall on bicycle handlebars. The diagnosis of intramural hematoma of the duodenum is generally not attempted early in patient evaluation because of the greater significance of other injuries. Six to twelve hours after the injury, the child may start to vomit. Barium study at this time may show complete or partial duodenal obstruction. Intramural and submucosal bowel-wall hemorrhage may completely obstruct the duodenum or produce a coiled-spring appearance.

Intramural hematoma may not be clinically apparent until 2 or 3 days after injury. Diagnosis usually dictates a conservative method of therapy.

Ruptured Diaphragm

Blunt trauma to the abdomen is the most common cause of rupture of the diaphragm, which results from a sudden increase in intra-abdominal pressure. The clinical picture is usually dominated by signs of abdominal injury. Diaphragmatic rupture occurs with much greater frequency on the left. The injury usually produces a large laceration in the posterolateral leaf of the diaphragm, allowing herniation of abdominal viscera—including stomach, spleen, colon, omentum, and sometimes small intestine.

Intestinal shadows, most commonly the stomach, which may become inverted and distended, are identified in the thorax. Abdominal content in the thorax may be mistaken for pneumothorax, pleural fluid, lung contusion, or eventration. A high index of suspicion is necessary for diagnosis. If rupture of the left hemidiaphragm (Fig 5–91) is suspected from the chest film, diagnosis is readily confirmed by introducing water-soluble contrast through a nasogastric tube. If the stomach has herniated into the chest, this herniation will be recognized. On the right side, ultrasound may be useful for confirmation. The diaphragm can be detected and the relationship of the liver parenchyma and fluid can be determined. Angiography may show vessels to the stomach, spleen, or omentum crossing the diaphragm.

Ultrasound, Nuclear Medicine, Magnetic Resonance Imaging, and Angiography in Blunt Abdominal Trauma

Multiple diagnostic tests, including abdominal paracentesis and lavage, ultrasound, computed tomography, isotopic scanning and intravenous urography, are widely used in assessment of blunt abdominal trauma. When these studies do not establish the presence or absence of severe visceral injury, angiography should be considered. Clinical judgment is crucial in selecting the next appropriate study. Nuclear medicine procedures are of substantial value in the study of patients with multiple abdominal trauma because of ease of performance, simplicity of technique, rapidity of procedure, ready availability, safety, and high accuracy. Multiple organ involvement in blunt abdominal trauma is not unusual. The spleen and liver can be scanned with a single tracer. The kidneys can be rapidly screened immediately thereafter. Injury to the right kidney is frequently associated with injury to the liver. Renal scanning has been a widely applied technique for detecting clinically important trauma. As a general rule, if the scan is normal, arteriography is not necessary, since the scan is quite reliable in surveying the traumatized kidney. However, angiography is usually more definitive and is often useful in assessing severe abdominal trauma.

Ultrasound examination can be of substantial value in detecting renal, splenic, hepatic, or pancreatic injury. With the current availability of mobile real-time equipment with excellent resolution, survey examinations can be quickly performed. Interfering bowel gas and difficulties in positioning severely injured patients are restricting factors. Computerized tomography is useful in acute trauma, especially if equipment is capable of rapid sequence scanning.

Choice of nuclear scanning, computerized tomography, or ultrasound will often depend on local expertise and equipment.

Selected cases of blunt abdominal injury and penetrating trauma can best be evaluated by angiography. When indicated, angiography should be performed without delay to ensure prompt and appropriate therapy. In some circumstances, patients in whom peritoneal tap reveals a large amount of blood are taken directly to surgery. However, when the patient's condition permits, angiography can be especially valuable in specifically delineating the problem preoperatively. Sometimes, surgery can be avoided with angiography if the bleeding can be controlled by transcatheter embolization. This technique is particularly useful in the pelvis.

The indications for abdominal arteriography are: (1) suspected vascular occlusion; (2) evidence of unexplained blood loss; and (3) results from peritoneal lavage, ultrasound, computed tomography, radionuclide scanning, conventional radiographic scout film, or excretory urogram that dictate the need for angiographic evaluation. These may be positive results of organ damage or negative results in which the clinical situation requires further evaluation. Angiography is of greatest value in trauma to the spleen, kidneys, liver, and aorta, and of less value in pancreatic and bowel injuries.

Angiography is a valuable technique for detecting dissection or rupture of the thoracic aorta, abdominal aorta, and mesenteric vessels, and it may be helpful in locating bleeding sites in massive retroperitoneal hemorrhage. The latter example is especially important if major pelvic trauma is the cause of bleeding. Selective angiographic study of solid viscera can precisely determine the site and extent of the damage before surgery.

Angiography can demonstrate hepatic injuries whether at the time of trauma or later (Fig 5–92). Laceration or hematoma deep within the liver sometimes cannot be fully identified surgically, and subcapsular hematoma may not be symptomatic immediately. Angiography gives the surgeon the most precise information about the nature and extent of injury and defines the major vascular anatomy of the liver. In selected cases, it may be the most definitive diagnostic study before surgery.

General considerations include the need to monitor the patient with multiple organ injury during the performance of the angiogram. If the patient is sent to the angiographic unit without an adequate team to carry out any type of required resuscitation, catastrophe is likely to follow. The hospital trauma team concept is most helpful here, since the angiographer can work most efficiently if the trauma team can manage the patient's general condition during the actual procedure. Obviously, angiography is contraindicated if the patient is in shock or requires resuscitation. The delay required to stabilize the cardiovascular system, develop an effective airway, immobilize fractures, and otherwise make the patient comfortable is time necessarily spent. If the angiographer is experienced in vascular embolization, diagnostic angiography may have a higher priority, because control of bleeding may preclude the need for immediate surgical intervention.

Magnetic resonance imaging (MRI) is making rapid technical advances. New applications are evolving very quickly.

However, for the emergency department patient, there are disadvantages which preclude the use of MRI in most patients. In order to have an MRI scan, the patient must be placed within the bore of a large magnet. The scans take a long time. Life support equipment should not be brought into the magnetic room. MRI, therefore, is not currently suitable for extremely sick patients.

We expect the applications of MRI to the emergency setting to expand as the technology improves and the limitations decrease.

Bladder and Urethra

Critically ill patients often have urinary catheters placed as soon as possible, frequently within the first few minutes in the hospital. The male with a urethral injury may suffer inestimable harm to the lower tract by the insertion of a urethral catheter. Urethral catheterization requires caution in patients with pelvic fractures because the procedure may convert a partial transection of the urethra to a complete transection or introduce infection. A tear in the urethra may be hidden by a catheter.

If catheterization is attempted with a ruptured upper urethra, a false passage may be made or the tear in the urethra may be made worse. Periurethral urine may be obtained, causing a significant delay in diagnosis. The contamination of the periurethral tissues occurring when the catheter is mechanically introduced from below is the most serious consequence. Such infection prevents extensive reconstruction of the severed urethra immediately, or even at a later date, and makes severe upper urethral stricture a virtual certainty. To forestall this occurrence, any evidence of urethral injury or of other serious pelvic fracture requires a retrograde urethrogram before other manipulation of the urinary tract. The traumatized male urethra can be examined using a tiny Foley balloon catheter or an infant feeding tube in the fossa navicularis.

The small Foley catheter is inserted into the distal urethra, the balloon is gently inflated with air, and 20 to 25 ml of water-soluble contrast (25% diatrizoate) is injected slowly from a sterile syringe. Oblique and lateral x-ray views are helpful in detecting small tears. If urethral damage is demonstrated, instrumentation is contraindicated and cystostomy must be performed. If no damage is seen, the catheter may be advanced into the bladder and cystography is then carried out. The urethrographic films must be studied prior to cystography, since extraperitoneal extravasation of contrast material from a ruptured bladder is not readily distinguishable from high posterior urethral rupture. Contrast from this procedure frequently enters the perivesical space. Retrograde cystourethrography should be performed in all instances, unless the patient's condition is so critical that urethral injury is of relative unimportance.

Under ideal conditions, retrograde cystourethrography may be performed under fluoroscopic control to observe the urethra in various degrees of obliquity. By this technique, small periurethral or perivesical tears that otherwise might be obscured by the contrast in the urethra are detected. Fluoroscopy, however, may not be feasible in emergency conditions.

A one-film urethrogram, although possibly providing a false negative examination, may be the only method possible in patients too severely injured to permit fluoroscopic examination. The urethrogram can be obtained in the emergency department with a mobile x-ray machine. The patient is placed in a 45-degree oblique position.

Bladder rupture is rare except in pelvic fractures and in alcoholics with overdistended bladders. Intraperitoneal rupture occurs from a direct blow to the dome of the distended bladder. Unless the bladder is greatly overdistended, rupture due to trauma is generally extraperitoneal. Extraperitoneal rupture is four times more common than intraperitoneal (Fig 5–93). Presence or absence of blood in the urine may not be a reliable indicator. A patient with a ruptured bladder may pass clear urine, whereas minor contusion may result in hematuria. Both conditions can be recog-

nized with introduction of contrast material.

Fifteen percent of patients with pelvic fractures sustain damage to the urethra or bladder. Of these, 60% have urethral trauma; 30%, bladder injury; and 10%, combined lesions. The classic signs of urethral injury are: (1) the prostate is not palpable on rectal examination (it floats free with high posterior urethral transection); (2) urethral bleeding is encountered or blood is seen at the urethral meatus; (3) the conscious patient cannot void although the bladder is palpable on abdominal examination; and (4) bloody urine is passed but clears terminally.

An alternative diagnostic approach is a high-dose excretory urogram. However, it should be recognized that, if the patient is in shock, the kidneys will not excrete the contrast agent. Additionally, a high-dose urogram may be a time-consuming procedure. It may be indicated to evaluate the kidneys and ureters of a patient with blunt abdominal or pelvic trauma; however, it does not provide an adequate method of studying the urethra and is not in itself adequate to rule out bladder lacerations.

A technique has been described for a "choke urethrogram" that may, under some circumstances, be applicable following the high-dose urogram in trauma patients. A Zipser clamp is applied to the urethra during voiding attempt, thus filling out the posterior urethra and demonstrating extravasation.

Extraperitoneal rupture of the urinary bladder may result in substantial accumulation of fluid in the extraperitoneal space, a potential space filled with adipose or loose aureolar tissue and limited superiorly by the pelvic peritoneal reflection, laterally by the levator ani and obturator internus muscles, and inferiorly by the urogenital diaphragm. The urinary bladder and prostate are contained within this potential space. The bladder and obturator muscles are commonly visible in anteroposterior radiographs of the pelvis.

An accumulation of blood or urine within the extraperitoneal perivesical space is recognizable by the effect of the fluid on the normal plain-film appearance of the bladder, the obturator internus muscles, and the pelvic small bowel loops. A narrow shadow is normally present along the lateral edges of the pelvic ring (ischium) and the soft tissues of the pelvis. This is continuous with the extraperitoneal fat extending over the dome of the urinary bladder. This fat shadow is obliterated on one side in extraperitoneal hematoma or ruptured urinary bladder from trauma (Figs 5–94 to 5–97). A small effusion, localized to one side of this perivesical space, will displace the urinary bladder to the opposite side. As the fluid collection increases and fills the perivesical space, it completely obscures the shadow of the bladder and displaces the

FIG 5–93.

Intraperitoneal rupture of urinary bladder. The film shows contrast injected through an indwelling catheter in the peritoneal cavity, indicating intraperitoneal rupture of the urinary bladder. There are multiple pelvic fractures, and the pubic symphysis is disrupted. The distribution of contrast in the peritoneal cavity gives good delineation of both lateral gutters *(closed arrows)*. There is some indication of the configuration of the right pelvic recess *(open arrow)*. The left recess is obliterated by a large extraperitoneal hematoma.

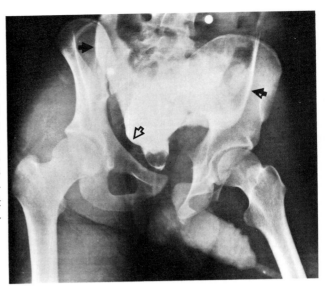

FIG 5–94.

Pelvic hematoma secondary to pelvic fractures. **A,** pelvis. There are nondisplaced fractures of both superior pubic rami *(large black arrows)*. There is slight deformity of the pubic symphysis *(open arrow)*. The peritoneal fat line over the obturator internus muscle is clearly visible on the left *(narrow arrows)* but is obliterated on the right. This finding suggests pelvic hematoma or extraperitoneal rupture of the urinary bladder. **B,** the urinary bladder is intact, but there is deformity on the right incident to a large pelvic hematoma *(diamond)*.

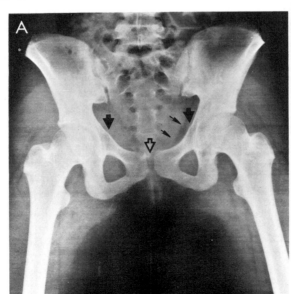

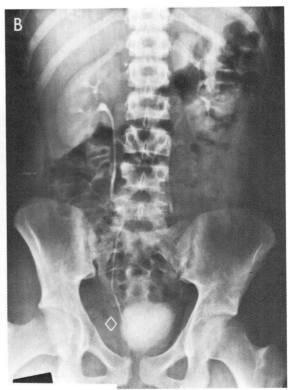

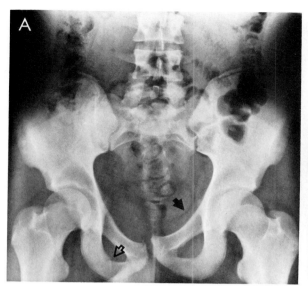
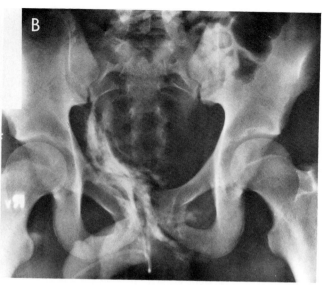

FIG 5–95.
Extraperitoneal rupture of urinary bladder. **A,** disruption of pubic symphysis; fracture of right inferior pubic ramus *(open arrow)*. Note that peritoneal fat shadow is obliterated on right but is well shown on left *(closed arrow).* **B,** contrast injected through a urethral catheter shows extraperitoneal extravasation of the contrast secondary to extraperitoneal rupture of the urinary bladder.

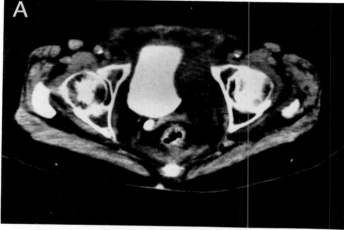

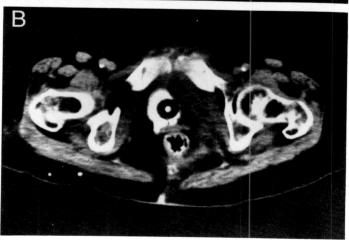

FIG 5–96.
Perivesical pelvic hematoma in a patient with multiple trauma and unexplained blood loss. Note distortion of the contrast-filled bladder which contains a Foley catheter. A fracture of the bony pelvis not seen on this image was demonstrated at conventional tomography performed later. Pelvic fractures not apparent on plain films may sometimes be seen on CT scans at bone window settings. Likewise, fractures shown on some plain film studies are not shown on CT.

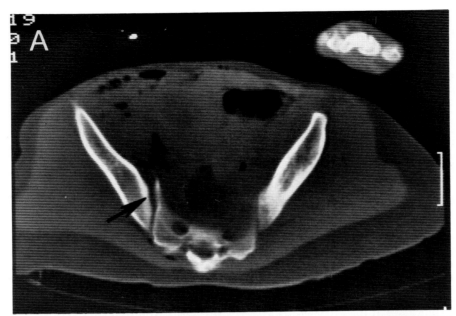

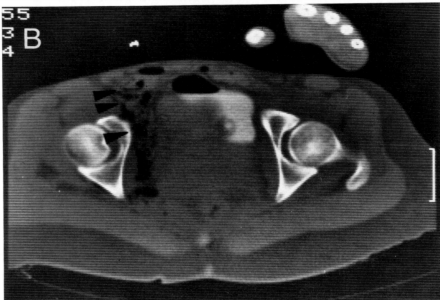

FIG 5–97.
A 25-year-old female automobile trauma victim. **A** and **B,** CT images of the pelvis at wide-window settings. IV contrast has resulted in bladder opacification **(B).** The bladder and its in-dwelling Foley catheter are displaced by a perivesical retroperitoneal hematoma. The patient's left hand and wrist are in the imaging field. Note widening of the right SI joint *(arrow).* The plain film also shows pubic diastasis and subcutaneous and retroperitoneal gas *(arrowheads).*

pelvic small bowel loops out of their normal position.

Pelvic fracture alone may be accompanied by massive and occasionally exsanguinating retroperitoneal hemorrhage. The perivesical space may serve as a reservoir for as much as 2,000 cc of fluid. Blood accumulating in the closed space causes a characteristic deformity of the bladder—the "teardrop." Eventually, the flank stripes will be obliterated by the dissection of fluid.

Pelvic hemorrhage is the most common cause of death, following pelvic skeletal injury. Exsanguination or renal failure secondary to shock is the usual mechanism. Hemostasis is best obtained by angiographic embolization.

The clinical significance of pelvic hemorrhage is that this bleeding is often clinically silent until the patient lapses into hemorrhagic shock. The signs of extraperitoneal hemorrhage, however, are usually evident in the initial radiograph of the pelvis. The clinician should therefore be aware of those pelvic injuries which are frequently associated with pelvic hemorrhage. There is a direct correlation between the severity of the pelvic skeletal injury and the magnitude of the hemorrhage. However, a significant hemorrhage can occur with only minimally displaced or innocuous-appearing fractures. An analysis of the types of pelvic fractures associated with various types of urethral and bladder injuries is not particularly useful because each patient should be evaluated for retroperitoneal hemorrhage and urinary tract injury. When diagnosis and management of these have been initiated, management of the pelvic fractures can be undertaken.

Injuries to the rectum, sciatic nerves, and blood vessels are less frequently associated with pelvic fractures and require specific evaluation for diagnosis. The pelvis can break in one place, but only if there is no displacement. Any time an anterior pelvic fracture is noted, the sacroiliac joint on the same side is suspect for injury. A sacral fracture as a component of pelvic fracture may be difficult to detect. One should look for disruptions of the sacral foramina, especially if there is a fracture of the fifth lumbar transverse process.

Renal Trauma

Renal trauma may result in renal contusion or laceration, renal artery or vein thrombosis, or transection of the renal pedicle. Clinical findings are hematuria, pain, guarding, spasm, bruises, and—if there is massive bleeding—possibly shock. Radiologic findings are scoliosis, enlargement of the kidney, obliter-

ation of renal and psoas margins, fullness of the flank, adynamic ileus, displacement of bowel loops by a retroperitoneal mass, and fracture of the spine and lower ribs.

Twenty to thirty percent of patients with blunt trauma to the kidneys have significant head, extremity, chest, or abdominal injuries, including specific liver, spleen, or bowel laceration and pelvic, spine, or pancreatic injury.

Of the renal injuries, simple contusion accounts for 60% and laceration for 30%, with the remaining 10% divided among shattered kidney with multiple fragments, vascular disruption or occlusion and ruptured renal pelvis. The kidney lies between the anterior and posterior layers of the renal (Gerota's) fascia. Blood from the lacerated kidney enters this inverted cone-shaped space. Perirenal hemorrhage is usually confined between the layers of Gerota's fascia which is unfused caudally, allowing blood to extend to the pelvis. The blood obscures the renal outline and infiltrates the perirenal fat.

Intravenous urography may be normal or may show an abnormal enlargement of the kidney with poor excretion, stretching, and displacement of the calyceal system by edema or blood within the renal parenchyma. Irregular collections of contrast medium within the renal parenchyma, associated with only minimal distortion of the collecting system, suggest that the renal laceration does not involve major vessels (Fig 5–98, A).

Extravasation of contrast material may be seen in renal laceration. In this situation, the compact retroperitoneal tissues would probably tamponade the hemorrhage and seal off the laceration. Renal vein thrombosis is characterized by enlargement of the kidney, and the involved kidney usually shows a prolonged nephrographic phase with diminished excretion of contrast on intravenous urography. Renal artery thrombosis is characterized by total absence of renal function on the affected side.

Nonvisualization of a kidney on excretory urography following trauma may result from renal laceration, renal artery thrombosis, or pedicle transsection. The latter is generally associated with obliteration of the renal and psoas shadows by extensive retroperitoneal hematoma. Nonfunction of a kidney on an excretory urogram is more significant than diminished function.

If the intravenous urogram shows markedly diminished function of a solitary kidney or nonfunction of either kidney, emergency angiography should be performed to demonstrate the status of the renal vascular supply, since the renal vessels can only be repaired

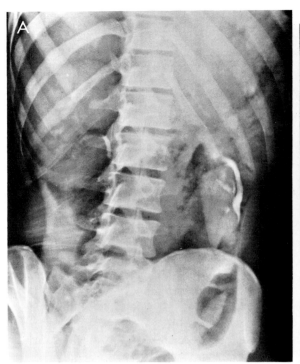

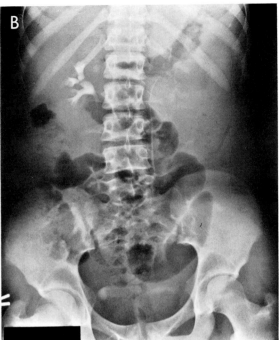

FIG 5–98.
Renal injury from blunt abdominal trauma. **A,**
excretory urogram—injury to both kidneys
(same patient as Figs 5–91 and 5–93). The
right kidney shows substantially diminished
function from contusion. The left kidney is
distorted and displaced. The patient was operated on for other injuries (intraperitoneal
rupture of the urinary bladder [Fig 5–93] and
rupture of the left hemidiaphragm [Fig 5–91]).
The kidneys were treated conservatively. The
patient made a rapid recovery. **B,** different
patient, excretory urogram. Note the diminished excretion of contrast by the left kidney.
Retroperitoneal hemorrhage displaces the left
ureter medially, obliterates the renal outline
and psoas shadow, and produces an ill-defined mass. **C,** same patient as **B,** selective
renal angiogram. The renal cortex is tran-
sected.

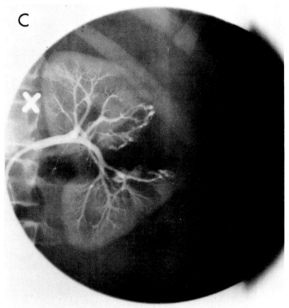

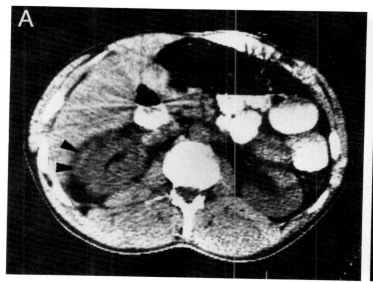

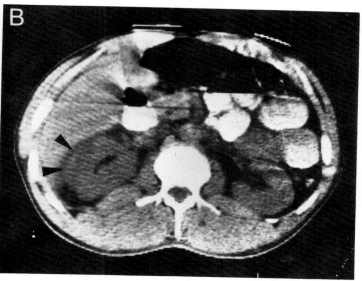

FIG 5–99.
This patient underwent CT scanning of the kidneys (**A** and **B**) following multiple trauma. An excretory urogram done in the emergency room showed a vague contour abnormality in the right kidney and a slight fall in hematocrit. The CT scan shows a crescentic density at the margin of the right kidney indicating a relatively small hematoma (*arrowheads*). Based on these relatively minimal findings, more invasive studies such as angiography were deferred.

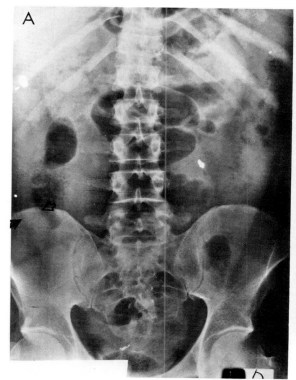

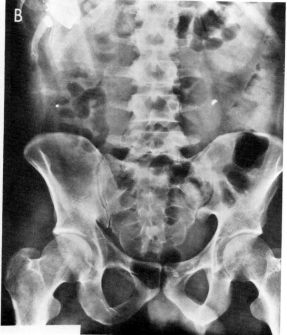

FIG 5–100.
Gunshot wound of abdomen. **A,** supine film. In addition to multiple metallic fragments, free blood in the peritoneal cavity is clearly visible in the right lateral gutter (*arrows*). There is, in all probability, blood in the left gutter as well, although the medial margin of this is not clearly visible. There are some ill-defined densities in the pelvis but no clear delineation of a dog ear sign. **B,** supine film after surgical exploration. Blood is no longer visible in either lateral gutter. Some of the metallic fragments remain in the patient.

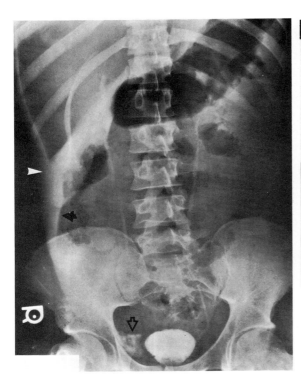

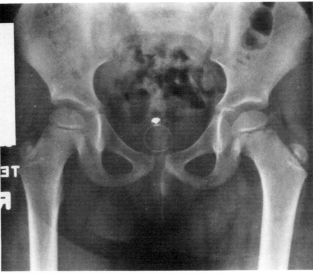

FIG 5–102 (top right).
Foreign body. Child with engagement ring in vagina.

FIG 5–101 (top left).
Stab wound of urinary bladder with perforation. Intravenous urogram shows extravasated contrast in the interstitial tissues to the right of the bladder *(open arrow)*, as well as in the right lateral gutter *(closed arrows)* and around the liver. The liver appears relatively lucent because it is surrounded by contrast material.

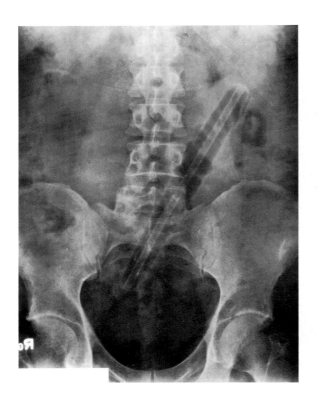

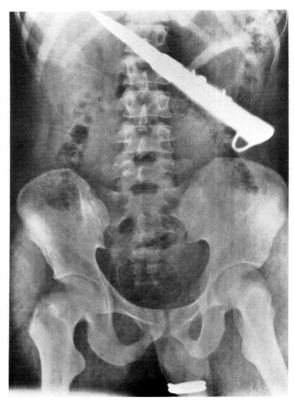

FIG 5–103 (far left).
Foreign body. Fishing cork introduced into rectum, found free in peritoneal cavity at surgery.

FIG 5–104 (near left).
Foreign body. Knife in epigastrium. Metal ring is at base of penis.

successfully for a few hours after injury. In fact, severe injury to a solitary kidney is generally an indication for angiography, since more aggressive therapy may be indicated in this circumstance.

Angiography is usually necessary specifically to diagnose renal vascular abnormality. Renal vascular lesions in blunt abdominal trauma (Fig 5–98, B and C) are substantially less frequent than contusion or disruption of the kidney. The anterior renal fascia separates the perirenal space from the anterior pararenal space of the transverse mesocolon.

Perirenal hemorrhage does not invariably obscure the adjacent psoas shadow. By compressing the perinephric fat layer, the hematoma usually reduces the fat muscle interface and renders the lateral margin of the psoas indistinct (Fig 5–99). Partial visualization of the psoas does not exclude perirenal hemorrhage. Perirenal hematoma is not an indication for immediate surgical repair, since retroperitoneal hemorrhage may occur from injury to kidneys, pancreas, retroperitoneal (bare) areas of duodenum and colon, and fractures of the spine and pelvis.

After an abdominal scout film is made, an excretory urogram with tomography is helpful in detecting retroperitoneal blood, if clinically feasible. This procedure is indicated in patients with hematuria to assess renal damage and to make sure there is a normally functioning kidney on the uninjured side. For the most part, renal damage can be managed with the urogram and follow-up of the patient. Urography is generally unsatisfactory in hypotensive patients because of failure of the kidneys to excrete the contrast.

In a hypotensive patient, angiography should be performed first. An abdominal film after angiographic contrast injection may give the same information as the urogram. Also, prompt angiography may lead to prompt therapy. An inflated balloon catheter in a transsected renal artery may be lifesaving to a patient who is hemorrhaging profusely.

Penetrating Trauma

Gunshot Wounds

Radiography is indicated in cases of gunshot wound of the abdomen to search for metallic foreign bodies (Fig 5–100). Surgical intervention is always necessary to repair bowel perforation or damage to other intra-abdominal organs. Blind exploration will be necessary if a known penetrating low-density material cannot be seen on plain films. Occasionally, when there have been multiple injuries, angiography may be used to decide which injury should be treated first. Hemorrhage may be controlled by angiographic catheter techniques.

Injury to the ureters from penetrating wounds is infrequent, probably because they are well protected anatomically by heavy adjacent bone and muscular structures. Fisher reports 9 ureteral injuries in 650 gunshot wounds to the abdomen.

Many patients with gunshot wounds are taken directly to the operating room. The optimal time for repair of the ureter is at the initial exploration.

The number of ureteral injuries ending in nephrectomy is greatly increased by delayed diagnosis and secondary repair. Up to 10% of patients have a normal urinalysis. As many as 25% are *not* diagnosed at the time of primary surgical intervention. Preoperative excretory urograms usually demonstrate the ureteral injury accurately. Therefore, an excretory urogram should be obtained if hematuria is present or if the path of the missile is near the urinary tract. Contrast extravasation at the site of ureteral injury is diagnostic. A large soft tissue mass may also be present, as the ureteral injury is usually in the midst of a large retroperitoneal hematoma. Similarly, perforations of the bladder may be demonstrated by extravasation of contrast material at the time of intravenous urography (Fig 5–101).

Injury to the ureter from blunt trauma is relatively infrequent, since the ureters are well protected anatomically by heavy adjacent bone and muscular structures. Most injuries occur when a pedestrian is struck by a motor vehicle. The pediatric age group seems more susceptible to ureteral injury, accounting for most of the case reports.

The presenting signs usually do not suggest urinary tract injury. In 10 of 15 cases, hematuria was either not present or reported as 2 to 5 RBCs per high power microscopic field. The later appearance of a flank mass is an indication for excretory urography, which will demonstrate extravasation of contrast material at the site of ureteral avulsion. Nearly all avulsions occur at or near the ureteropelvic junction.

If clinically feasible, excretory urography should be performed in a patient with hematuria because the procedure is up to 91% accurate in demonstrating ureteral injury.

Contrast extravasation at the site of ureteral injury is diagnostic. A large soft tissue mass may also be present as the ureteral injury is usually in the midst of a large retroperitoneal hematoma.

The complication rate and number of ureteral injuries ending in nephrectomy are greatly increased by delayed diagnosis and secondary repair.

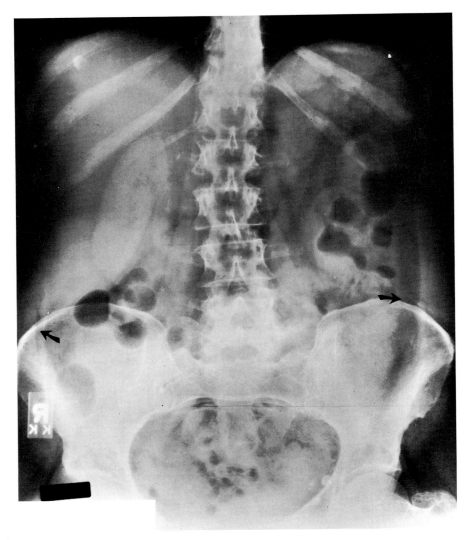

FIG 5–105.

Abdominal anatomy—normal variations (same illustration as Figs 5–3 and 5–7,**A**).

Bone structure	Normal (note slight scoliosis).
Lung bases	(Bright light) normal.
Opacities	Calcified granuloma, liver.
	Metallic artifact, left hemidiaphragm.
	Multiple phleboliths, left hemipelvis.
Major organs	Liver to iliac crest.
	Spleen: vaguely visible, left upper quadrant.
	Kidneys: both well delineated by surrounding fat.
	Bladder: not clearly visible.
Flank stripes	*Black arrows.* Stripe is narrow on right, wide on left.
Psoas shadows	Well defined (better on right).
Gas in bowel	Colon: Cecal gas adjacent to flank stripe. The potential space of the right lateral gutter is seen between the cecal gas and very narrow right flank stripe; this is the maximum normal width of the lateral gutter. Lateral gutter also visible on left between descending colon and left flank stripe. Colon gas also visible in splenic flexure, sigmoid, and rectum.
	Small bowel: none seen.
	Stomach: faint shadow in left upper quadrant (below spleen, medial to splenic flexure).
Gas outside bowel	None seen.
Masses	None seen.

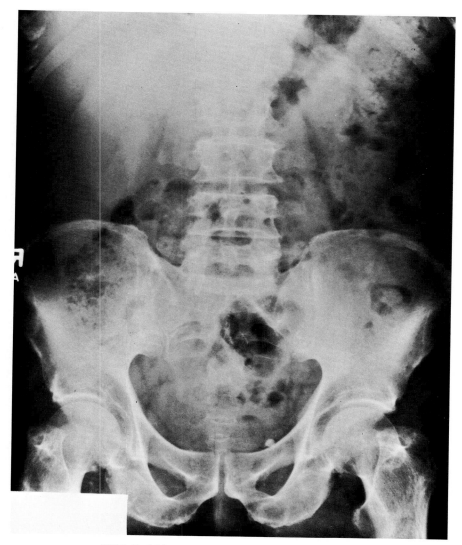

FIG 5–106.
Abdominal anatomy—normal variations.

Bones	There is a lucency in intertrochanteric regions bilaterally. Further evaluation suggested.
Lung bases	Not on film.
Opacities	Calcified costal cartilage in right upper quadrant at corner of film. There is minimal costal cartilage calcification in this patient; however, any amount of costal cartilage calcification is normal at any age. Very extensive rib cartilage calcification may be seen in some individuals (see Fig 5–4,**A**).
	Phlebolith above left superior pubic ramus.
Major organs	Liver projects to iliac crest.
	Spleen not visible.
	Kidneys well shown.
	Bladder very faint; note fat delineating bladder margin on right.
Flank stripes	Narrow; can be identified on both right and left at level of iliac crests.
Psoas shadows	Left well defined; right poorly defined.
Gas in bowel	Colon: note fecal material mixed with gas scattered through colon. This is the principal feature that usually makes colon recognizable. Visible superimposed on sacrum and in pelvis.
	Small bowel: none.
	Stomach: clearly visible in left upper quadrant.
Gas outside bowel	None.
Masses	None.

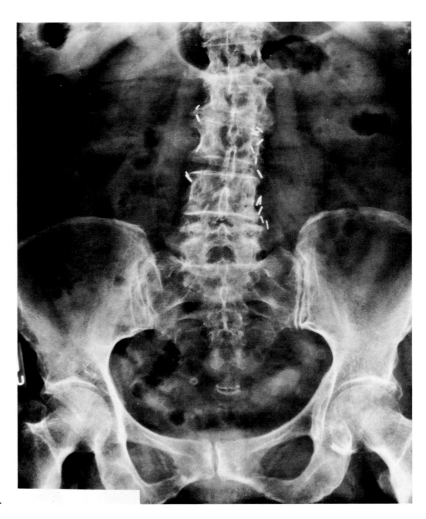

FIG 5–107.
Abdominal anatomy—normal variations.

Bones	Spine scoliotic. Narrow intervertebral spaces and osteophytic lipping of margins on a degenerative basis. Bones may be slightly demineralized. This is difficult to evaluate because variations in x-ray technique cause variations in apparent bone density. However, edges of the vertebral bodies and iliac crests are of relatively greater density, favoring osseous demineralization. This is especially apparent at the junction of the sacrum and coccyx.
Lung bases	Not on film.
Opacities	Costal cartilage in upper quadrant is barely included on film on left. There is a small adjacent artifact.
	Phlebolith to right of coccyx. Unusually high in position. Note lucent center.
	Surgical clips along both sides of spine.
	Film marker adjacent to right ischium.
	Vague curvilinear shadow projected along inferior margin of left femoral head, possibly in joint capsule.
	Tiny calcific density in lower part of the left pubic symphysis. A slightly larger one is present along the inferior margin of the right pubic symphysis. These are most likely phleboliths but could be small benign bone islands of no consequence.
Major organs	Liver edge visible at right costal margin. Hepatic flexure gas superimposed. Note how much smaller apparent liver size is in comparison to previous two patients.
	Spleen not visible.
	Kidneys rather high in abdomen.
	Bladder very low in position, behind pubic bones, indicating relaxation of pelvic floor.
Flank stripes	Clearly shown on both sides. The flank stripe on the right is very narrow; a small amount of bowel gas is adjacent. Stripe on the left is very wide; opacity medial to it is fluid in the descending colon. This is a trap when evaluating for blood in the peritoneal cavity. One can be sure of the presence of blood in the lateral gutter only if it is seen between the flank stripe and colon gas. Occasionally, gas in small bowel will be slightly separated from the flank stripe, giving the false impression of fluid in the lateral gutter. This patient is a good example of normal flank anatomy in that there is a very small amount of small bowel gas medial to the fluid in the descending colon, which emphasizes the latter structure.
Psoas shadows	Well shown, extending well down over iliac crests on both sides.
Gas in bowel	Colon: gas scattered through colon in peripheral abdomen. Haustrations and fecal content are not prominent, making differentiation between colon and small-bowel gas extremely difficult in this patient.
	Small bowel: small amount of gas is scattered through small bowel. None of the small bowel is distended, and there are no definite characteristics.
	Stomach: projected in upper central abdomen. The stomach appears inverted. Differentiation between stomach and transverse colon gas in this patient is uncertain.
Gas outside bowel	None.
Masses	Vague oval shadow in the left hemipelvis, most likely fluid in the sigmoid colon.

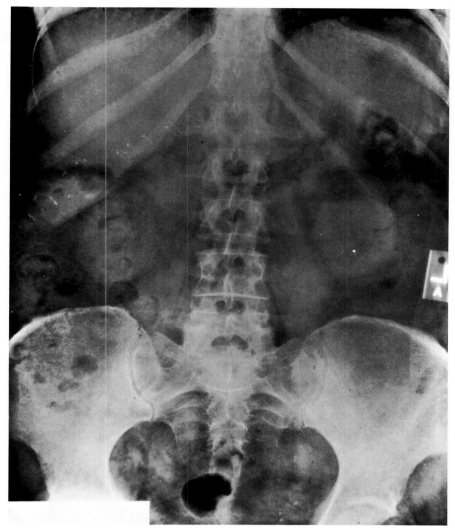

FIG 5–108.
Abdominal anatomy—normal variations (same illustration as Fig 5–5,**A**).

Bones	Normal.
Lung bases	Barely visible on left; no pleural fluid detected.
Opacities	Phleboliths, left hemipelvis.
	Sutures, right upper quadrant.
	Artifact, lower pole of left kidney.
	Film marker on left; tape produces a vertical line or shadow projecting over the iliac crest.
Major organs	Liver edge partially obscured by colon content.
	Spleen slightly enlarged.
	Kidneys normal.
	Bladder not on film.
Flank stripes	Right, not on film, left obscured by marker tape.
Psoas shadows	Left clearly shown, right partially obscured.
Gas in bowel	Colon: fecal material clearly identifies colon, prominent rectal bubble. Note fecal material in sigmoid colon.
	Small bowel: none.
	Stomach: projected obliquely across upper pole of left kidney.
Gas outside bowel	None. Vague gas shadow projected just below left hemidiaphragm is most likely in gastric fundus.
Masses	None.

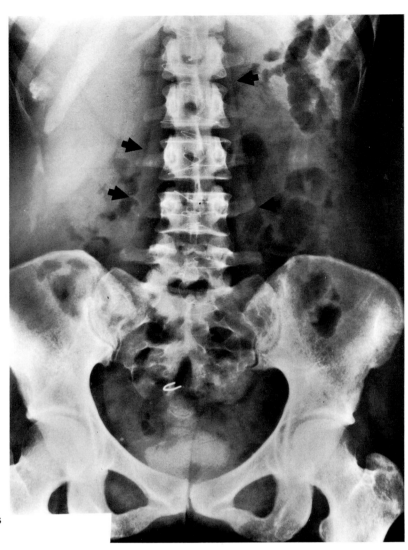

FIG 5–109.
Abdominal anatomy—normal variations
(same illustration as Fig 5–6).

Bones	Slight scoliosis.
Lungs	Not on film.
Opacities	Calcified costal cartilage well shown on right, rather obscure on left.
	Surgical clip projected over sacrum.
	Phlebolith, right hemipelvis
	Tiny density (artifact), left hemipelvis.
Major organs	Liver edge halfway between ribs and iliac crest.
	Spleen not visible.
	Kidneys: right kidney very high, superimposed on liver adjacent to upper lumbar spine; left obscured by bowel gas.
	Bladder well defined.
Flank stripes	Narrow and faint on both sides. On right can be seen extending along lateral liver edge, where free air localizes on a left lateral decubitus abdomen film.
Psoas shadows	*Black arrows.*
Gas in bowel	Colon: scattered in picture-frame distribution.
	Small bowel: gas in left abdomen. Note bent finger and valvulae conniventes. This pattern is consistent with the "nonspecific abdomen." Minimal small-bowel gas in nondistended loops may at times also be present in normal patients.
	Stomach: obscured by superimposed small bowel gas.
Gas outside bowel	None.
Masses	None.

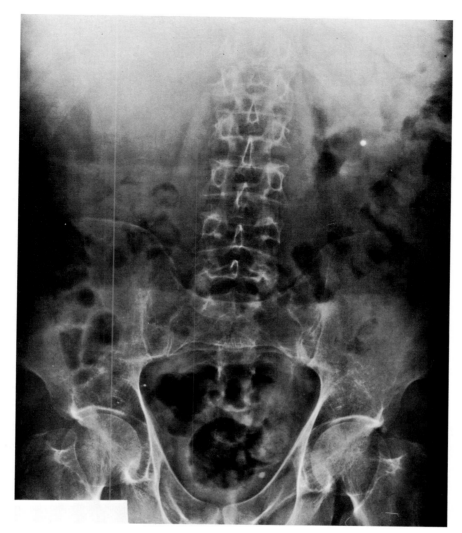

FIG 5–110.
Abdominal anatomy—normal variations.

Bones	Demineralized; note sharp margins of vertebral bodies, iliac crests, and hip joints.
Lung bases	Not included.
Opacities	Birdshot in left central abdomen (seen in patients who eat wild game).
	Phlebolith, left hemipelvis.
Major organs	Liver projects over iliac crest.
	Spleen not visible.
	Kidneys rather obscure, due to paucity of body fat. Right kidney is visible along the right psoas margin superimposed on liver shadow; left can be seen in left upper quadrant. The birdshot is over the lower pole.
	Bladder obscured by fecal content in colon; right edge is visible.
Flank stripes	Very narrow and poorly delineated, due to paucity of body fat.
Psoas shadows	Visible on both sides.
Gas in bowel	Colon: gas and fecal material scattered throughout. The transverse colon is low in position (projected along iliac crests). Some haustrations are visible.
	Small bowel: none.
	Stomach: gas visible medially and above birdshot.

Foreign Bodies

The human species has a propensity for inserting various objects into body orifices. Most physicians with substantial emergency department experience have seen all manner of foreign bodies introduced into the body in various ways (Figs 5–102 to 5–104). Each is an individual consideration for diagnosis and treatment.

As a general rule, ingested foreign bodies are best left to pass through the intestinal tract naturally unless some special circumstance dictates surgical intervention.

Except for metallic objects, foreign bodies are extremely difficult or impossible to demonstrate intra-abdominally, because the thickness of the abdominal tissues obscures any low-density material.

Normal Variants, Calcifications, Oddities, and "Aunt Minnies"

The six cases illustrated here (Figs 5–105 to 5–110) point out the great variation in normal anatomy. The reader is encouraged to use them to develop a systematic approach to film analysis.

Calcifications and Opacities

Radiology is not learned by memorizing lists, but rather by recognizing patterns. The following calcifications and opacities are offered as a checklist of recognizable patterns.

Costal cartilages
Vascular (aneurysm, atherosclerosis)
Mesenteric lymph nodes
Gallstones
Kidney cysts and neoplasms
Urinary stones (kidney, ureter, bladder)
Pancreatic stones
Enteroliths (coproliths)
Granulomatous foci in lung, liver, spleen
Parasites (calcified or in bowel)
Diaphragm (asbestosis)
Hepatic (hematoma, echinococcal cyst, cavernous hemangioma)
Cystic duct
Pancreatic trauma (necrosis, pseudocyst)
Adrenal (tumor, granuloma)
Infarcts of spleen and kidney
Abscess wall (subphrenic, intra-abdominal)
Dermoid, teratoma

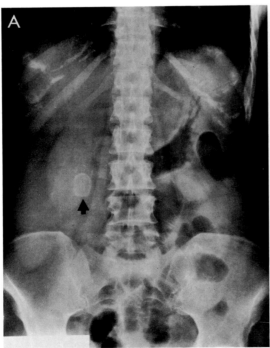 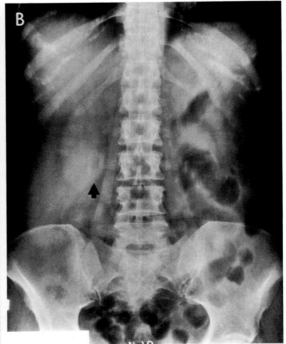

FIG 5–111.
A, gallstone *(black arrow).* **B,** same patient. Gallstone obscured by breathing motion during x-ray exposure.

It is important to be aware that motion unsharpness can obscure gross detail.

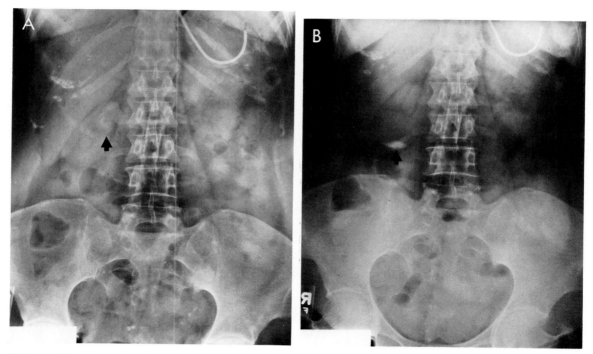

FIG 5–112.
Milk of calcium bile. **A,** supine film. Calcium in gallbladder is obscure *(black arrow).* **B,** upright film. Calcium in gallbladder forms amorphous layer.

FIG 5–113.
Pancreatic calcification in head *(lower arrow)* and tail *(upper arrow).*

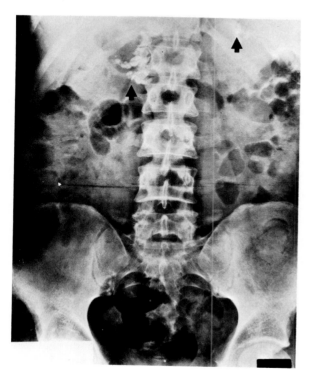

FIG 5–114.
Calcified right multicystic kidney.

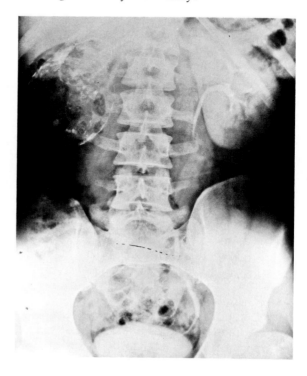

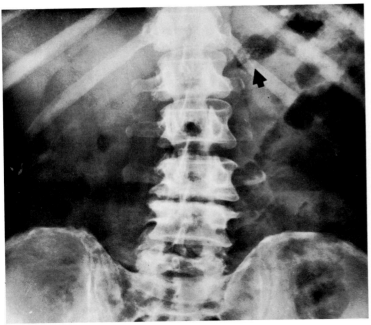

FIG 5–115.
Calcified adrenal gland *(arrow)*. Also note phlebolith or calcified granuloma above gas in stomach. It is most likely in the spleen.

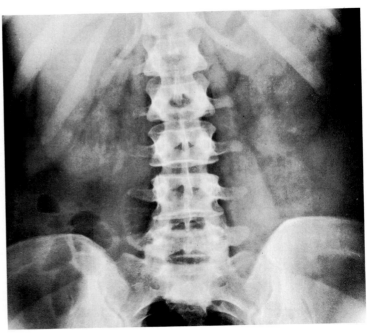

FIG 5–116.
Nephrocalcinosis. The calcifications in both kidneys are very tiny.

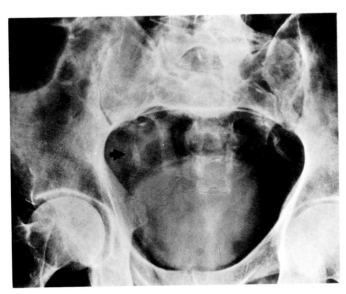

FIG 5–117 (left).
Calcified pelvic arteries *(arrows)*.

FIG 5–118 (right).
Calcified abdominal aortic aneurysm projecting to the right of the lower lumbar spine *(arrow)*. Aneurysms usually present as a shell-like, curvilinear, calcific density. Two thirds are detected along the left margin

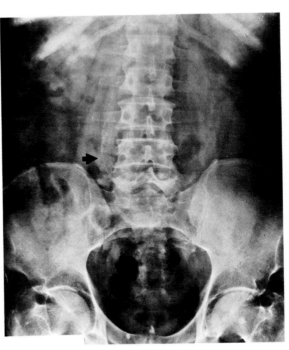

of the spine. A lateral view of the lumbar spine is often helpful in identification. If you suspect aneurysm because of a palpable mass or bruit, abdominal sonography is the method of choice for diagnosis.

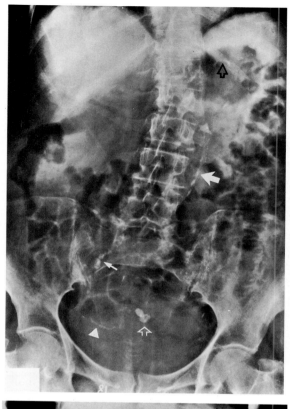

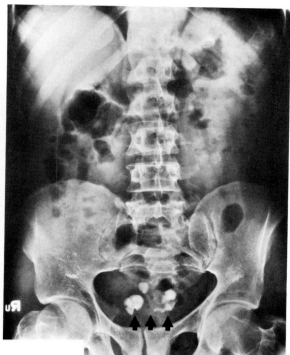

FIG 5–119 (top left).
Calcified abdominal aorta *(large white arrow)*, iliac arteries *(small white arrow)*, and splenic artery *(open black arrow)*. Calcified bladder stones *(open white arrow)*. Calcified fallopian tube *(triangle)*. Note that both walls of the abdominal aorta are visible. The urinary bladder is quite distended.

FIG 5–120 (top right).
Multiple bladder stones *(arrows)*. Bladder stones are always faceted if multiple, round or oval if single.

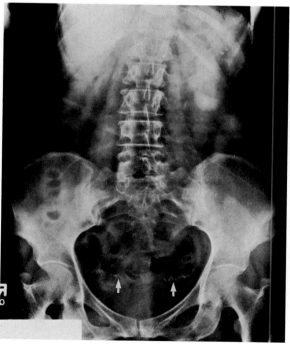

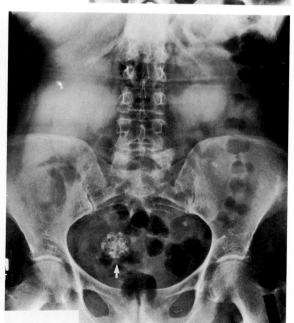

FIG 5–121 (bottom left).
Calcified fallopian tubes *(arrows)*. Calcified seminal vesicles in the male are virtually identical in appearance. Both are more common in diabetic patients.

FIG 5–122 (bottom right).
Calcified uterine fibroid. A typically calcified uterine fibroid resembles a popcorn ball.

FIG 5–123 (top left).
Ovarian dermoid (teratoma). A right pelvic mass *(arrows)* is characterized by amorphous calcification surrounded by radiolucent fat. The calcifications at times have the appearance of teeth. The fat layer is not always present.

FIG 5–124 (top right).
Intra-abdominal surgical sponge. Surgical sponges are marked with an opaque thread in order to make them visible by x-ray examination.

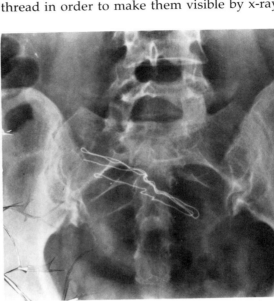

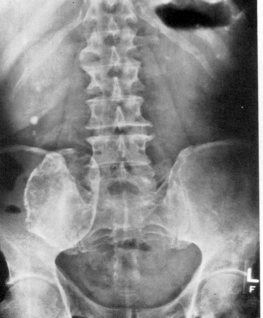

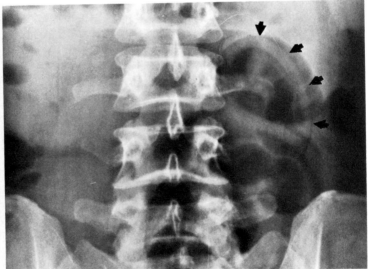

FIG 5–125 (bottom left).
Old calcified surgical sponge. A calcified right lower quadrant mass was found at autopsy to be a calcified surgical sponge left in abdomen at time of chole-cystectomy, 18 years earlier. At that time surgical sponges were not marked with opaque thread; thus it went undetected. Also note multiple right renal calculi.

FIG 5–126 (bottom right).
Ascaris in small bowel *(arrows)*. If the patient is given barium, the ascaris may ingest it, confirming the diagnosis. This is the same patient seen in Fig 5–5,B (which also shows the ascaris).

FIG 5–127 (top left).
Doughnut pessary in vagina *(arrows)*.

FIG 5–128 (top right).
Gas in the gallbladder; emphysematous cholecystitis *(arrows)*.

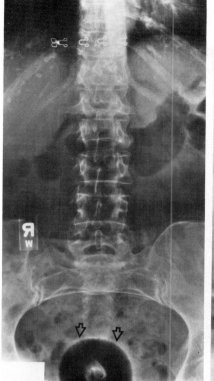

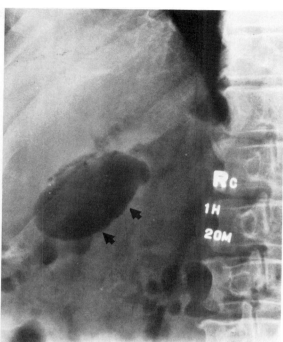

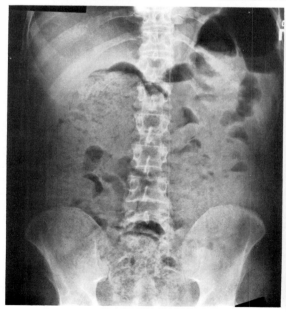

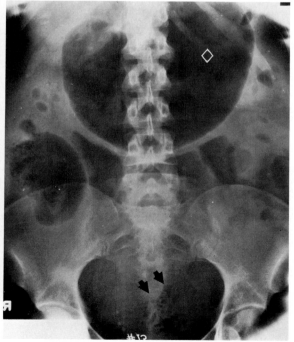

FIG 5–129 (bottom left).
Massive fecal accumulation in colon.

FIG 5–130 (bottom right).
Gastric distention. The patient was admitted to the emergency department in a diabetic coma. Note acute gastric distention *(diamond)*. *Arrows* point to a cluster of gas bubbles in the pelvis incident to vaginitis em-physematosa (seen in diabetics). On this single film, the gas bubbles cannot be differentiated from colon content. Gas in the vaginal wall was confirmed by a lateral view (not shown).

Abdomen—Calcifications and Opacities / **341**

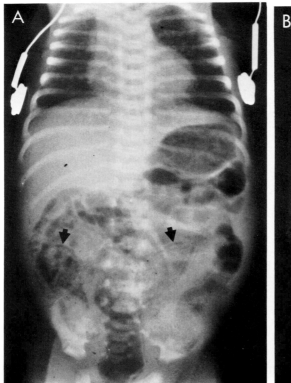

FIG 5–131.
Pneumatosis intestinalis in necrotizing enterocolitis. Note air *(arrows)* in the wall of the small intestine (best seen in lateral view). Pneumatosis intestinalis may also occur in a benign, asymptomatic form in adults and may produce asymptomatic pneumoperitoneum. This form does not require surgery.

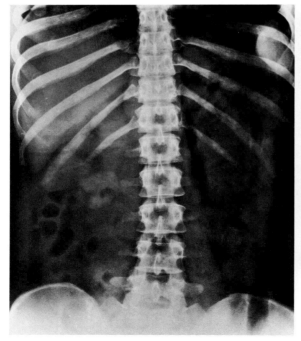

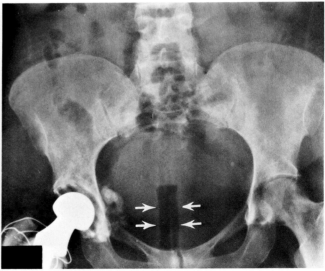

kidney. There is also some intraperitoneal gas detectable at the liver margin. In this patient, both are iatrogenic following an unsuccessful pelvic pneumogram. Pelvic pneumography for ovarian evaluation has been replaced by pelvic ultrasound.

FIG 5–132 (bottom left).
Retroperitoneal dissection of gas. Note gas surrounding the left

FIG 5–133 (bottom right).
Vaginal tampon *(arrows).*

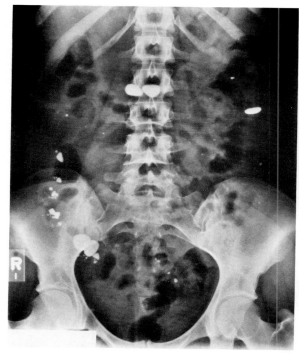

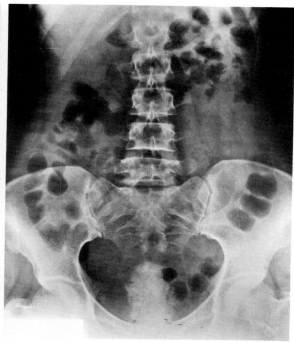

FIG 5–134 (top left).
Enteric-coated pills, some partially disintegrated.

FIG 5–135 (top right).
Iodoform packing in vagina.

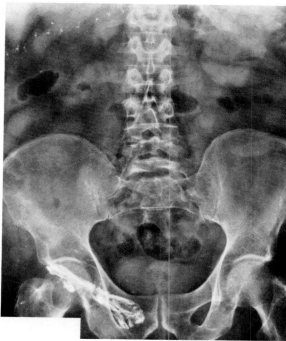

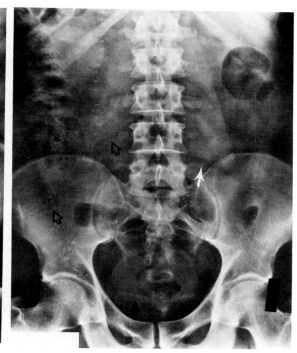

FIG 5–136 (bottom left).
Tantalum mesh in right inguinal region used for inguinal hernia repair. Sutures in right upper quadrant from prior cholecystectomy.

FIG 5–137 (bottom right).
Note the suture material to the right of the midline. There are several linear artifacts projected over the right abdomen due to folds in the patient's gown or in the sheet on the x-ray table

(open arrows). An interesting artifact is a butterfly-like shadow projected above the pubic symphysis representing the patient's buttocks on the x-ray table *(black arrows)*. There is another soft tissue shadow projected transversely above the sacroiliac joints across the fifth lumbar vertebra. This is also due to the soft tissues of the patient's buttocks *(white arrow)*. This is the same patient shown in Figure 5–17,**A.** Note the sentinel loop in the left upper quadrant (bent-finger sign).

Uterine myoma
Pregnancy
Gluteal fat necrosis
Prostate
Bismuth in gluteus muscles
Birdshot in bowel
Surgical vascular clips

Wire sutures
Barium in colon diverticula
Various foreign materials
Figures 5–111 through 5–137 illustrate some of the more important or confusing abdominal opacities and radiolucencies.

Suggested Reading

Abrams HL: *Abrams Angiography: Vascular and Interventional Radiology*, ed 3. Boston, Little, Brown & Co, 1983.

Callen PW: *Ultrasonography in Obstetrics and Gynecology*, ed 2. Philadelphia, WB Saunders Co, 1988.

Fleischer AC, James AE: *Principles and Practice of Sonography*. Philadelphia, WB Saunders Co, 1988.

Johnsrude, IS, Jackson DC, Dunnick NR: *A Practical Approach to Angiography*, ed 2. Boston, Little, Brown & Co, 1987.

Keats TE: *Atlas of Normal Roentgen Variants That May Simulate Disease*, ed 4. Chicago, Year Book Medical Publishers, 1988.

Keats TE, Smith TH: *Atlas of Normal Developmental Roentgen Anatomy*, ed 2. Chicago, Year Book Medical Publishers, 1988.

Margulis AR, Burhenne J: *Abdominal Imaging (Alimentary Tract Radiology)*, vol 3. St Louis, CV Mosby Co, 1983.

Meyers MA: *Dynamic Radiology of the Abdomen, Normal and Pathologic Anatomy*. New York, Springer-Verlag, 1988.

Putman CE, Ravin, CE: *Textbook of Diagnostic Imaging*. Philadelphia, WB Saunders Co, 1988.

Toombs BD, Sandler CM: *Computed Tomography in Trauma*. Philadelphia, WB Saunders Co, 1987.

Rosenberger A: *Trauma Imaging in the Thorax and Abdomen*. Chicago, Year Book Medical Publishers, 1987.

Sarti DA: *Diagnostic Ultrasound*, ed 2. Chicago, Year Book Medical Publishers, 1986.

Swischuk LE: *Emergency Radiology of the Acutely Ill or Injured Child*, ed 2. Baltimore, Williams & Wilkins Co, 1986.

Normal Variants

Theodore E. Keats, M.D.

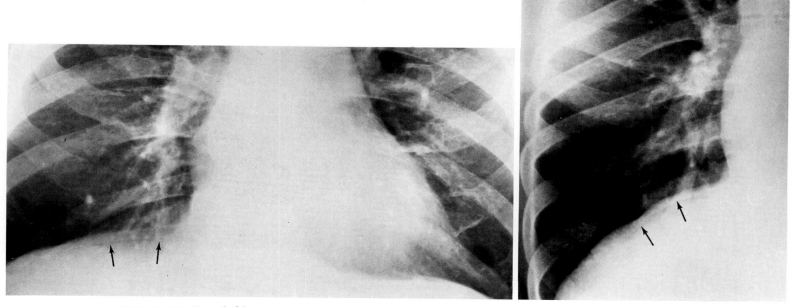

FIG 5–138 (top left).
Simulated pneumoperitoneum. This is usually the product of fat beneath the diaphragm.

FIG 5–139 (top right).
Simulated pneumoperitoneum produced by overlapping shadows of the rib and diaphragm. (Ref: Martinez LO, Raskin MM: Fat under the diaphragm simulating pneumoperitoneum. *Br J Radiol* 1974; 47:308.)

FIG 5–140 (bottom).
Simulated pneumoperitoneum produced by fat around the lateral and superior aspects of the liver.

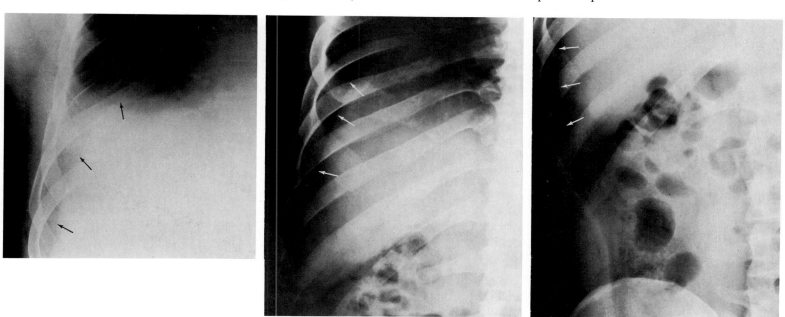

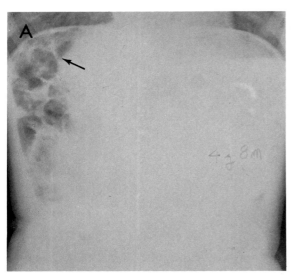

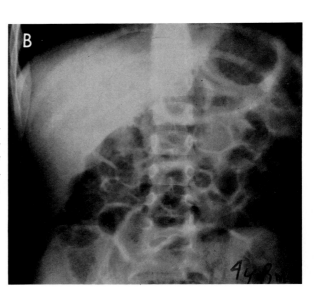

FIG 5–141.
Colonic interposition between the liver and diaphragm in a 4-year-old boy **(A)** and its spontaneous reduction on the same day **(B)**.

FIG 5–142.
Colonic interposition on the right, simulating pneumoperitoneum.

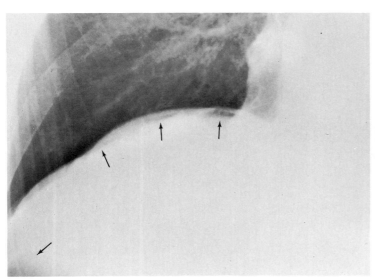

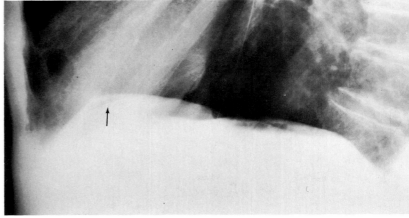

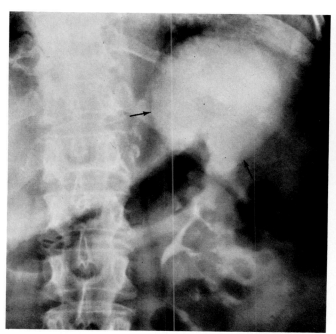
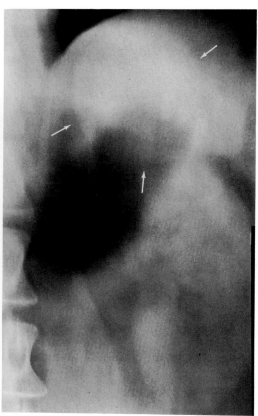

FIG 5–143.

In the supine position, the fluid-filled fundus of the stomach simulating a mass lesion. On the left, plain film; on the right, laminagram. This pseudotumor may opacify on angiography and further obscure its proper identification. (Ref: Bjorn-Hansen RW, O'Brien DS: Aortographic opacification of the gastric fundus simulating neoplasm. *Am J Roentgenol* 1967; 100:408.)

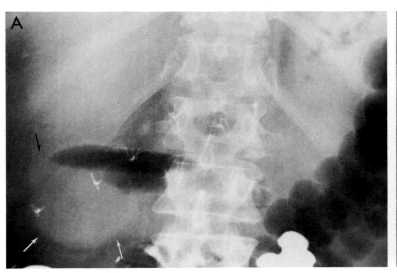

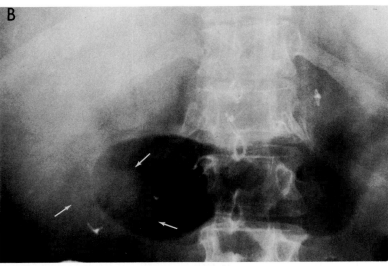

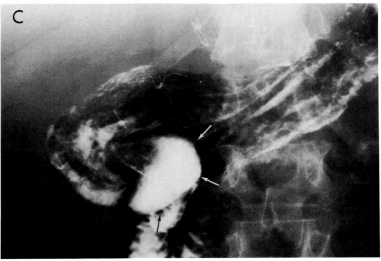

FIG 5–144.
A, the fluid-filled duodenal bulb may present as a right upper quadrant mass in the prone position. **B,** supine position shows mass less distinctly. **C,** barium examination shows the mass effect to be due to the duodenal bulb.

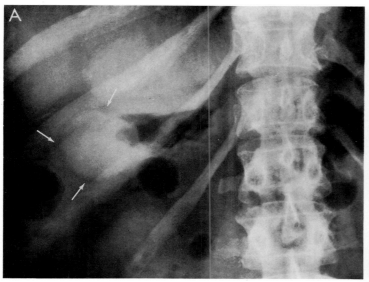

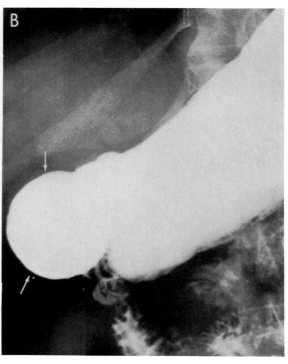

FIG 5–145.
A, in the prone position the fluid-filled gastric antrum may also simulate a right upper quadrant mass. **B,** antrum filled with barium in same position as **A.** (Ref: Balthazar E: Right upper quadrant pseudotumor, a fluid-filled viscus. *Radiology* 1974; 112:11.)

FIG 5–146.
Ring-shaped calcified costal cartilage, simulating gallstones.

FIG 5–147.
Calcified costal cartilage in the left upper quadrant, simulating a renal calculus.

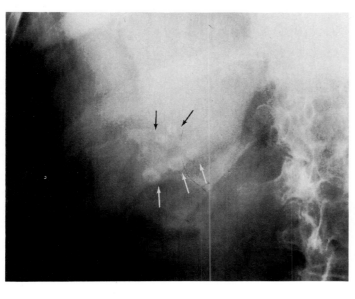

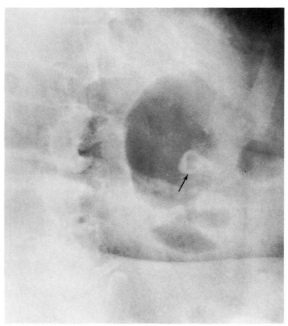

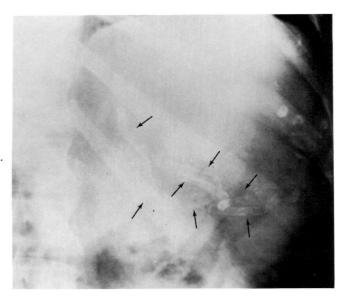

FIG 5–148.
Calcification in a tortuous splenic artery.

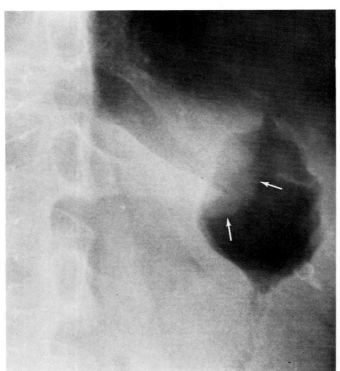

FIG 5–149.
The left lobe of the liver presenting into the gastric air bubble (proved at surgery), simulating a neoplasm.

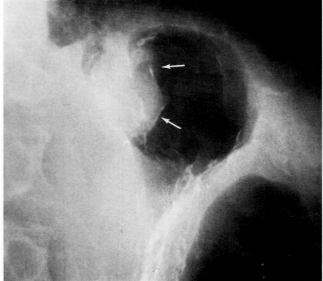

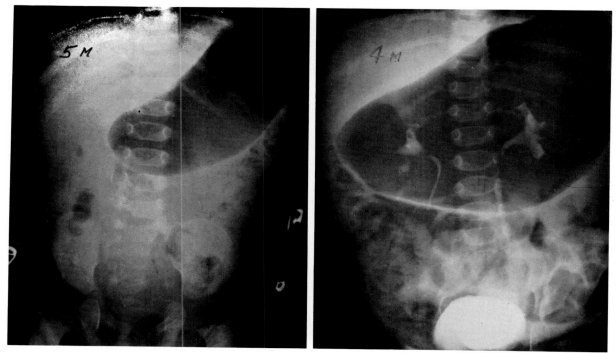

FIG 5–150.
Demonstration of normal degrees of distention of the infantile stomach.

FIG 5–151.
Three examples of the pylorus of the stomach, simulating a fissured biliary calculus. In **B** and **C** the air in the duodenal bulb simulates emphysematous cholecystitis with stone.

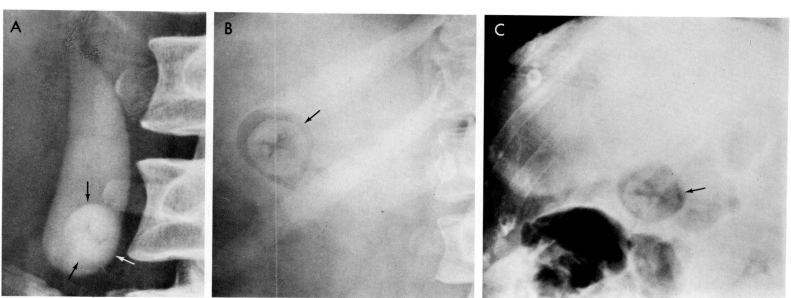

FIG 5–152.
The shadows of the levator ani muscles *(arrow)*. The obturator internus muscles are also seen *(notched arrow)*. (Ref: Levene G, Kaufman JA: The diagnostic significance of roentgenologic soft tissue shadows in the pelvis. *Am J Roentgenol* 1958; 79:697.)

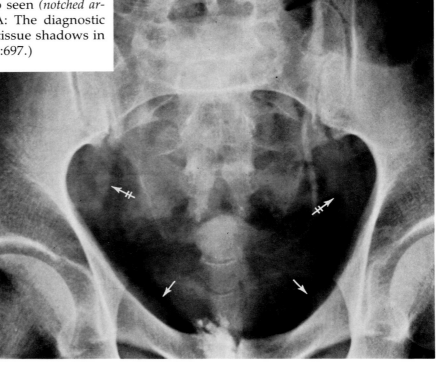

FIG 5–153.
Examples of calcification of the sacrospinal ligaments.

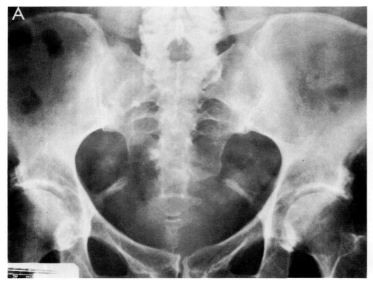

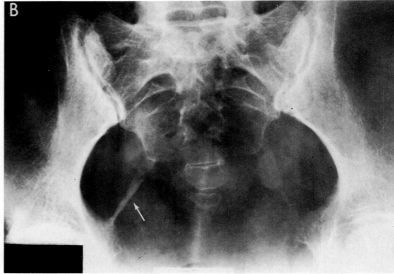

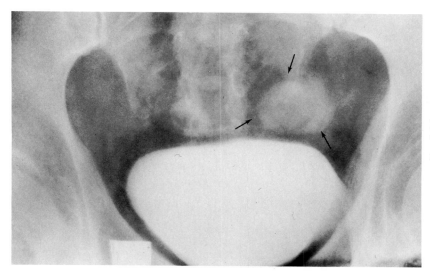

FIG 5–154.
The sigmoid colon simulating a pelvic mass.

FIG 5–155.
Calcification of the sacrotuberous ligaments.

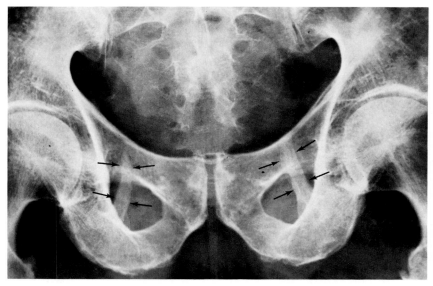

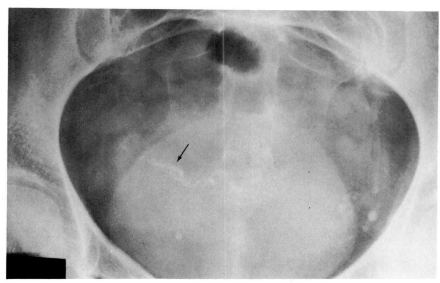

FIG 5–156.
Calcification in the uterine arteries in an elderly woman.

FIG 5–157.
Calcification of the fallopian tubes in an elderly woman.

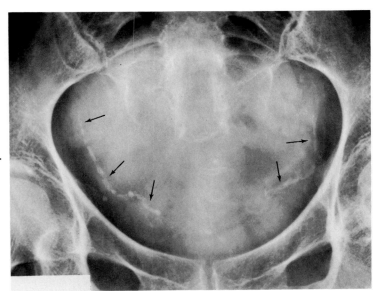

FIG 5–158.
Apparent absence of one psoas muscle. This is seen in many normal individuals and is not necessarily of significance. (Ref: Elkin M, Cohen G: Diagnostic value of psoas shadow. *Clin Radiol* 1962; 13:210.)

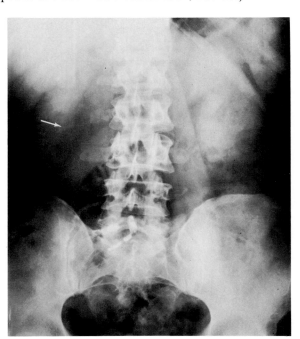

FIG 5–159.
The low-lying left kidney. The left kidney lies at a level lower than the right in 5% of normal individuals and is, therefore, not necessarily indicative of displacement. (Ref: McClelland RE: A low-lying left kidney. *J Urol* 1956; 75:198.)

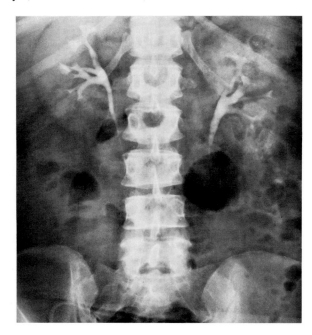

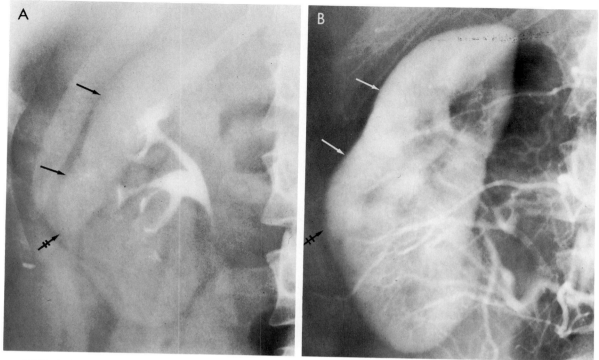

FIG 5–160.
The hepatic impression *(arrow)* upon the right kidney that produces a "bump" in its midportion *(notched arrow)*. **A,** urogram; **B,** angiogram. (Ref: Doppman JL, Shapiro R: Some normal renal variants. *Am J Roentgenol* 1964; 92:1380.)

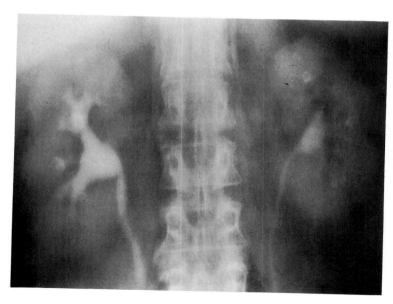

FIG 5–161.
Fetal lobulation of the kidneys.

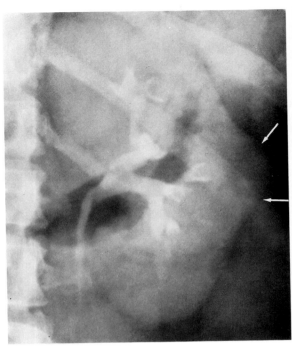

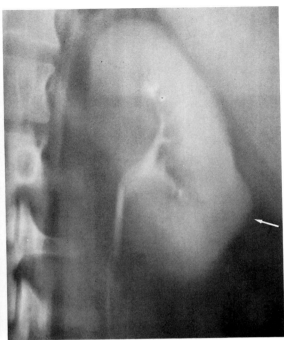

FIG 5–162.
Two examples of the dromedary left kidney, an anatomical variation that simulates a mass lesion. (Ref: Harrow BP, Sloane JA: The dromedary left kidney. *Am J Roentgenol* 1962; 88:148.)

FIG 5–163.
The gastric fundus simulating a suprarenal mass. **A,** before ingestion of barium; **B,** after ingestion of barium. (Ref: Martire JR, Goldman SM: Left suprarenal pseudotumor. *Radiobiologiia* 1977; 17:12.) This pseudotumor may opacify on angiography and further obscure its proper identification. (Ref: Bjorn-Hansen RW, O'Brien DS: Aortographic opacification of the gastric fundus simulating neoplasm. *Am J Roentgenol* 1967; 100:408.)

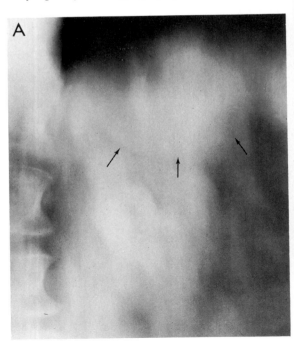

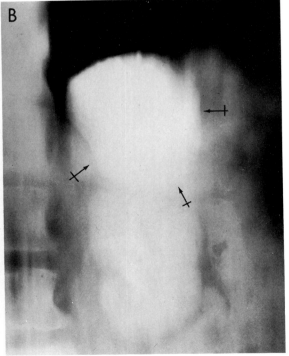

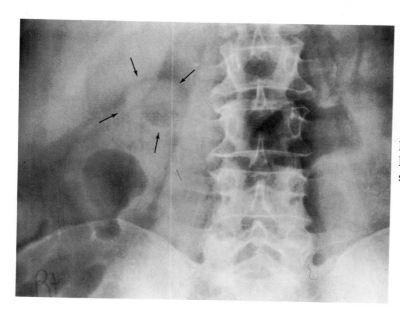

FIG 5–164.
Fluid-filled duodenal bulb, simulating a suprarenal mass.

FIG 5–165.
Two examples of renal pseudotumors produced by the spleen. (Ref: Madayag M, et al: Renal and suprarenal pseudotumors caused by variations of the spleen. *Radiology* 1972; 105:43.)

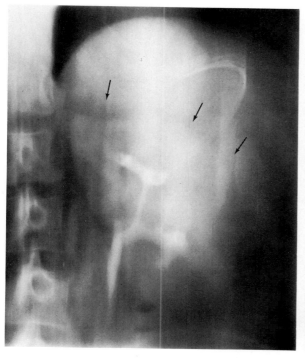 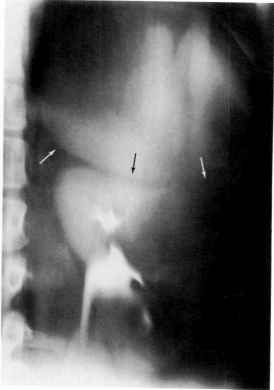

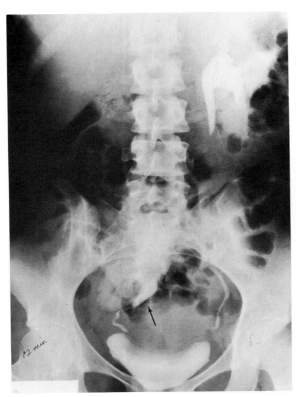

FIG 5–166.
Pelvic kidney.

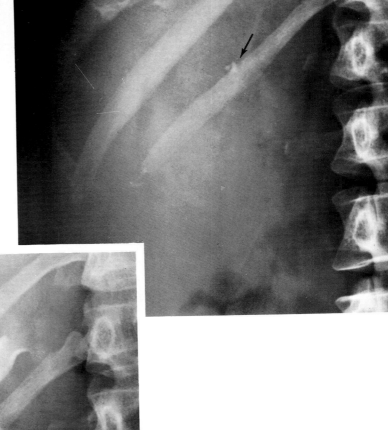

FIG 5–167.
A, costal cartilage calcification, simulating renal calculi. **B,** the calcification is obscured by the contrast material in the urogram.

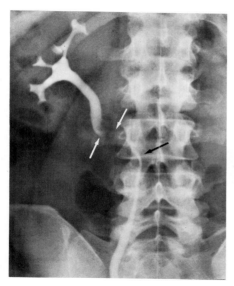

FIG 5–168.
The retrocaval ureter, coursing around the posterior aspect of the inferior vena cava. (Ref: Emmett JL, Witten DM: *Clinical Urography,* ed 3. Philadelphia, WB Saunders Co, 1971, p 1327.)

FIG 5–169.
Medial deviation of the distal ureters as a normal variant due to iliopsoas hypertrophy, and not secondary to retroperitoneal fibrosis. (Ref: Saldino RM, Palubinskas AJ: Medial placement of the ureters: A normal variant which may simulate retroperitoneal fibrosis. *J Urol* 1972; 107:582.)

FIG 5–170.
Asymmetry of the pelvic ureters in normal females, with medial deviation of the distal right ureter, is seen as a normal variation. (Ref: Kabakian HA, et al: Asymmetry of the pelvic ureters in normal females. *Am J Roentgenol* 1976; 127:723.)

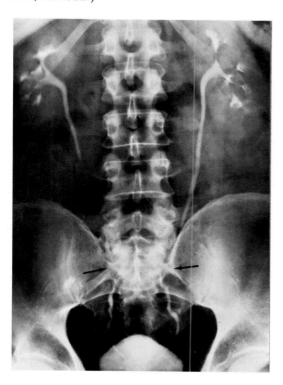

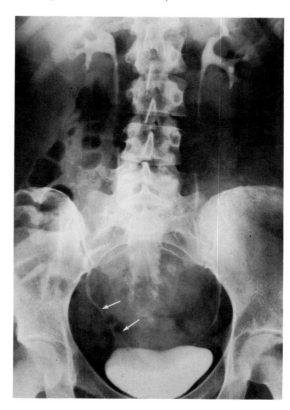

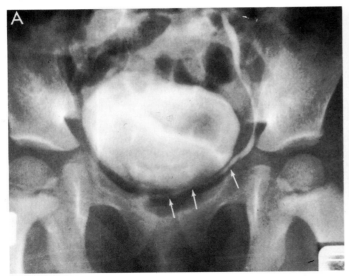

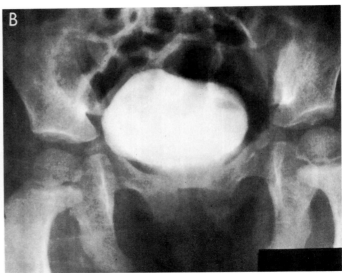

FIG 5–171.
A, a pseudoectopic ureter seen in the prone position, in which the contrast material in the bladder gravitates toward the head into the dependent anterior dome and leaves the trigone area filled with nonopa- cified urine. The distal ureters appear to extend below the bladder. **B,** supine film does not show the same effect seen in **A.** (Ref: Riggs W, Jr, Seibert J: Pseu- doectopic ureter on prone urogram. *Radiology* 1973; 106:391.)

FIG 5–172.
Two examples of the ureteral jet phenomenon. A stream of opaque medium leaving the ureter may simulate an anomalous configuration of the ureter. Note the impaction of the jet on the bladder wall in **A** *(notched arrow).* (Ref: Kalmon EH, et al: Ureteral jet phenomenon. Stream of opaque medium simulating anomalous configuration of ureter. *Radiology* 1955; 65:933.)

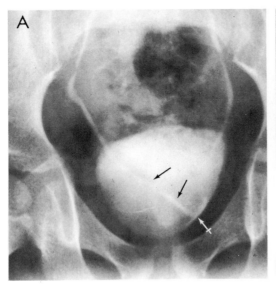

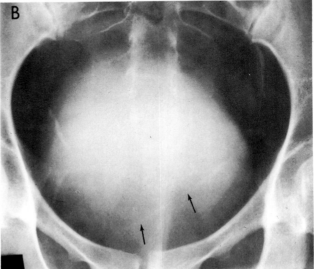

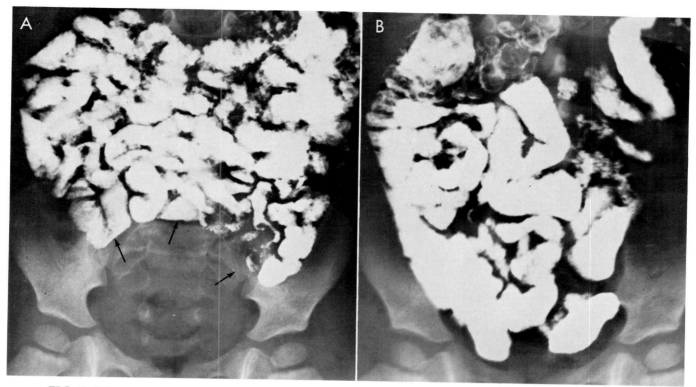

FIG 5–173.
A, normal distention of the bladder in a 2-year-old, displacing the small bowel; **B,** after voiding.

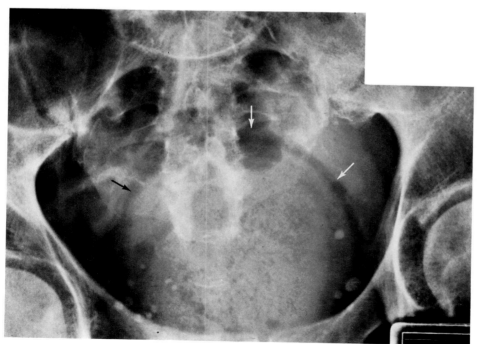

FIG 5–174.
Perivesical fat producing an appearance simulating emphysematous cystitis.

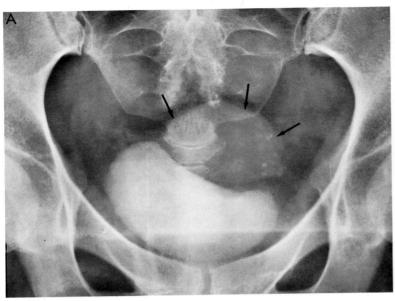

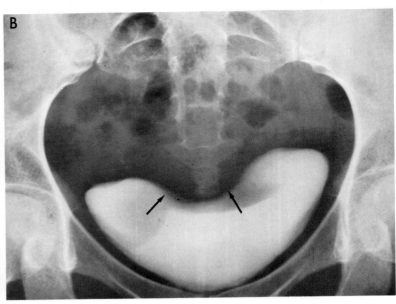

FIG 5–175.
The uterine impression on the bladder. **A,** the shadow of the uterus is seen indenting the bladder. **B,** the shadow of the uterus is not seen above the impression on the bladder.

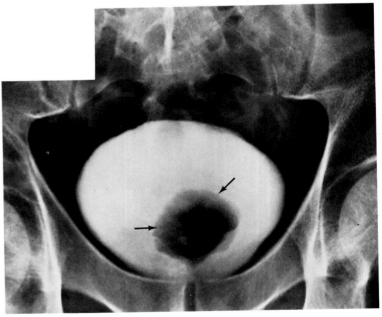

FIG 5–176.
Gas in the rectum seen as a radiolucency within the contrast-filled bladder, simulating the filling defect of a bladder neoplasm.

6
Pelvis and Hips

Hans O. Riddervold, M.D.
Thomas Lee Pope, Jr., M.D.

The pelvis and hips are commonly injured in trauma and can be an especially difficult region to evaluate clinically. Thus, the x-ray examination is heavily relied upon in making clinical judgments and deciding upon subsequent therapy.

The principal cause of morbidity and mortality in pelvic injuries is hemorrhage, as the retroperitoneal space may harbour up to 2,000 cc of blood without obvious radiographic abnormality on the plain films. Death from pelvic hemorrhage has been estimated to occur in as many as 30% of cases, although interventional angiography with embolization has markedly reduced this figure.[1-3] Urethral or bladder damage is another significant injury associated with pelvic trauma. It is estimated that this type of injury occurs in 20% of patients with pelvic arch fractures, and many experts think that all patients with pelvic trauma should be evaluated for bladder and urethral injury.[4] Of course, an adequate retrograde cystoure-throgram should be performed on all such patients before the insertion of a Foley catheter.[5, 6] Only in this way can one ensure against creating false passages or doing further damage by blind insertion of the catheter. Remember, an intravenous urogram and voiding cystourethrogram do not constitute a proper urethral examination.

Unfortunately, pelvic pain from fractures may not be reliably localized by the patient's symptoms or physical examination, and proper evaluation should include films of the lumbosacral spine and hips, as pain may be referred from these areas to any region of the pelvis. Also, roentgenograms of the pelvis should be closely examined for secondary signs of soft tissue injuries such as hematomas and intraperitoneal fluid.[7] Furthermore, in every pelvic roentgenogram the periphery of the plain film may often be dark and should, therefore, be hot-lighted. Small unsuspected fractures may otherwise be missed. On plain films of the pelvis, however, overlapping bowel gas may partially obscure bony pathology, and relatively hidden areas such as the sacrum and coccyx will not be adequately visualized.

As with any other anatomic area, computed tomography (CT) offers the best morphologic and anatomic depiction of normal anatomy and pathology. It is particularly useful in detecting or excluding intra-articular bony fragments, determining the overall appearance of acetabular surfaces, and delineating associated soft tissue injuries.[8-11] CT is a more time-consuming examination and may not be feasible in the unstable patient, so the plain films must be scrutinized for findings of anterior compression, lateral compression, vertical shear, or complex patterns of injury. Together with the clinical findings, this information may enable one to aid the surgeon in determining rapid corrective procedures.[12] If a fracture is seen on plain films and the patient is stable, we often recommend CT to identify abnormalities which may not be seen on the plain film studies.

Technique

Our routine is to obtain anteroposterior (AP) and frog-leg views of the pelvis, including the proximal aspects of both hips on each view. We also try to include the lower lumbar spine on all pelvic views obtained in trauma cases. Angled views of the pelvis, made by turning the x-ray tube 25 to 30 degrees caudally, are complementary views in the acute setting.[13] The angled view is particularly useful in showing the degree of inner displacement or rotation of fractures involving the pelvic brim or acetabulum. Oblique views are also useful in assessing the acetabular-femoral relationship. Their importance in evaluating acetabular fractures has been stressed by Judet; hence these projections are referred to as "Judet views."[14]

Fluoroscopy, tomography, nuclear medicine, and ultrasound may all be adjuncts to plain film in evaluating pelvic trauma, but we do not often use them in the acute setting because of the wide availability and sensitivity of CT.

FIG 6–1.

Normal adult pelvis. *A* = femoral neck; *B* = ischial spine; *C* = acetabulum; *D* = inferior ramus; *E* = superior ramus; *F* = lower lumbar spine; *G* = intertrochanteric region of left femur; *H* = greater trochanter of right femur; *I* = lesser trochanter of the right femur. *Arrow* points to vascular calcification, and *arrowheads* designate sacroiliac joints.

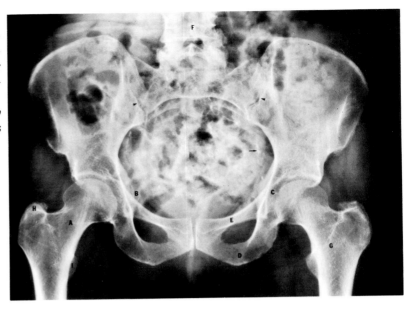

FIG 6–2.

Normal pediatric pelvis. *Arrowheads* = epiphyses of greater trochanters; *small arrows* = femoral head epiphyses; *large arrows* = unfused acetabulum. Ischial pubic synchondroses have fused.

FIG 6–3.

Coned-down AP pelvic view of a 34-year-old involved in an automobile accident shows fractures of the superior pubic ramus on the right and fractures of the inferior rami of the ischii bilaterally *(arrowheads)*. The *arrow* points to a large hematoma displacing the bladder superiorly.

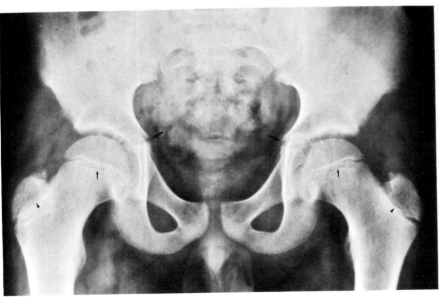

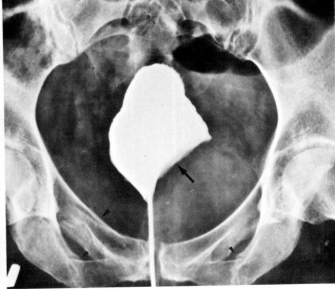

Anatomy

In this chapter we will stress plain film findings, as these views will be the ones the emergency room physician will be required to screen. We will also point out certain situations in which CT may be necessary. As previously mentioned, most pelvic fractures in a clinically stable patient should be evaluated with CT to look for other unsuspected fractures and associated soft tissue injury.

The general plain film anatomy of the adult pelvis is familiar to most emergency physicians (Fig 6–1). Careful attention should be paid to the commonly injured regions such as the femoral neck, iliac spine, acetabulum, inferior ramus of the ischium, and superior pubic ramus. In all cases of trauma, the lower lumbar spine should also be surveyed for possible injury.

Normal pediatric pelvic anatomy differs slightly from that of the adult. The location of the epiphyseal plates and synchondroses should be kept in mind (Fig 6–2). In most patients, the synchondroses should be fused at about age 10.

Pathology

Pelvic traumatic injuries are usually associated with significant soft tissue changes and hemorrhage is the most important of these. Plain film evidence of hemorrhage is usually manifest by displacement of the bladder by a large hematoma. Usually, however, the bladder must be fully filled with contrast to appreciate this alteration (Fig 6–3). When active hemorrhage is suspected, angiography followed by pelvic embolization may be necessary (Fig 6–4). Of course, as previously noted, CT clearly defines the bony and soft tissue injuries in the pelvis and should be used extensively (Figs 6–5 to 6–7).

In approximately 20% of patients with pelvic arch fractures, the urethra or bladder is injured. These structures may also be injured by separation of the symphysis pubis associated with separation of one sacroiliac joint. In such cases, it is mandatory that a technically-acceptable retrograde urethrogram be done before insertion of a Foley catheter. Of course, if the patient has more serious life-threatening injuries, a Foley or suprapubic catheter may need to be inserted immediately, without evaluation, to monitor the patient's output. Figures 6–8 and 6–9 demonstrate "poor" and "good" techniques in retrograde urethrography. Injury to the urethra can be much more extensive than is clinically suspected (Fig 6–10).

Fractures of the pelvis can be grouped according to a 1965 classification by Peltier:[15]

Fractures not affecting weight-bearing
  Avulsion fractures
  Isolated fractures of the iliac wing
  Pubic rami fractures—unilateral or bilateral
Fractures affecting weight-bearing
  Sacral fractures—isolated or combined
  Acetabular fractures
    Posterior rim—with or without dislocation
    Roof or floor—with or without central dislocation
  Separation of symphysis pubis
  Fractures of hemipelvis

This system takes into consideration factors either affecting or not affecting the weight-bearing surfaces. It should be remembered that the pelvis is a ring and that breaks commonly occur in two or more places. There may be two or more fractures, or there may be fractures and dislocations at one of the sacroiliac joints or the symphysis pubis. These combinations are important since they are potentially serious injuries.

Isolated fractures of the major pelvic bones usually pose no specific diagnostic challenge (Figs 6–11 and 6–12). However, avulsion injuries are quite common and may be difficult to diagnose. In suspected cases, the film should always be "hot-lighted," as the fracture may be hidden in a dark area. The most frequent sites of such injury are the anterior superior iliac spine (insertion of the sartorius muscle), anterior inferior iliac spine (insertion of the rectus femoris muscle), and ischial tuberosity (insertion of hamstring muscle group)(Figs 6–13 to 6–15).

Fractures of the sacrum are not observed as commonly, but deserve special attention. The sacrum may be hidden by bowel gas and is not as clearly seen on plain radiographs as other bony structures in the pelvis. Fractures of this anatomic area are being recognized with increasing frequency as we perform CT on more patients with pelvic trauma. On the plain radiograph, the most important landmarks are the curved anterior sacral foraminal lines. Any disruption or discontinuity of these lines should suggest fracture, and CT should be performed (Figs 6–16 and 6–17).[16–18] Another important point is that sacral fractures are seldom isolated. If a sacral or pelvic fracture is identified, other fractures should be diligently sought (Figs 6–18 and 6–19). Nuclear medicine bone scanning may rarely be used to detect sacral fractures unsuspected from the plain films.[19] The coccyx is commonly injured, but the diagnosis rests chiefly on the clinical findings of point tenderness on rectal examination. Radiographs are unnecessary in most cases, since the risk of high gonadal radiation dose is probably greater

FIG 6–4.
A, coned-down left-hip view of a 22-year-old involved in automobile accident shows marked comminution of the trochanteric region of the left hip. **B,** the hip was disarticulated, and the patient continued to bleed. Arteriography was performed and showed extravasation of contrast *(arrows).* **C,** embolization with Gelfoam and Gianturco coils *(arrows)* stopped the bleeding.

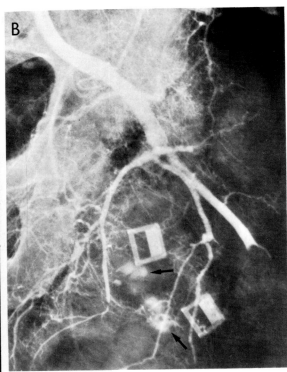

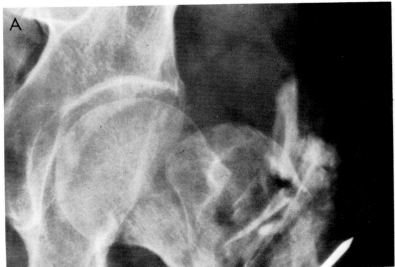

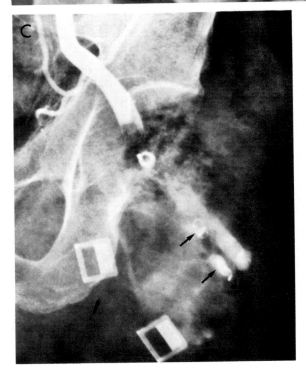

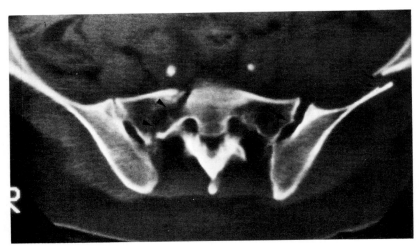

FIG 6–5.
Computerized tomographic view through the pelvis of a 42-year-old female involved in an automobile accident shows fractures of the left ilium *(small arrows)* and right sacrum *(arrowheads),* and diastasis of the left sacroiliac joint *(large arrow).* (Courtesy of Dr. Victor Haughton, Medical College of Wisconsin, Milwaukee.)

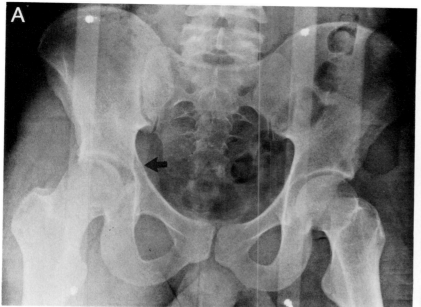

FIG 6–6.
A, AP pelvis of 25-year-old injured in an automobile accident shows subluxation of right femoral head with a possible associated acetabular component *(ar-* *row).* **B,** coned-down view from CT confirms comminuted fracture of the posterior column with two intraarticular bony fragments. CT is helpful in these situations.

FIG 6–7.
A, AP pelvis of 23-year-old involved in motor vehicle accident shows obvious fractures of right superior and inferior pubic rami. No other injuries are dem- onstrated. **B,** coned-down view of sacrum from CT shows comminuted fracture not detected on plain film *(arrows).*

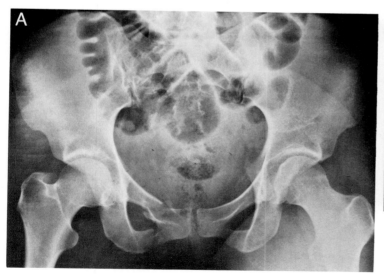

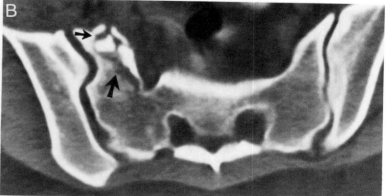

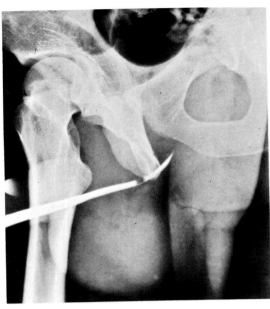

FIG 6–8.
"Poor" technique in retrograde urethrography, with only the penile urethra being demonstrated. There is no demonstration of the posterior urethra or bladder.

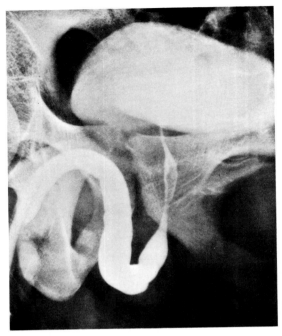

FIG 6–9.
"Good" technique in retrograde urethrography showing the entire extent of the urethra and the bladder.

FIG 6–10.
A, AP view of pelvis of a 21-year-old male involved in an auto accident shows markedly distracted bilateral fractures of the pubis and ischium. Dislocation of left sacroiliac joint, with fracture of left ilium is also noted. **B,** retrograde urethrography shows marked distortion of the posterior urethra, with extravasation of contrast.

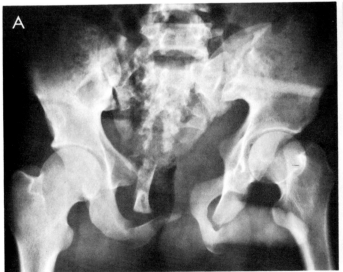
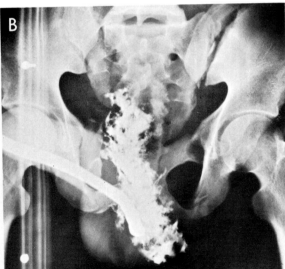

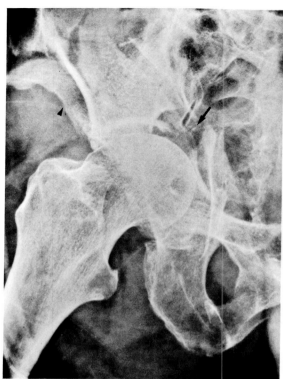

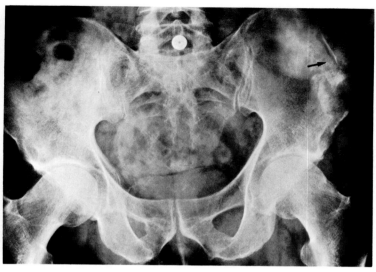

FIG 6–11 (top left).
Right-hip view of 55-year-old female involved in an auto accident shows comminuted fracture of the right ilium *(arrowhead)* and central fracture of the acetabulum *(arrow)*. The latter may be a cause of bladder rupture.

FIG 6–12 (top right).
AP pelvic view of 45-year-old male involved in a motorcycle accident. Fractures of the left ilium are noted *(arrow)*.

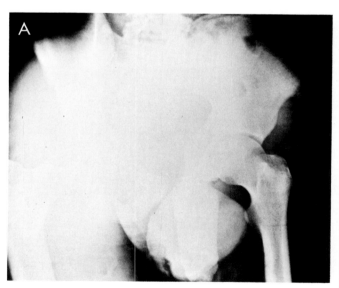

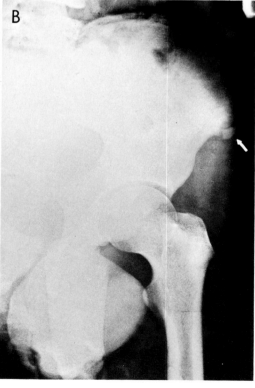

FIG 6–13.
A, oblique view of pelvis of 21-year-old runner who collapsed crossing the finish line was interpreted as normal. (Original film was very dark; print is markedly improved.) **B,** close-up of same film, showing avulsion fracture of the anterior superior iliac spine *(arrow)*. Always remember to "hot-light" the periphery of dark pelvic films to look for pathology.

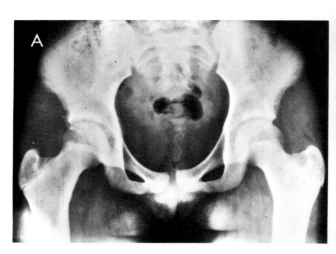

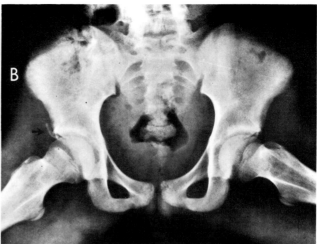

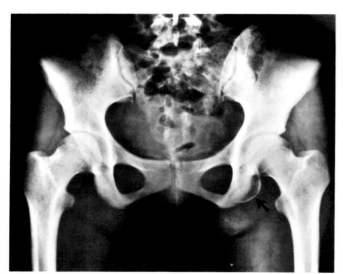

FIG 6–14 (top left and right).
A, AP pelvic view of young woman with right-hip pain interpreted as normal. **B,** frog-leg view of same patient shows fracture of the anterior inferior iliac spine to much better advantage *(arrow).*

FIG 6–15 (left).
Avulsion of the ischial tuberosity in 16-year-old complaining of pain while running.

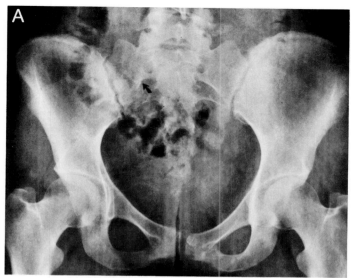

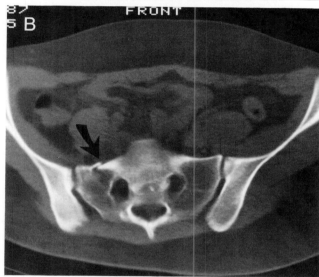

FIG 6–16.
A, AP pelvis of 19-year-old female injured in automobile accident. Note disruption of sacral foraminal line *(arrow)*. **B,** CT confirms minimally displaced sacral fracture *(arrow)*. **C,** also shown are small fractures of both pubic rami *(arrows)*.

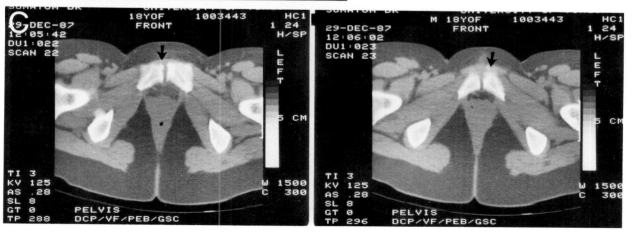

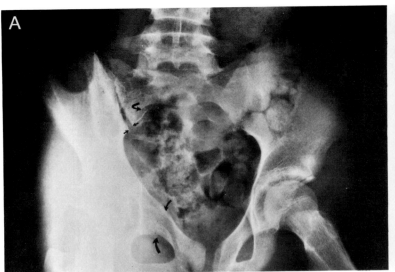

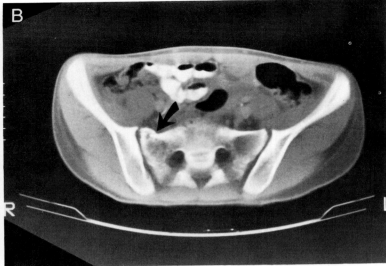

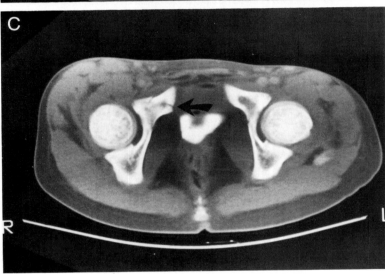

FIG 6–17.
A, oblique AP pelvis in 13-year-old injured in automobile accident shows superior pubic ramus fracture *(slightly curved arrows)*, widening of right SI joint *(small arrows)*, and discontinuity of arcuate lines on the right *(curved arrow)*. **B,** CT confirms the sacral fracture *(arrow)*. **C,** lower CT cut shows right pubic ramus fracture *(arrow)*.

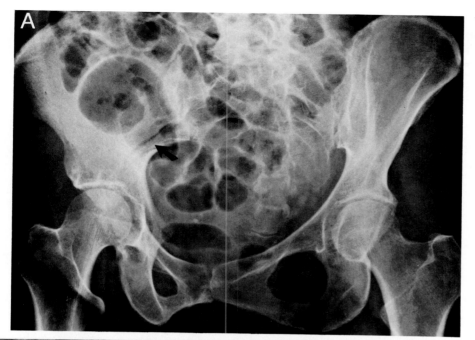

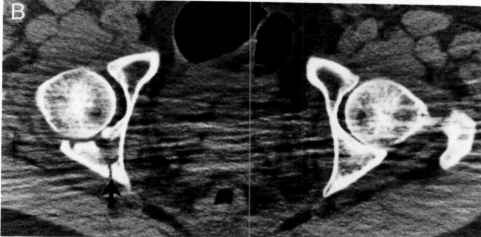

FIG 6–18.
A, AP pelvis of 49-year-old involved in automobile accident shows linear fracture of innominate bone *(arrow)*. **B,** CT shows fracture extended down into posterior column of acetabulum *(arrow)*. **C,** higher cut from CT shows associated fracture of left sacrum *(arrow)*. Fractures of the sacrum are seldom isolated pelvic injuries.

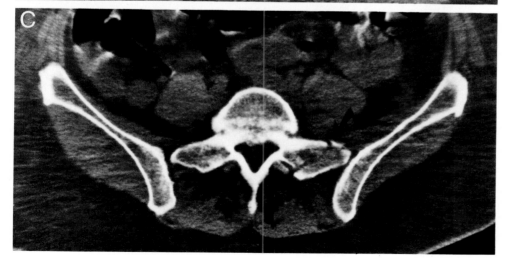

FIG 6–19.
A, sacral view of 22-year-old with clinically suspected sacral fracture *(arrow).* **B,** lateral lumbar spine with long film of same patient shows compression fracture of T-12 *(arrow)* missed on initial interpretation. Always look for other fractures when one is seen.

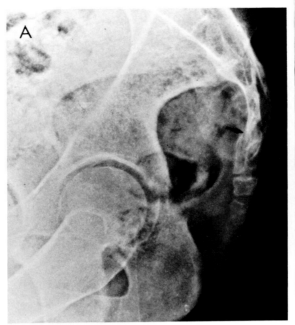

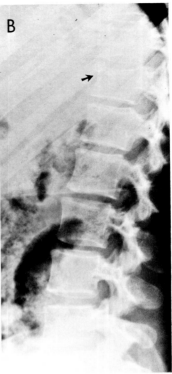

FIG 6–20.
Right-hip view of 16-year-old runner shows sclerotic line through inferior aspect of femoral neck, representing a stress fracture *(arrowhead).*

FIG 6–21.
Displaced intertrochanteric fracture in 75-year-old female.

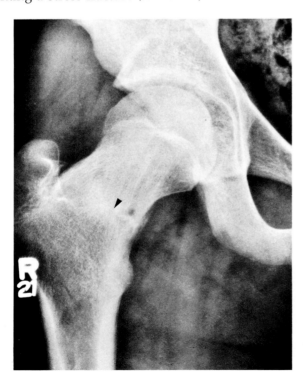

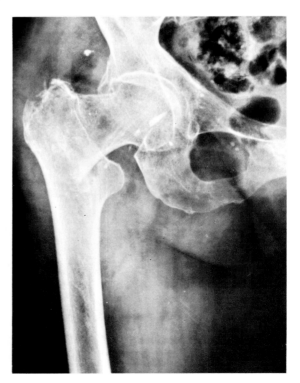

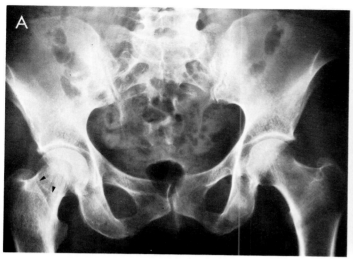

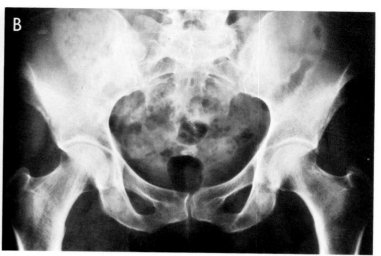

FIG 6–22.
A, AP pelvic view of 45-year-old woman taken at another hospital and read as femoral neck fracture *(arrowheads).* **B,** repeat study at our institution with feet and legs rotated inward shows no asymmetry of the femoral necks and no fracture. Good technique when obtaining AP pelvic views is necessary to avoid misdiagnosis.

FIG 6–23.
A, AP pelvic view of 72-year-old who fell and had left hip pain. This film was initially read as normal, but note sclerosis of left femoral neck. *Arrow* points to impacted fracture of the left femoral neck. **B,** attempted frog-leg view of left hip shows small line of sclerosis, indicating fracture *(arrows).* Impacted fractures are often missed and may be very difficult to diagnose unless special projections, tomography, or nuclear scanning are used in questionable cases.

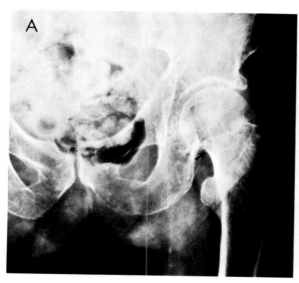

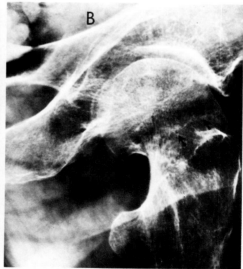

Pelvis and Hips—Pathology / **379**

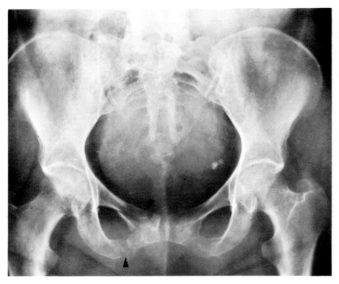

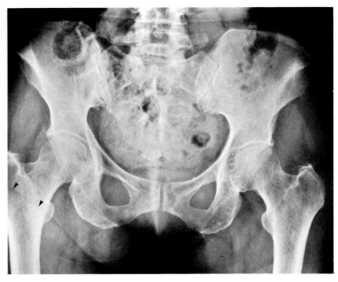

FIG 6–24.
AP pelvic view of 38-year-old woman who fell, striking right hip. Only the right hip was requested before this study and was initially read as normal. This AP pelvic view shows fractures of the inferior and superior rami on the right *(arrowheads).* An AP pelvic view should probably be obtained on all patients with traumatic hip pain.

FIG 6–25.
AP pelvic view of 59-year-old after injury shows a skin fold overlying the intertrochanteric region of the right femur *(arrowheads).* This should not be mistaken for a fracture line.

FIG 6–26.
A, AP pelvic view of 77-year-old female who fell and had right hip pain. The lucency marked by the *arrow* was read in the emergency room as representing a

skin fold. **B,** AP view the following day shows displaced intertrochanteric fracture of the right femur. In retrospect, the fracture was present on the previous film and overlooked because of the skin fold.

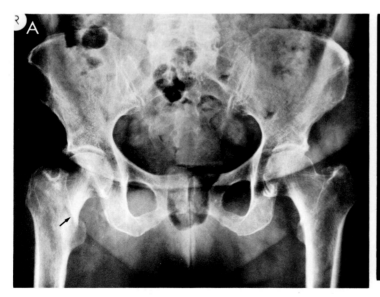

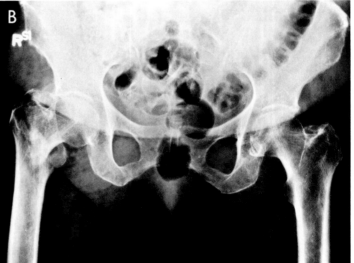

FIG 6–27.
A, right hip view of 73-year-old female who fell 4 days prior to this film, which was read as normal. **B,** nuclear bone scan shows increased uptake *(arrow)* 5 days after injury. In retrospect, fracture was present on plain film *(arrowhead)*. Impacted fractures may be difficult to diagnose, and ancillary techniques may often be necessary.

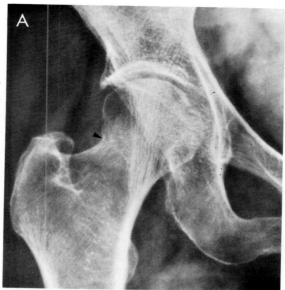

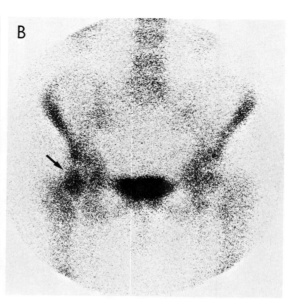

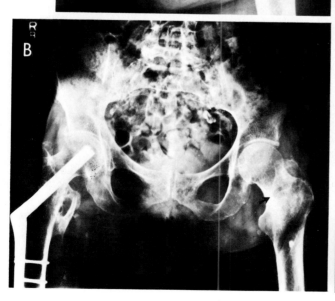

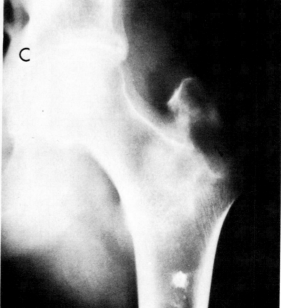

FIG 6–28.
A, AP view of left hip in 63-year-old patient involved in an accident. Film was originally very dark and was read as normal, but the *arrow* points out an area of concern. **B,** repeat AP pelvic view with better technique 3 weeks later shows same area *(arrow)* still too unclear for diagnosis. **C,** tomography shows a fracture of the left greater trochanter *(arrow)*. This sequence indicates the importance of tomography in cases of continued pain accompanied by subtle abnormality on plain films.

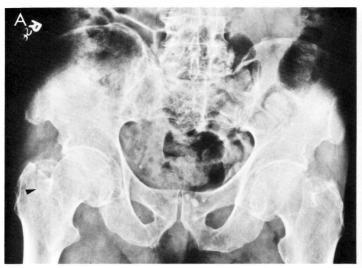

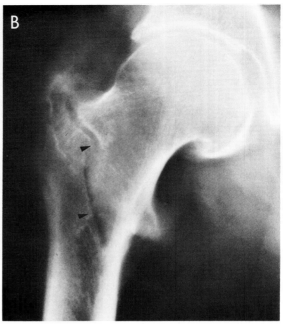

FIG 6–29.
A, AP pelvic view of 88-year-old patient involved in fall. Questionable intertrochanteric fracture of the right hip was noted *(arrowhead)*. **B,** tomography the following day showed the intertrochanteric fracture to much better advantage *(arrowheads)*.

FIG 6–30.
A, AP pelvic view of 78-year-old female who fell. In the emergency room, a question of left femoral neck fracture was raised. However, the marked degenerative disease did not allow a definitive diagnosis. **B,** tomography of the left hip showed no fracture.

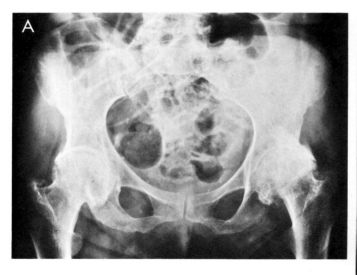

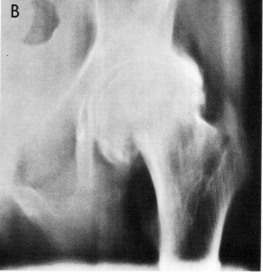

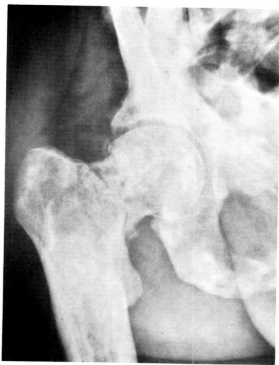

FIG 6–31.
A, 77-year-old male with metastatic prostate, both osteolytic and osteoblastic types. Femoral neck fracture
with varus deformity was pathologic in origin.

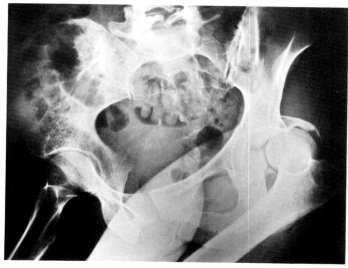

FIG 6–32.
Traumatic dislocation of left hip with comminuted
acetabular fracture. These hip dislocations are often
associated with fractures of the acetabulum.

FIG 6–33.
A, AP pelvic film of 35-year-old patient involved in
auto accident was originally read as normal. **B,** left

hip view shows fracture fragment of posterior aspect
of acetabulum *(arrowheads).*

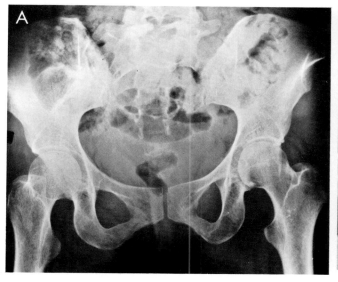

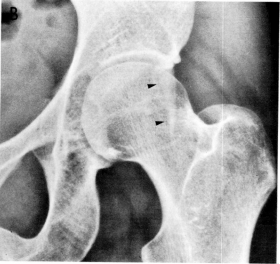

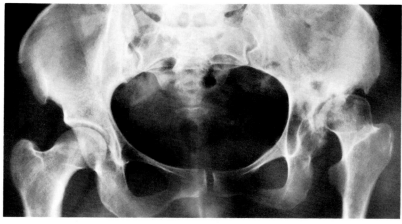

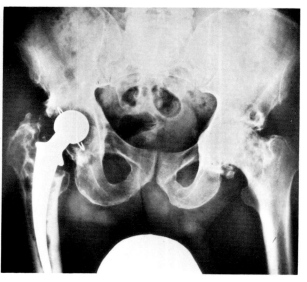

FIG 6–34 (top left).
Congenital dislocation of the left hip with "false" acetabulum and degenerative changes. This should not be confused with acute pathology.

FIG 6–35 (top right).
A, 70-year-old male complaining of right-hip pain after right total hip replacement. Note marked lucency surrounding the total hip prosthesis, indicating infec-

tion and loosening. Also note marked degenerative disease of left hip. The distal aspect of the femoral prosthesis should be seen on all patients.

FIG 6–36.
A, left-hip view of 77-year-old female obtained in January 1979 shows postsurgical changes. **B,** a film ob-

tained 1 year later shows a nondisplaced fracture of the inferior ramus *(arrowhead)*. The patient had fallen, striking her left hip.

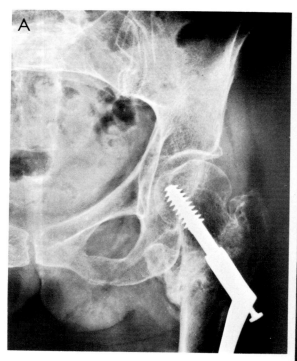

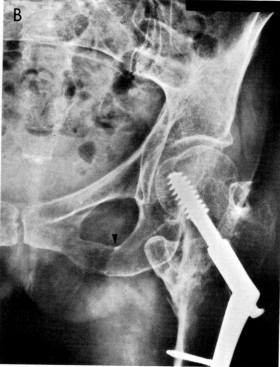

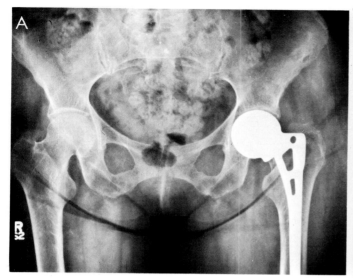

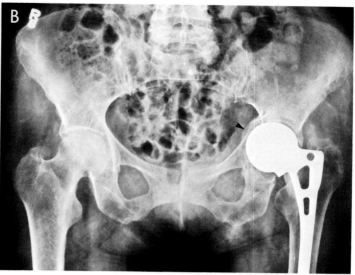

FIG 6–37.
A, AP pelvic view of 68-year-old female 2 months af- ter left total hip replacement. **B,** injury 1 year later shows central fracture of the acetabulum *(arrowhead)*.

FIG 6–38.
A, 58-year-old man after right total hip replacement with a history of "popping." This film was interpreted as showing only postoperative changes. **B,** a radio- graph taken after the patient produced the "popping" shows dislocation of the femoral component from the acetabular component. History may be very impor- tant in diagnosing certain injuries.

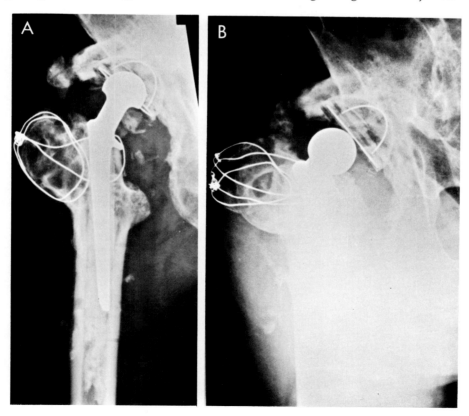

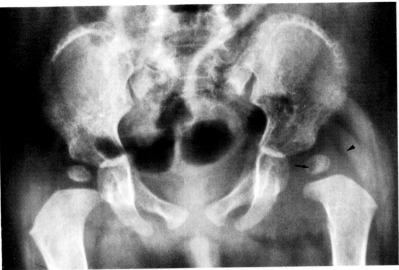

FIG 6–39.
AP pelvic film of 14-month-old with a limp and posturing of left hip. Lucency in femoral epiphysis on the left *(arrow)* with associated effusion *(arrowhead)* indicates infection. The femoral head is partially dislocated by the large effusion. Rachitic changes are noted.

FIG 6–40.
A, AP pelvic view of 12-year-old boy with right knee pain. Both knees were normal, but pelvis shows slipped capital femoral epiphysis on the left and a questionable slippage on the right. **B,** frog-leg view of pelvis confirmed bilateral slippage. Pain in lower femur and knee may be referred from the hips.

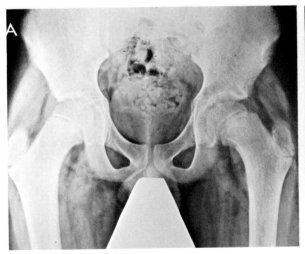
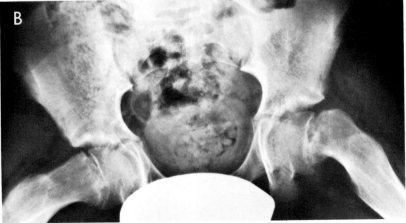

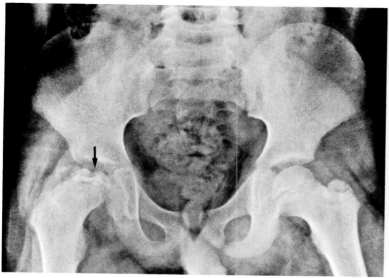

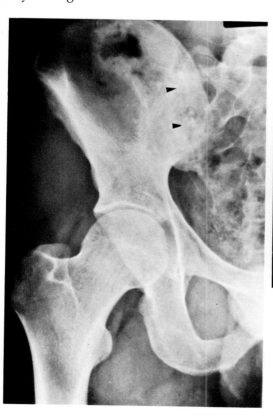

FIG 6–41.
AP pelvic film of 7-year-old male shows changes of Legg-Calvé-Perthes disease (aseptic necrosis) in the right hip *(arrow)*. There was no history of trauma.

FIG 6–43.
Right-hip view of 22-year-old female with Crohn's disease. Sacroiliitis denoted by *arrowheads*. Always look for nontraumatic causes of hip pain in the emergency setting.

FIG 6–42.
AP pelvic view of 42-year-old known alcoholic shows radiographic changes of ischemic necrosis in both femoral heads, with sclerosis and lucencies.

FIG 6–44.
A 70-year-old female with extensive lytic metastases from breast cancer.

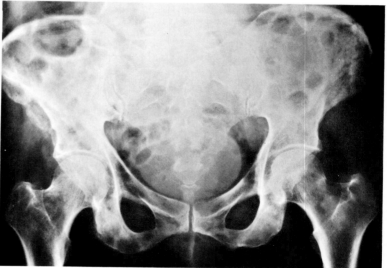

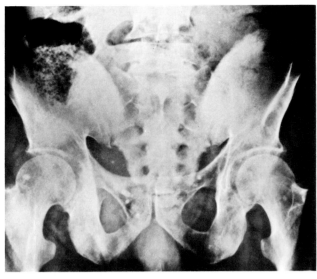

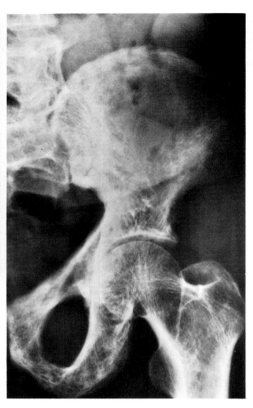

FIG 6–45 (top left).
A 71-year-old male with extensive osteoblastic metastases from prostatic carcinoma.

FIG 6–46 (top right).
A 62-year-old male with Paget's disease, showing prominent trabeculae and thickening of the iliopectineal line. Paget's disease may mimic metastatic disease.

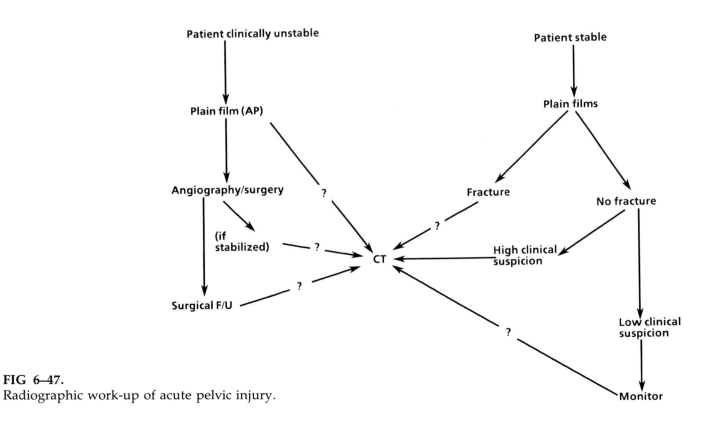

FIG 6–47.
Radiographic work-up of acute pelvic injury.

than the potential yield from the examination.

The hip, in addition to being the most commonly injured region in the pelvis, also manifests a significant amount of nontraumatic pathology. Of course, as with any other area of the skeleton, meticulous history-taking and physical examination may aid in localizing the injury to this anatomical area and help delineate the extent of such injuries.

Fractures of the hip most commonly occur in the neck and intertrochanteric regions. In the younger patient, the femoral neck is a potential site of stress fractures (Fig 6–20). However, femoral neck fractures are most commonly seen in elderly women, often after only mild trauma, such as a fall or slip. These fractures may be widely displaced (Fig 6–21). In many cases, an impacted fracture may be virtually invisible. In such instances, it is important to obtain the AP view with the feet and legs rotated inward to avoid foreshortening of the femoral neck, an appearance which may mimic an impacted fracture (Fig 6–22). Impacted fractures may only be evident by a thin sclerotic line through the neck (Fig 6–23). There is a pitfall in only radiographing the hip in traumatized patients with hip pain since referred pain from other injuries may mimic hip fracture. Therefore, we routinely obtain an AP pelvic view in such cases (Fig 6–24).

In the obese patient with a panniculus, the overlying skin fold of the pannus should not be confused with a fracture. This fold may lie directly over the neck or intertrochanteric region and simulate a true fracture (Fig 6–25). Likewise, just because there is a skin fold overlying this region, do not assume there is no fracture (Fig 6–26).

Plain films may, even in retrospect, be normal in certain impacted femoral neck fractures. These cases may require nuclear bone scanning (Fig 6–27).

In any hip fracture, tomography may often be helpful (Figs 6–28 and 6–29). Extensive degenerative disease may mask possible pathology on plain films. In such cases, tomography or CT is also indicated (Fig 6–30). Always remember that all femoral neck fractures are not straightforward ones. This anatomical area is a favorite region for metastases and, in all cases, the radiograph should be searched for other bony evidence of secondary deposits (Fig 6–31).

Hip dislocations are common, particularly in automobile accidents. These injuries are often associated with acetabular fractures (Figs 6–32 and 6–33). In fact, tomography or CT may be required to define the full extent of this lesion. Of course, congenital dislocations should not be mistaken for acute trauma (Fig 6–34).

Evaluation of the postoperative total hip replacement is a common situation encountered in the emergency room. Evidence of infection of the prosthesis should be carefully sought (Fig 6–35). Also, other traumatic pelvic injuries may occur in these patients (Figs 6–36 and 6–37). Finally, partial dislocation of total hip replacement does occur. In such patients, a history of "popping" may be the clue to the diagnosis (Fig 6–38).

All radiographs of patients with hip pain should be scrutinized for soft tissue changes and more subtle radiographic evidence of pathology. For instance, septic arthritis may be manifested radiographically by joint effusion and lateral subluxation (Fig 6–39). A slipped capital femoral epiphysis may be masked on the AP view, yet show up on the frog-leg projection. This entity is bilateral in 30% to 40% of cases (Fig 6–40). Aseptic necrosis, a common cause of hip pain, may be more obvious in children than in adults (Figs 6–41 and 6–42). Of course, sacroiliac disease may also cause back and hip pain (Fig 6–43). Finally, always look for nontraumatic causes of pelvic pain. Metastases, particularly from the breast in the female and the prostate in the male, are commonly observed in the pelvis (Figs 6–44 and 6–45). Moreover, Paget's disease involving the pelvis may mimic metastatic disease (Fig 6–46).

In summary, plain films of the pelvis are the mainstay of screening the acutely injured patient. However, CT should be liberally used to supplement plain radiography when the plain films are normal but the clinical suspicion of fracture or soft tissue injury is high or there is an obvious fracture on plain films. CT is the best examination for delineating the overall pathology in this anatomic region (Fig 6–47).

References

1. Matalon TSA, Athanasoulis CA, Margulis MN, et al: Hemorrhage with pelvic fractures: Efficacy of transcatheter embolization. *AJR* 1979; 133:859.
2. Lang EK: Transcatheter embolization of pelvic vessels for control of intractable hemorrhage. *Radiology* 1981; 140:331.
3. Kam J, Jackson H, Ben-Menachem Y: Vascular injuries in blunt pelvic trauma. *Radiol Clin North Am* 1981; 19:171.
4. Sadler CM, Phillips JM, Harris JD, et al: Radiology of the bladder and urethra in blunt pelvic trauma. *Radiol Clin North Am* 1981; 19:195.
5. Reynolds BM, Nalsano NA, Reynolds FX: Pelvic fractures. *J Trauma* 1973; 13:1011.
6. McLaughlin AP, Pfister RC: Double catheter technique for evaluation of urethral injury and differentiating urethral from bladder rupture. *Radiology* 1974; 110:716.
7. Harris JH, Jr, Loh CK, Perlman HC, et al: The roentgen diagnosis of pelvic extraperitoneal effusion. *Radiology* 1977; 125:543.
8. Gilula LA, Murphy WA, Tailor CC, et al: Computed tomography of the osseous pelvis. *Radiology* 1979; 132:107.
9. Shirkhoda A, Brashear HR, Staab EV: Computed tomography of acetabular fractures. *Radiology* 1980; 134:683.
10. Harley JD, Mack CA, Winguest RA: CT of acetabular fractures: Comparison with conventional radiography. *AJR* 1982; 138:413.
11. Gill K, Buckholz RW: The role of computerized tomographic scanning in the evaluation of major pelvic trauma. *J Bone Joint Surg* 1984; 66A:34.
12. Young JWR, Burgess AR, Brumback RJ, et al: Pelvic fractures: Value of plain radiography in early assessment and management. *Radiology* 1986; 160:445.
13. Pennal GF, Tile M, Waddell JP, et al: Pelvic disruption: Assessment and classification. *Clin Orthop* 1980; 151:12.
14. Judet R, Judet J, Letourrel E: Fractures of the acetabulum: Classification and surgical approaches for open reduction. *J Bone Joint Surg* 1964; 46A:1615.
15. Peltier LF: Complications associated with fractures of the pelvis. *J Bone Joint Surg* 1965; 47A:1060.
16. Northrop CH, Eto RT, Lopp JW: Vertical fracture of the sacral ala: Significance of noncontinuity of the anterior superior sacral foraminal line. *AJR* 1975; 124:102.
17. Laasonen EM: Missed sacral fractures. *Ann Clin Res* 1977; 9:84.
18. Montana MA, Richardson MC, Kilcoyne RF, et al: CT of sacral injury. *Radiology* 1986; 161:499.
19. Schneider R, Yacovone J, Ghelman B: Unsuspected sacral fractures: Detection by radionuclide bone scanning. *AJR* 1985; 144:337.

Suggested Reading

Harris JH, Jr, Harris WH: *The Radiology of Emergency Medicine,* ed 2. Baltimore, Williams & Wilkins, 1981.

Orkin LA: The diagnosis of urologic trauma in the presence of other injuries. *Surg Clin North Am* 1953; 33:1473.

Reynolds BM, Nalsano NA, Reynolds FX: Pelvic fractures. *J Trauma* 1973; 13:1011.

Rogers LF: Radiology of Skeletal Trauma, vols. 1 and 2. New York, Churchill Livingstone, 1982.

Thaggard A, III, Harle TS, Carlson V: *Bony Pelvis and Hip. Roentgenology of Fractures and Dislocations.* Seminars in Roentgenology. New York, Grune & Stratton, 1978.

Normal Variants

Theodore E. Keats, M.D.

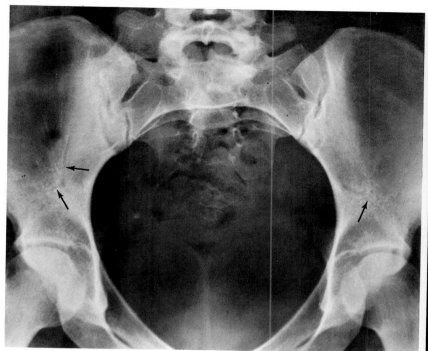
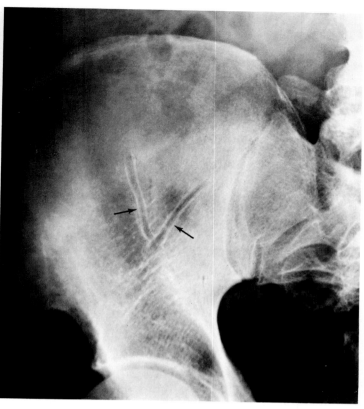

FIG 6–48.
Examples of the grooves for the nutrient arteries of the ilium.

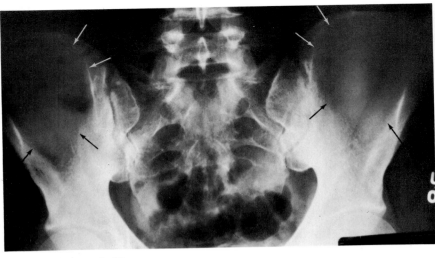

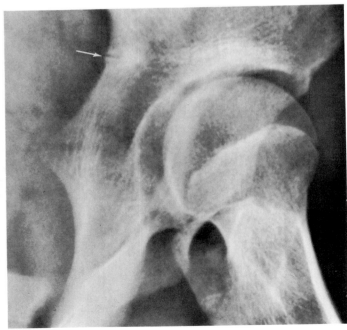

FIG 6–49 (top left).
Normal lucency of the iliac fossae, which may resemble a cystic lesion in bone.

FIG 6–50 (top right).
Normal sclerosis and irregularity of the sacroiliac joints in a 14-year-old boy, resembling the changes of ankylosing spondylitis.

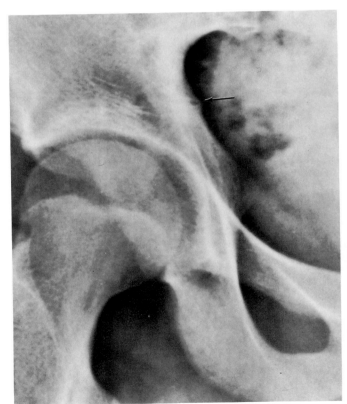

FIG 6–51.
Remnants of the synchondrosis between the ilium and ischium in a 12-year-old girl.

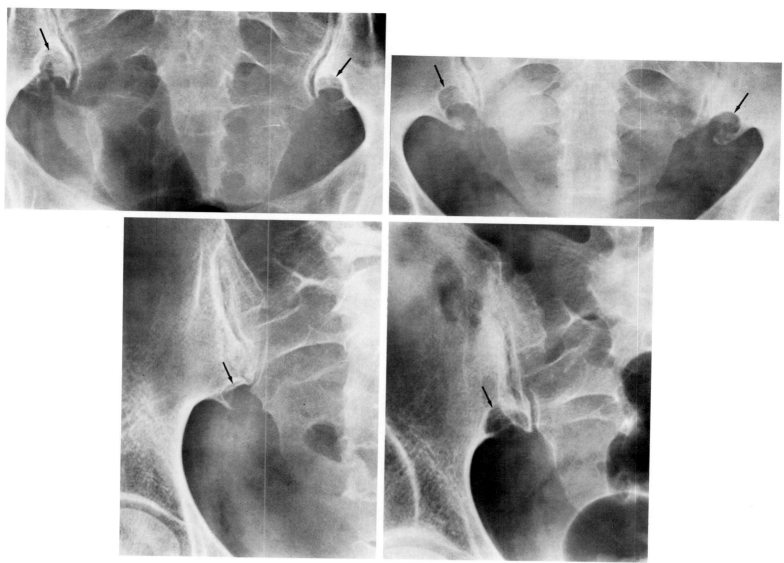

FIG 6–52.
Examples of preauricular (paraglenoidal) sulcus. This groove transmits the superior branch of the gluteal ar-tery and supplies insertion for a portion of the sacro-iliac ligament. It is apparently a characteristic of the female pelvis and is not necessarily symmetric.

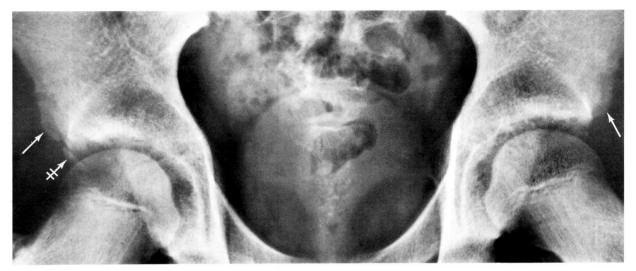

FIG 6–53.
Ossification center for the anteroinferior iliac spine *(arrows)* and acetabular rim *(notched arrow)* in a 13-year-old boy.

FIG 6–54.
A, irregularity of the anteroinferior iliac spine in an adolescent boy. This represents a "tug" lesion at the insertion of the rectus femoris muscle and should not be mistaken for the changes of neoplasm. **B,** enlargement of area of interest. Note that the muscle planes are not disturbed. (Ref: Murray RO, Jacobson HG: *The Radiology of Skeletal Disorders,* ed 2. New York, Churchill Livingstone, 1977, p 274.)

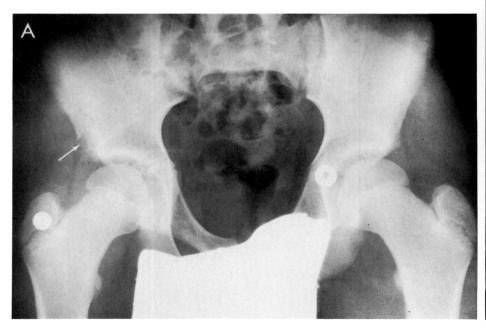

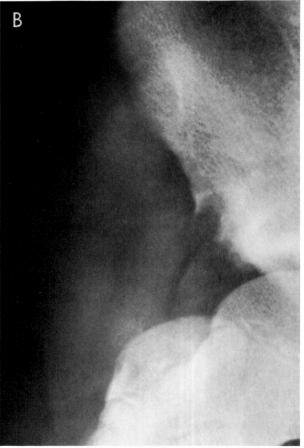

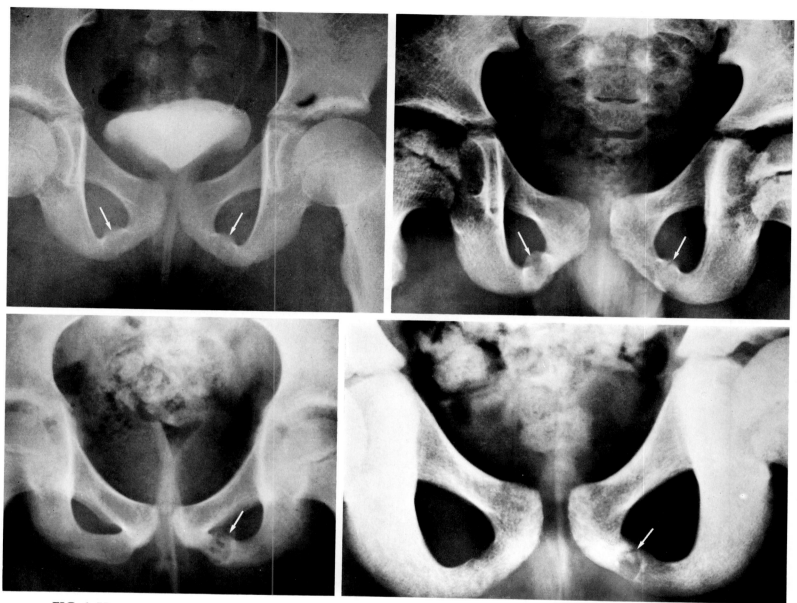

FIG 6–55.
Normal variations and asymmetry in closure of the ischiopubic synchondrosis. These are normal phe- nomena which should not be mistaken for evidence of osteochondrosis.

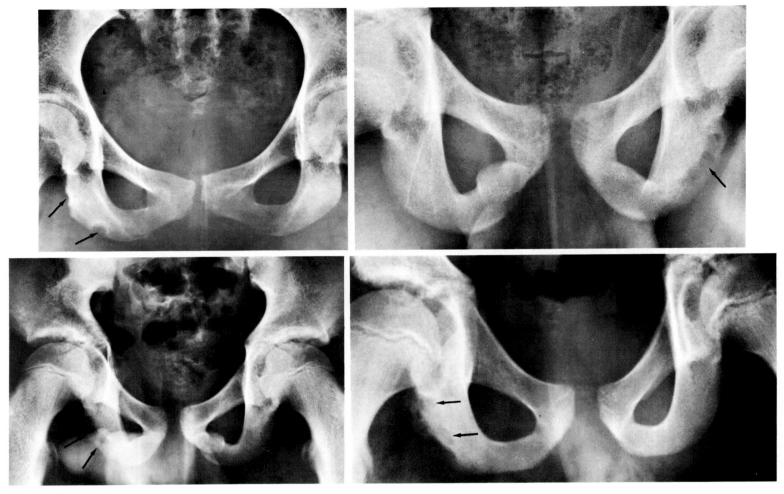

FIG 6–56.
Normal irregularities of ossification of the ischia in adolescent children. These changes are usually asymmetric and disappear with increasing age. They result from the tug of the adductor muscles.

FIG 6–57.
Normal irregularities of the margins of the symphysis pubis in a 12-year-old girl.

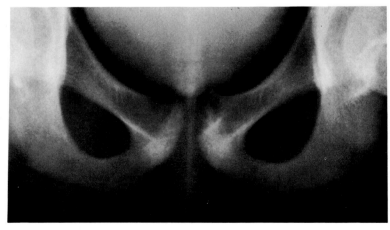

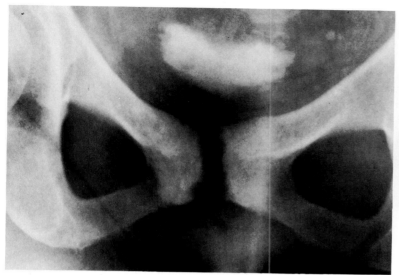

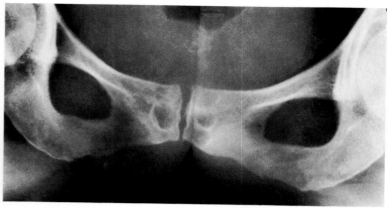

FIG 6–58.
Postpartum changes in the symphysis pubis.

FIG 6–59.
Normal malalignment of the symphysis pubis in a 14-year-old girl. The lower margin of the symphysis is a more reliable indicator of the level than the upper margin. (Ref: Vix VA, Ryu CY: The adult symphysis pubis: Normal and abnormal. *Am J Roentgenol* 1971; 112:517.) Note also the accessory ossification center in the margin of the left side of the symphysis. Such accessory centers are common in the juvenile symphysis *(arrow)*.

FIG 6–60.
Accessory ossification centers in the superior portions of the acetabula (os acetabuli marginalis superior) in a 14-year-old boy *(arrows)*. Note also additional ossification centers in the acetabula at lower level *(notched arrows)*. These centers usually fuse solidly with the contiguous portions of the ilium. (Ref: Caffey J: *Pediatric X-Ray Diagnosis*, ed 8. Chicago, Year Book Medical Publishers, 1985, p 334.)

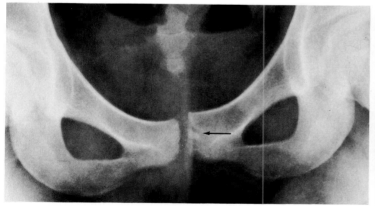

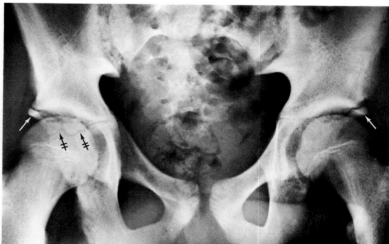

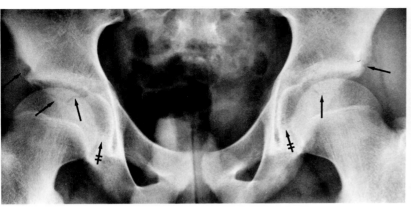

FIG 6–61.
Partial union of secondary ossification center of the acetabulum in the adolescent *(arrows).* Note also the wide medial aspect of the joint space at this age *(notched arrows).*

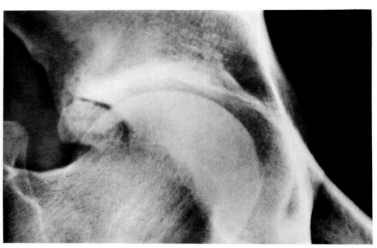

FIG 6–62.
An os acetabuli marginalis superior which has persisted as a separate ossicle into adult life.

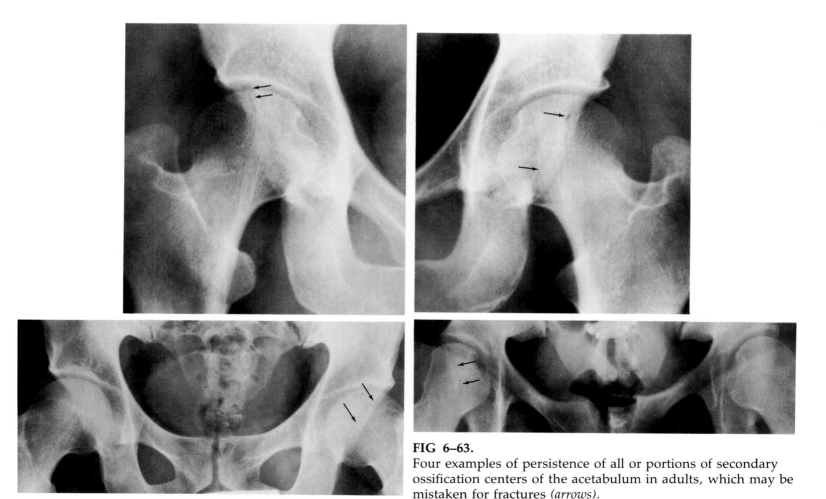

FIG 6–63.
Four examples of persistence of all or portions of secondary ossification centers of the acetabulum in adults, which may be mistaken for fractures *(arrows).*

7
Extremities

K. K. Wallace, Jr., M.D.

Anatomical Considerations

Skeletal development and form influence the diagnosis of bone injury and disease. As each area is discussed, a brief description of the growth centers and anatomy will be presented. Excellent material on the subject of anatomic variation is presented elsewhere in this volume. These descriptions will emphasize points which are important in the patterns of skeletal injury. Fractures may be manifest only by a deformity of the normal contour of the bone. Sometimes, as in plastic fractures, there is no demonstrable fracture line. Figure 7–1 demonstrates a metacarpal fracture manifest almost entirely by deformity. Subtle shifts in the relationships of the bones may be the only sign of dislocation. Normal structures may be mistaken for pathology. Suffice it to say that one should be familiar with both bone anatomy and the patterns of bone growth, particularly with respect to the growth centers.

Comparison Views

In interpreting skeletal radiographs, the routine use of comparison views of the opposite side is an attractive expedient. This practice should, however, be discouraged for several reasons. If the radiographs show the affected side to be clearly fractured, the comparison views are unnecessary. The pattern of bone growth may not be identical on the opposite side (Fig 7–2), and therefore the comparison view could be misleading. Since the patient in whom this problem arises is a child, it is especially important to avoid unnecessary radiation exposure. The bilateral comparison examination will require considerably more time. There will be additional cost, if not to the patient, then to some health care provider.

In some cases, doubt arises as to the integrity of a particular structure. Thorough knowledge of anatomy and development will reduce these cases to a minimum. Also, there are several alternatives to a complete examination of the opposite side. Comparison with other epiphyseal lines in the same area may reveal a difference in the relative width of the epiphyseal plates, which itself is significant. The patient may have had a previous examination showing the area of concern. It is not rare for an accident-prone person to have previous films of the same area in the file, or a previous film of a related area may show the area of concern. For example, a chest film may show the

shoulder or an abdominal radiograph, the hip. Furthermore if there is a concern, the problem is usually evident on only one projection. That single view may be made of the opposite side, thereby making judicious use of radiographic exposure.

Vascular Grooves

Normally-occurring vascular grooves may cause diagnostic problems. There are two features of vascular grooves that differentiate them from fracture lines. Since the cortex forms the surface of the bone within the groove, as well as the outside surface, it provides a fine line of increased density on either side of the radiolucent vascular canal. Such a cortical border on a fracture line would be a clear indication of nonunion and would be unlikely to cause a diagnostic problem. Moreover, since a fracture line represents an actual, albeit small, diastasis of the bone, it will be more radiolucent than a vascular groove of the same diameter (Fig 7–3).

Patterns of Bone Injury

One must be mindful of several patterns of bone injury in order to be able to diagnose extremity injuries accurately. In any given area, certain fractures and dislocations occur more frequently than others. These fractures and dislocations may be modified by the mechanism of injury, such as direct or indirect trauma. The age of the patient will also have some influence on the injury produced. For example, the same mechanism that produces a clavicular fracture in a child may cause a fracture of the surgical neck of the humerus in an adult. Special attention should be paid to areas known to be predisposed to fracture.

In the forearm and in the leg, there are two parallel bones which are relatively rigidly secured to one another directly by ligaments or indirectly through another structure. If an injury shortens or dislocates one of the bones, the other bone will frequently become fractured or dislocated. Therefore, it is advisable to examine the entire length of both bones in the arm and the leg. If not done routinely, supplementary views should be obtained if such an injury exists.

If one sees an undisplaced fracture with the fracture line meeting the cortex at an acute angle, one should project the line entirely across the bone. In this manner, one may be alerted to a much more severe fracture than was originally suspected (Fig 7–4).

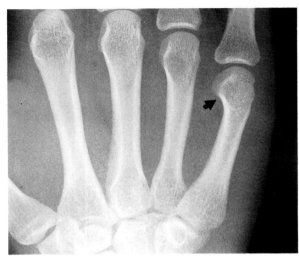

FIG 7–1.
Fracture of the fifth metacarpal manifest almost entirely by a deformity of the shape of the bone.

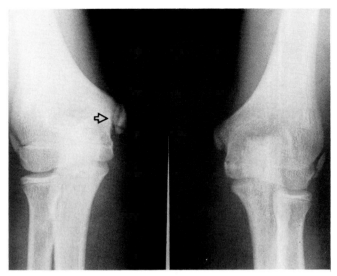

FIG 7–2.
Normal elbows. Notice that there is a bipartite center for the medial condyle of the humerus only on one side.

FIG 7–3.
A, vascular groove in the scapula. Notice the thin line of increased density bordering the radiolucent line, which is lighter than the region in which there is no bone. **B,** fracture of the scapula in a similar location.

There is no increased density at the margin of the radiolucent line. Although this line is narrower than the vascular groove, it is as dark as the portion of the film not interrupted by bone.

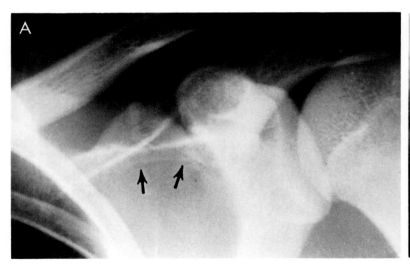 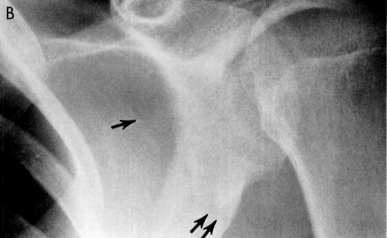

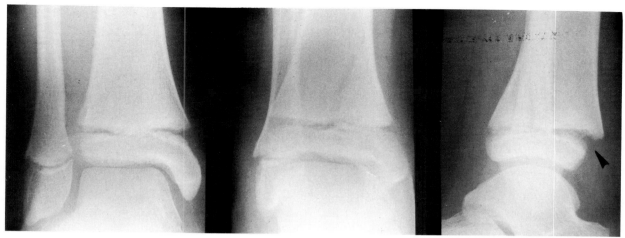

FIG 7–4.
Fracture of the metaphysis of the tibia. On the frontal and oblique views, this appears to be a relatively innocuous undisplaced fracture. On the lateral it is shown to be a fracture into the epiphyseal plate with displacement of the epiphysis.

FIG 7–5.
Salter-Harris classification of epiphyseal fractures.

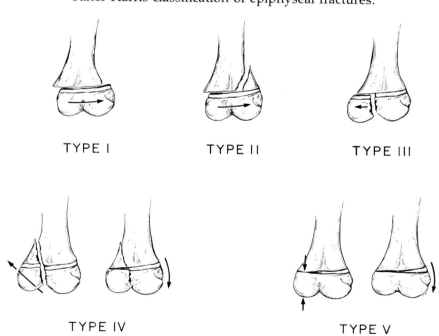

TYPE I   TYPE II   TYPE III

TYPE IV   TYPE V

The Salter-Harris classification, devised to assist in establishing prognosis, is employed to describe fractures of the epiphysis. As the classification number increases, the prognosis worsens. Salter-Harris I is a fracture of the epiphyseal plate alone without associated fracture of the metaphysis or epiphyseal center. Salter-Harris II is a fracture of the metaphysis with extension through the epiphyseal plate. Salter-Harris III is a fracture of the epiphyseal center with extension into the epiphyseal plate with or without displacement of the epiphysis. Salter-Harris IV is a fracture through the epiphysis, the plate and the metaphysis. A Salter-Harris V fracture is a crushing fracture of the epiphyseal center (Fig 7–5).

Patterns of Bone Repair

Even with careful radiographic technique and interpretation, some fractures may not be visible initially. The ribs are notorious in this regard. In cases of suspected rib fracture, delayed filming after 7 to 10 days will demonstrate early evidence of healing and permit the diagnosis of fracture. After a fracture occurs, the margins of the fracture absorb. This absorption will widen the radiolucent fracture line. New bone is then produced at the margins of the fracture beneath the periosteum (Fig 7–6). These radiopaque shadows also accentuate the fracture. Therefore, if a fracture is not visible but is suspected, a delayed examination may establish the diagnosis. Ten days is usually sufficient time for the radiographic signs to appear, and the patient is not overtaxed by immobilization without a diagnosis.

Radiographic Technique

Accurate radiologic diagnosis requires good radiographic technique. A lengthy discussion of this subject is not appropriate here. In a radiology department, sets of routine examinations have been designed and specified so that, generally, an examination stated on the consultation request will automatically call for a specific view or group of views. These are selected to demonstrate the area of concern to best advantage with the least exposure. Because the anatomical part is three-dimensional, it is important to have at least two projections, preferably at right angles to one another. These are often supplemented by one or more oblique views (Fig 7–7). The carpal navicular bone, the patella, and the calcaneus present special problems. As will be shown later, fractures of these bones may not be demonstrated well, if at all, on the general routine examinations of these areas. Moreover, none of these views may project the plane of the fracture so that it can be seen. In these cases, high clinical suspicion or supplementary radiographic signs may make additional projections, such as oblique views, necessary. In the discussion of each individual extremity, a brief discussion of the appropriate views will be presented. It is important, however, to have a general appreciation of those views that constitute a reasonable examination of a given area.

The quality of each radiograph should be assessed. The projections obtained should be appropriate to the area. Films that are overexposed may fail to demonstrate existing pathology (Fig 7–8). Moreover, motion artifact may also result in loss of detail and missed fractures (Fig 7–9).

Special Radiologic Procedures

Modern radiology comprises many different diagnostic modalities. Although this section emphasizes conventional radiography, other modalities may provide additional information. More sophisticated procedures are generally used when conventional radiography leaves unanswered questions, particularly if the diagnosis remains uncertain or if therapy depends on additional definition of the injury or disease. These modalities are rarely used to evaluate the peripheral skeleton in an emergency setting.

Stress Views

A stress view may be employed to gain graphic evidence of disruption of the ligaments. In obtaining a stress view, there is a risk of traumatizing an already injured structure or aggravating an existing condition. The patient is exposed to more radiation, as is the technologist. Pain may prevent the use of sufficient stress for diagnosis (see Fig 7–48). For these reasons, stress views should be undertaken only when the outcome will significantly affect the course of therapy. Stress should be applied by someone aware of all these factors in order to achieve a high level of confidence in the result.

Arthrography

By injecting contrast into various joints one may obtain information on cartilages, ligaments and other joint structures. Arthrography is generally used in cases of chronic skeletal problems involving joints.

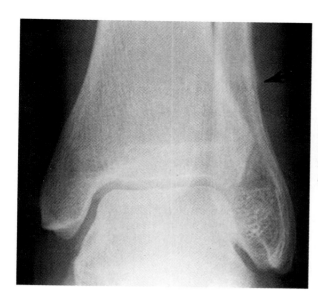

FIG 7–6.
Initially invisible fracture of the fibula is manifest by small area of callus formation and subperiosteal new bone.

FIG 7–7.
Fracture of the third metacarpal bone is almost invisible on the frontal and oblique views. It is clearly visible in the lateral projection.

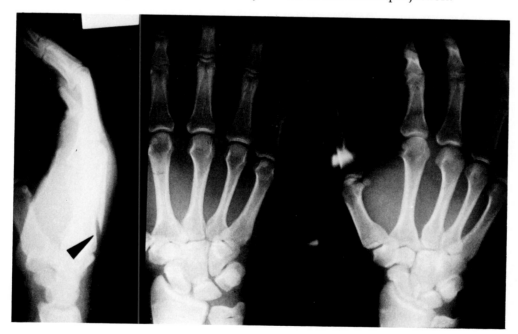

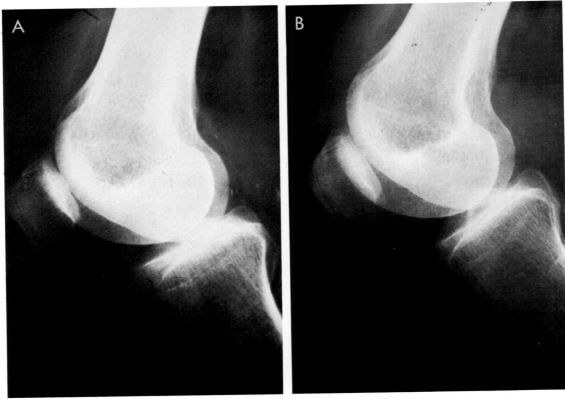

FIG 7–8.
Radiographic technique. **A,** fracture of the patella is almost invisible on the overexposed film. **B,** a film with the proper exposure clearly shows the fracture.

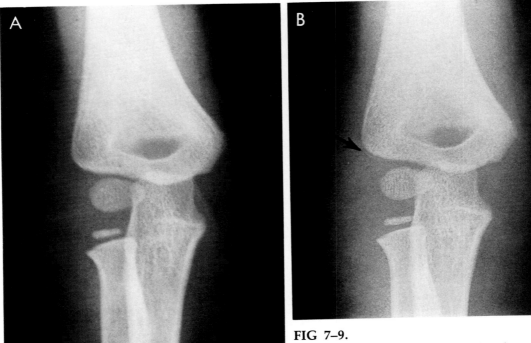

FIG 7–9.
Radiographic technique. **A,** detail on initial film is slightly compromised by motion. **B,** repeat view reveals minimal supracondylar humeral fracture initially obscured.

Angiography

Arteriography is employed in an emergency setting to assess the integrity of the vascular system after injury. It is also used to define cases of acute vascular insufficiency. Venography may be used to evaluate venous thrombosis.

Ultrasound

Diagnostic ultrasound is used to assess cases of suspected deep venous thrombosis. It is less invasive but also less accurate than contrast venography.

Tomography

Conventional (noncomputed) tomography can confine the examination to a defined plane by obscuring superimposed structures. This feature is particularly useful in larger bones and in complex areas. Tomography requires a cooperative patient as well as additional time and radiation exposure.

Radionuclide Scanning

Radiopharmaceuticals are administered to seek out actively metabolizing bone. This material preferentially seeks areas of more active metabolism such as healing fractures. Almost invariably a fracture will become positive on scans within a very few days and remain positive for months. A positive area is not, however, specific for fracture. Although radionuclide scanning is usually employed in cases of questionable findings in the spine or hip, it may be used in any bone. These procedures involve total body radiation and require several hours to perform.

Computed Tomography

Computed tomography (CT) combines an x-ray machine with computer technology to create a cross-sectional display of the body part. Its unique ability to produce axial views makes CT useful in assessing skeletal trauma. CT provides excellent contrast resolution useful in delineating pathology.

Magnetic Resonance Imaging

Magnetic resonance imaging's (MRI) excellence in demonstrating soft tissues will make it increasingly important in skeletal evaluation. Normally invisible cartilagenous, tendinous, and ligamentous structures can be evaluated, and MRI can examine in any plane. CT and, in particular, MRI, require a high degree of patient cooperation. Many technical considerations make it difficult to examine severely injured or ill patients using MRI.

General Considerations

Certain influences may be distracting in the evaluation of radiographic examinations. An obvious lesion may divert attention from a more subtle one. Marks placed on the film may have the same effect. In any event, permanent marks should not be made since they are distracting. They also destroy the teaching value of the film, and they may be embarrassing if directed to a normal structure or diagnostic error.

High intensity lights are helpful in evaluating soft tissues and other dark portions of radiographs. They are not, however, an appropriate substitute for proper exposure. Magnifying lenses are not often necessary. They enlarge the grain of the film to a perceptible level and therefore add little detail on conventional film. Spotlights and magnifying lenses are useful in concentrating one's attention on a small area.

Clinical Examination of the Patient

Before any radiographic examination is requested, the injured area should be defined and an examination ordered adequate to cover the site of injury without exposing additional tissue unneccessarily. Special views may be requested if the injury involves one of those special structures that are not shown clearly on a routine examination. In evaluating the radiographic examination, one must first be sure that the films do indeed include the area of concern. Clinical examination will show that portion of the radiographic examination to which one should direct the most stringent attention. The radiographic examination must be correlated with the signs and symptoms of the patient. Indeed, failure of the radiographic examination to explain the clinical picture may be an indication for obtaining supplementary views.

Radiographic examinations are performed to obtain additional objective information regarding the patient's condition. Although the result of the radiographic examination should be correlated with the clinical information, one should not be unduly influenced by the clinical findings. Overreliance on clinical information may result in radiologic overdiagnosis. It is equally important to recognize that it is hazardous to attempt radiologic diagnosis without any clinical information. The search pattern should conform to the clinical situation.

The following checklist covers the basic elements

required to interpret extremity radiographs. Following this checklist or any other systematic approach will decrease the likelihood of error. Most errors of interpretation occur when some portion of the systematic approach is deliberately or accidentally disregarded. To be sure, clinical emergencies may dictate shortcuts, but those shortcuts should be avoided if at all possible. As one proceeds, the significance of the various items in the checklist will become evident. Most of the points in the outline are in the preceding general material on extremity trauma. Careful adherence to these basic principles will be rewarded with greater diagnostic accuracy.

Checklist

1. Are these the films of the patient in question? Are they of the correct side?

2. Do the radiographs demonstrate the area in question? There may have been a failure in communication.

3. Have the proper projections been obtained? One should consider whether the injury site may be in a structure, such as the patella, carpal navicular, or calcaneus, that requires a special projection.

4. Are the radiographs properly exposed? Is detail adequate?

5. Are the structures in proper relation to one another? Is there any unusual contour to any of the bones? Are there any sharp angles or abrupt changes in contour?

6. Trace the cortical margin of each individual bone completely. Search the interior of each bone. Look through each bone at others that may be superimposed. Particular emphasis should be placed on the localized area of clinical concern and on areas known to be predisposed to injury.

7. Look for ancillary soft tissue signs. If they are present, repeat your search and consider obtaining additional views or follow-up.

8. If there is an obvious lesion, disregard it until you have looked at the remainder of the film. Concentrating on an obvious lesion can distract attention from other findings. Similarly, a mark placed to demonstrate one finding may divert attention from a significant abnormality.

9. Write down your opinion. The findings should explain the clinical picture. If not, you may wish to obtain additional views or require follow-up. The record of what was seen can be invaluable for others who subsequently attend the patient. Moreover, we are more painstaking in our work if we know that it is going to be committed to a permanent record.

Shoulder

The shoulder actually comprises two joints and portions of three bones. This structure, together with an almost unrestricted range of motion, makes it susceptible to a variety of different injuries.

Anatomy

During development, there are growth centers for the head and the greater tuberosity of the humerus. At 6 years of age, the two fuse to form a single epiphyseal center for the proximal humerus. There is an epiphysis for the acromion process and one for the coracoid process of the scapula. In addition, there is a center for the rim of the glenoid of the scapula. This center may remain unfused into early adulthood, an appearance that may suggest an avulsion fracture. The epiphysis for the clavicle is at the medial end. These structures are illustrated in Figure 7–10.

Radiography

Often the shoulder is examined in frontal projections with the humerus in extreme internal and external rotation. These projections provide right-angle views of the humerus but not of the other structures of the shoulder. As a note of caution, it should be pointed out that rotation of the humerus may aggravate a fracture or, occasionally, reduce a dislocation. In the presence of a fracture or dislocation, movement may be restricted and conventional views may not be obtainable.

In trauma patients, we have adopted the use of a pair of oblique views. These provide true frontal (see tangential glenoid view, Fig 7–13,B) and lateral (scapular Y) views of the glenohumeral joint (Fig 7–11). These views can be made without manipulating the humerus. Views at right angles to the coronal plane may be obtained in two ways. A transthoracic view shows the shoulder in a lateral projection. Because the plane of the glenohumeral joint is rarely projected parallel to the sagittal plane, this view will not provide an accurate lateral view. Usually, the joint faces anteriorly at an angle of approximately 30 degrees. The transthoracic view is difficult to interpret because of superimposition of the ribs and the vertebrae. An axial or axillary view is another projection at 90 degrees to the coronal plane and inevitably requires more manipulation than any other view. In non-trauma states, the frontal view in external rotation, together with the axillary view, provides the most useful information.

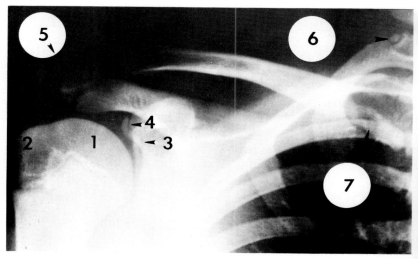

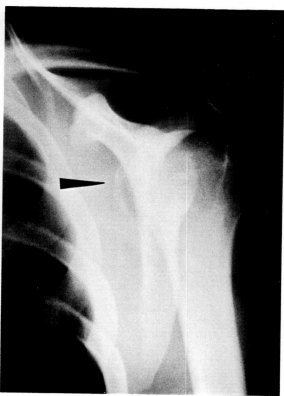

FIG 7–10 (top left).
Normal shoulder of an 11-year-old male. Notice the fused centers for the head *(1)* and greater tuberosity of the humerus *(2)*, the centers for the rim of the glenoid *(3)*, the coracoid process *(4)*, the acromion process *(5)*, and the transverse process of the first thoracic vertebra *(6)*. The rhomboid fossa *(7)* is a normal anatomic variation.

FIG 7–11 (top right).
Avulsion fracture of the anterior rim of the glenoid of the scapula seen on the scapular Y view of the shoulder.

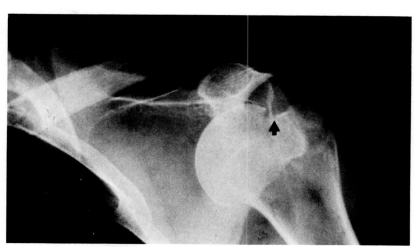

FIG 7–12.
Anterior (subcoracoid) dislocation of the shoulder on conventional frontal view. Head of the humerus is displaced medially. Notice the increased distance from the humeral head to the acromion process and the impaction fracture deformity *(arrow)*.

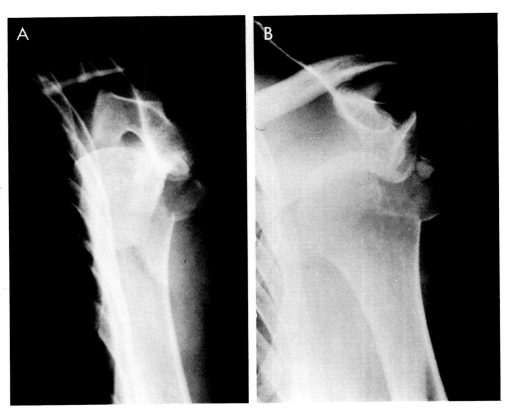

FIG 7–13.
Anterior (subcoracoid) dislocation of the humerus with a comminuted fracture of the greater tuberosity. **A,** scapular Y view. **B,** tangential view.

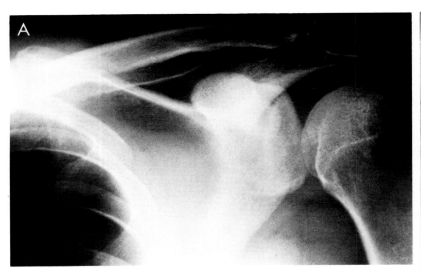

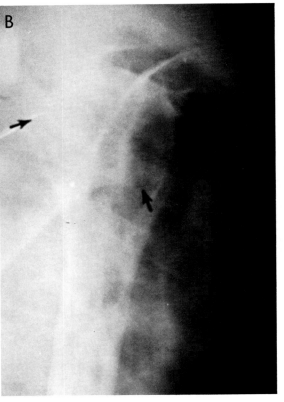

FIG 7–14.
Posterior dislocation of the shoulder. **A,** in the frontal projection, the head of the humerus is displaced laterally. **B,** on the transthoracic view, the head *(single arrow)* is shown to be posterior to the rim of the glenoid *(three arrows).*

Dislocations

The angle of the plane of the glenohumeral joint with respect to the sagittal plane has been described. Demonstration of this plane is most important in determining whether the humeral head is dislocated and the type of dislocation. Because, in the frontal projection, the anterior rim of the glenoid is more medial than the posterior, the anteriorly dislocated humeral head will move medially as well. Instead of a small ellipse of the head overlapping the glenoid, a greater portion of the head will be superimposed. Occasionally, the head may be entirely medial to the glenoid in the frontal projection. Since the head will then lie directly beneath the coracoid process, an anterior dislocation is frequently called subcoracoid. The distance from the humeral head to the acromion process, normally approximately 10 mm, will increase (Fig 7–12.) This situation is obvious on the paired oblique views with the humeral head overlapping the glenoid on the tangential view and anterior to the glenoid on the Y view (Fig 7–13).

Patients with dislocations of the shoulder will often have impaction fractures of the humeral head which result from impingement of the head upon the glenoid (Sachs-Hill deformity). Posterior dislocations of the humerus are much less common, constituting fewer than 5% of shoulder dislocations, and are more difficult to diagnose. It has been stated that as many as half are missed initially. Since in the frontal projection the posterior rim of the glenoid is more lateral than the anterior rim, a posteriorly-dislocated humeral head will move into a more lateral position than its usual location. The distance from the coracoid process to the humeral head, which is usually 15 mm, will increase. In the frontal projection, the distance from the anterior rim of the glenoid to the humeral head, which is usually 8 mm, will also increase (rim sign). As opposed to the normal slight overlap, one may see "daylight" through the glenohumeral joint in the frontal projection. The humerus will be in internal rotation: indeed, it is said that, if the humerus can be externally rotated, a posterior dislocation does not exist. There may be an impacted fracture of the anterior portion of the articular surface of the humerus that produces a double outline of the humeral head (trough sign). In the transthoracic projection, the humeral head will be seen posterior to the glenoid (Fig 7–14). On the Y view, the head of the humerus will be posterior to the glenoid. On the tangential view, the humeral head and the glenoid will overlap (Fig 7–15).

Scapula

Radiography

The scapula should be examined in the lateral as well as the frontal projection. The lateral view should be obtained in a 60-degree anterior oblique projection with the arm elevated as far as possible.

Fractures

Fractures of the scapula are almost always caused by direct trauma and are usually visible as radiolucent lines. The cortex of all three borders should be carefully traced and the continuity of the spine of the scapula should be established. Scapular fractures may present as radiopaque lines that may be confused with normal scalloping (Figs 7–16 and 7–17).

Clavicle

Because of its location, the clavicle is unavoidably superimposed on the ribs and other structures in the frontal projection. Because of the proximity of the scapula to the chest wall, it is impossible to obtain the desired films in two projections at right angles to one another. In addition to the frontal projection, a second view is obtained by angling the tube-caudad in the PA position or cephalad in the AP position. The resulting view will project the clavicle clear of the adjacent structures (Fig 7–18). A view of the sternoclavicular articulation is obtained by angling either the patient or the radiographic tube in an oblique position. In some cases we have evaluated these structures in axial projections by CT. The acromioclavicular joint is examined by first making an erect nonstress view (which is reviewed for possible fracture) followed by a view in the same position with the patient holding in his hand as much weight as possible (Figs 7–19 and 7–20).

Dislocations and Subluxations

In evaluating suspected acromioclavicular separation, it is important to first review a nonstress-bearing view because a fracture of the lateral end of the clavicle can have the same clinical appearance. In this clinical setting, it is far more common for young children to have a fracture of the clavicle than an acromioclavicular separation. It is important to use as much stress as is tolerable because good conditioning or muscle spasm may hold the structures together

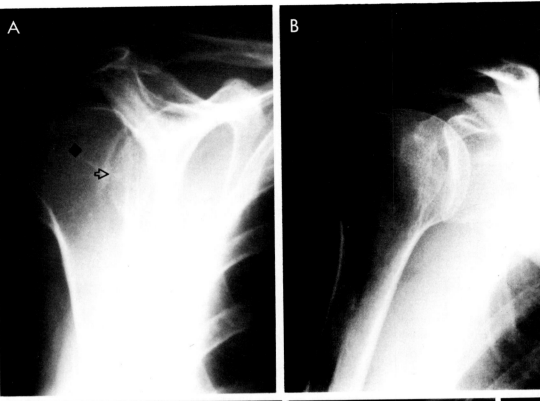

FIG 7–15.
Posterior dislocation of the shoulder. **A,** scapular Y view of humeral head *(diamond)* and glenoid rim *(arrow).* **B,** tangential view showing overlapping of dislocated humeral head.

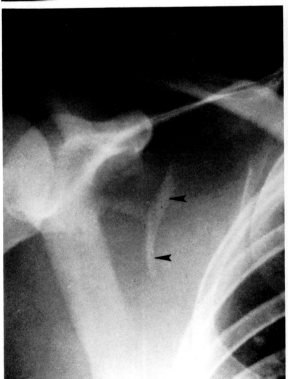

FIG 7–16.
Fracture of the scapula manifest by radiopaque line, which indicates impaction or overlap of the fragments.

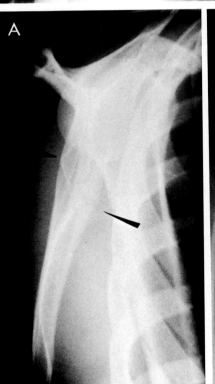
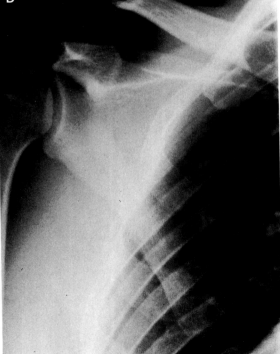

FIG 7–17.
Fracture of the scapula shown on lateral view **(A),** but not on frontal view **(B).**

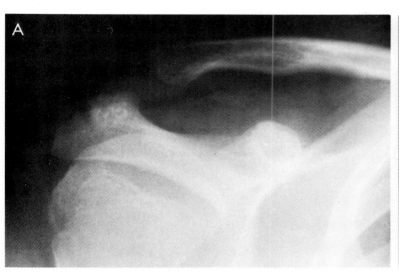

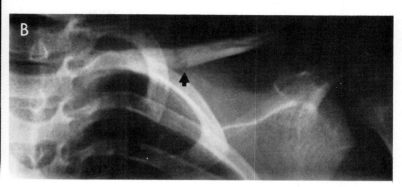

FIG 7–18.
Clavicular fracture not seen on regular frontal view because of superimposed structures **(A)**. The clavicular view shows the fracture clearly **(B)**.

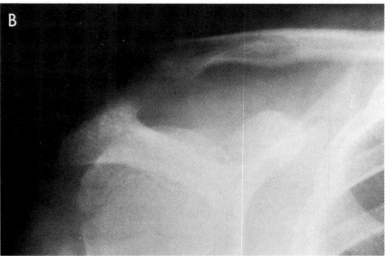

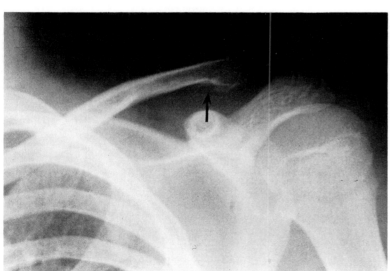

FIG 7–19 (middle left and right).
Acromioclavicular separation. **A,** on the initial examination, there is equivocal widening of the joint. **B,** a stress-bearing view confirms the diagnosis.

FIG 7–20 (bottom left).
Fracture of the clavicle shown on the initial examination of patient with suspected acromioclavicular separation. Stress view is unnecessary.

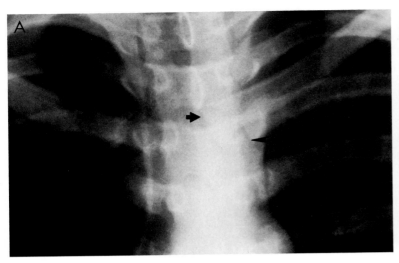

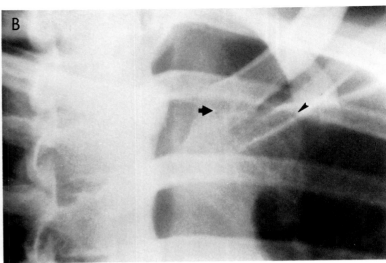

FIG 7–21.
Dislocation of the medial end of the clavicle. In the frontal projection, left clavicle *(arrow)* overlaps the sternum *(arrowhead)*. On the oblique view the clavicle is displaced posteriorly from the articular surface of the sternum.

FIG 7–22.
Fracture of the supracondylar portion of the humerus *(arrowhead)* manifest almost entirely by posterior displacement of the capitulum. A line projected from the anterior cortex of the humeral shaft should intercept a substantial portion of the capitulum *(arrow)*. The normal side shown for comparison **(B).**

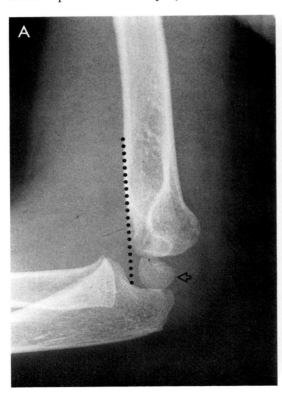

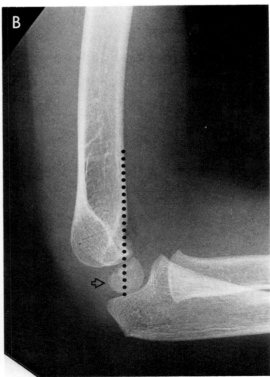

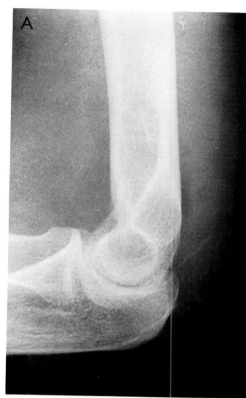

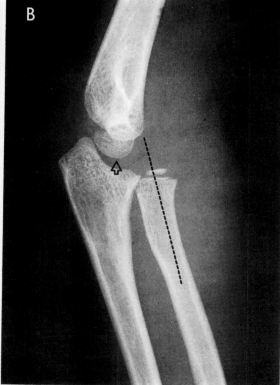

FIG 7–23.
Fracture of the olecranon process of the ulna. **A,** there is a small irregularity of the posterior ulna *(arrow)*. **B,** tangential view confirms fracture not visible on frontal view.

FIG 7–24.
Dislocated radial head. In both projections the head and shaft of the radius do not align with the capitulum, the largest growth center in the elbow of a child.

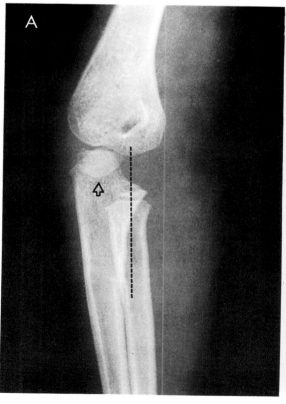

even though the ligament has been torn. Since the superior border of the clavicle may normally be higher than the acromion process, one should note that the inferior cortex of the acromion, together with the inferior cortex of the clavicle, usually makes a continuous line. In some individuals, the line of the inferior margin of the clavicle may lie at a higher or lower level, making comparison with the opposite side essential. When dislocation of the sternoclavicular joint occurs, the clavicle is almost always displaced anteriorly. When posterior dislocation occurs, it must be regarded as a most serious injury because of the potential damage to the vital structures in the upper mediastinum (Fig 7–21).

Elbow

Anatomy

The elbow comprises two different joints, a hinge joint between the trochlear portion of the humerus and the ulna, and a rotating hinge joint between the radius and the capitulum of the humerus. The capitulum and the trochlear portion of the humerus are at approximately a 45-degree angle to the shaft of the humerus, so that a line projected down the center of the medullary canal of the humerus falls posterior to these structures. A line along the anterior cortex of the humerus should intersect the middle of the ossification center of the capitulum (Fig 7–22). The elbow joint capsule will be discussed below. The distal attachment of the capsule occurs at the radial head. The elbow region is extremely complex from the standpoint of epiphyseal growth. There are growth centers for the radial head and the olecranon process of the ulna. The first secondary growth center to appear in the humerus is that for the capitulum. Later, centers appear for the medial and lateral condyles and the trochlear portion (see Fig 7–2).

Radiography

Frontal and lateral views will usually suffice for examination of the elbow. Because of the multiplicity of growth centers and their variable appearance, comparison views are more frequently necessary than for any other extremity area. Because subtle fractures can occur, oblique views are used to supplement the routine projections. Tangential views may be used for injuries of the posterior aspect of the elbow (Fig 7–23) or in patients who cannot straighten the elbow.

Dislocations

The relationship of the notch of the olecranon process of the ulna to the trochlear portion of the humerus is an obvious one, and dislocations are easily recognized. Dislocations of the radius may, however, be subtle and easily overlooked. A useful criterion for this diagnosis is the axis of the radial shaft. In all projections, a line drawn through the center of the shaft of the radius should pass through the center of the capitulum (Fig 7–24).

Dislocation of the radial head is a component of Monteggia's fracture, which will be discussed below. Dislocation of the radial head through the orbicular ligament is believed to be the etiology of so-called nursemaid's elbow. This dislocation is usually produced by sharp traction on the forearm of very young ambulatory children. Often the dislocation reduces spontaneously or by manipulation before radiographic examination. Before reduction, the dislocation can be diagnosed by using the radial line.

Posterior Humeral Fat Pad Sign

The fat pads around the elbow are useful indicators of trauma. On both the anterior and posterior surfaces of the distal humerus, there are cavities which contain fat. The posterior pad is not normally seen on lateral radiographs. A small portion of the anterior pad is usually visible as a thin, triangular shadow. The elbow joint capsule attaches immediately adjacent to the lower edge of these pads. If the elbow joint capsule becomes distended by hemorrhage or effusion, it will force the fat pads upward and outward. The posterior humeral fat pad, which is normally invisible, becomes visible and constitutes the posterior humeral fat pad sign. At the same time, the anterior pad becomes more visible than normal. One should not become distracted by the various configurations of the anterior pad. Remember that it is necessary only to consider the posterior pad which, if visible, always indicates abnormality.

In a trauma setting, almost all elbows with a positive posterior humeral fat pad sign will have a fracture. Therefore, without a visible fracture, one must assume that a subtle fracture is present and look more closely or obtain additional views, such as obliques (Fig 7–25). If the fracture is not immediately visible, there is usually a radial head fracture in an adult or a supracondylar fracture in a child (Fig 7–26). If no fracture is detected, one should inform the patient that an occult fracture is highly possible and that follow-up is desirable.

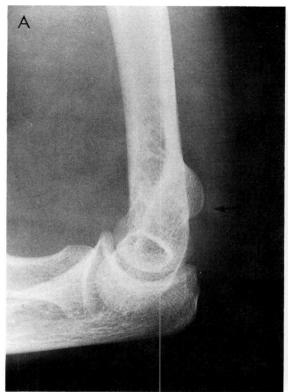

FIG 7–25.
A, elbow injury with positive posterior humeral fat pad sign *(arrow).* No definite fracture on frontal view. **B,** oblique view shows radial head fracture.

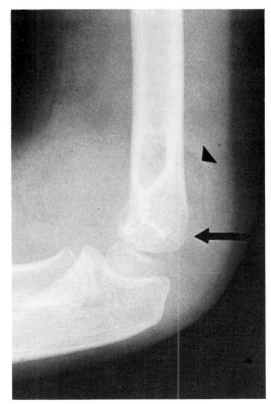

FIG 7–26.
Positive posterior humeral fat pad sign in a 6-year-old child. Close inspection reveals a deformity of the posterior cortex, indicating supracondylar humeral fracture.

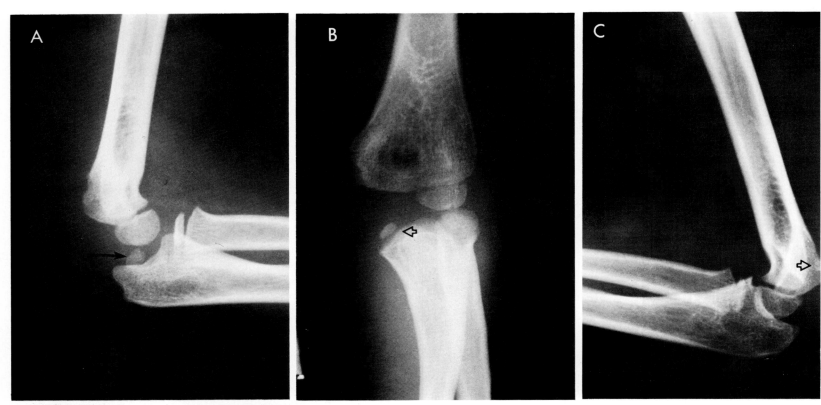

FIG 7–27.
A and **B,** avulsion fracture of the ossification center of the medial epicondyle of the humerus. The avulsed growth center is displaced into the joint, which is widened. Normal side is shown for comparison (**C** and **D**).

FIG 7–28.
Fracture of the coronoid process of the ulna.

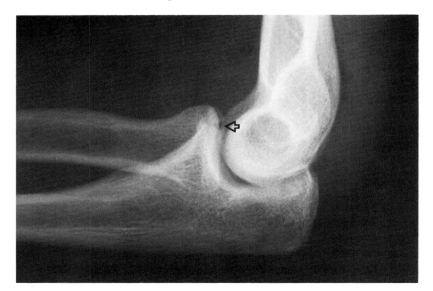

Fractures

Avulsion fracture of the ossification center of the medial epicondyle of the humerus is a common injury in children and is easily overlooked. Because this injury may lacerate the joint capsule, the fat pad sign may not be positive. However, there will usually be marked soft tissue swelling at the medial aspect of the joint, and the center will be displaced from its normal location (Fig 7–27). In these cases, a comparison view of the opposite side will be helpful.

Fracture of the coronoid process of the ulna (Fig 7–28) may occur independently of dislocation of the elbow joint. Often, the fragment can only be seen by looking through the superimposed radius on the lateral view.

Forearm

Anatomy

The relationships of the proximal radius and ulna to the humerus have been described in the section on the elbow. There is a small flange just distal to the semilunar notch of the ulna which articulates with the medial aspect of the radial head. The radial tuberosity on the medial side of the radius just distal to the head is the site of attachment of the biceps. When seen en face, it can give the misleading appearance of a radiolucent lesion in the radius (Fig 7–29).

Except for a small intracapsular articulation between the ulna and the radius, the osseous articulation of the wrist is between the radius and the proximal row of carpal bones. The distal ulna articulates with the radiographically-invisible triangular fibrocartilage. The ulna is rigidly attached to the humerus at the elbow, and the radius is rigidly attached to the proximal row of carpal bones at the wrist. The radius and the ulna are thus attached to one another at both ends. This is the anatomical basis of an important consideration in evaluating fractures of the forearm. If an angulated fracture of one of the paired bones effectively shortens one bone, the other bone must be shortened by fracture or dislocation.

Development

The epiphysis for the olecranon appears at approximately the 10th year and fuses at about the 16th year. The center for the radial head appears around the 4th year and fuses at about the 20th year. Ossification begins in the radial head in the 5th year, with fusion at the 17th year. The center for the distal radius appears in the 2nd year and fuses at approximately the 20th year.

Radiography

Frontal and lateral views of the forearm virtually always suffice. Because of the paired bone relationship, it is important to see both ends of both bones, especially if there is an angulated fracture of one.

Fractures

In addition to the more common fractures of both bones, there are two fractures which involve a fracture of one bone and a dislocation of the other. Monteggia's fracture is a break of the proximal or midulna with dislocation of the radial head (Fig 7–30). Galeazzi's fracture is a fracture of the distal or midradius with dislocation of the distal end of the ulna. In children one may see a fracture of one or both bones manifested merely by a bowing deformity. These fractures may be overlooked unless one is suspicious enough to obtain comparison views of the opposite side. The lateral projection is particularly useful in this regard.

Wrist

Anatomy

One should carefully trace the relationship of the bones of the wrist on each examination. Failure to do so is a frequent cause of error. It is especially important to note that on a properly positioned lateral radiograph the posterior cortices of the radius and ulna are parallel to one another and have a straight or gently curving contour. The distal articular surface of the radius faces slightly in a palmar direction, almost at a right angle to the axis of the shaft. On the lateral view, the axis of the radius should pass through the center of the proximal and distal rows of carpal bones and the shafts of the medial four metacarpal bones. It is particularly important to note whether the lunate, which is easily identifiable, is properly placed on the articular surface of the radius and whether the capitate articulates within the concavity of the lunate (Fig 7–31,A). Gilula has emphasized that the cortices of the rows of carpal bones form parallel arches (Fig 7–31,B).

Development

Skeletal maturation of the distal radius and ulna is described in the section on the forearm. The epiphysis of the radius and ulna close simultaneously at about the 20th year. The ossification centers for the carpal and metacarpal bones appear through the early years. The time of appearance provides a convenient means of assessing skeletal maturation.

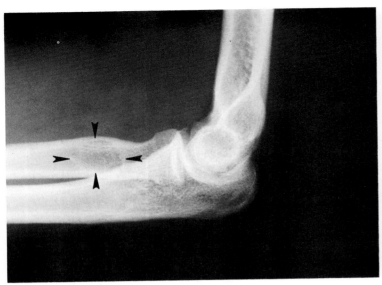

FIG 7–29.
Normal elbow. The radial tuberosity seen en face simulates destructive lesion.

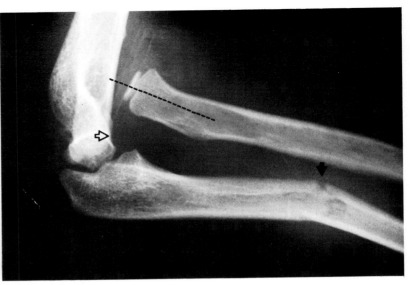

FIG 7–30.
Monteggia's fracture. The ulna is shortened by an angulated ulnar fracture. The radius has accommodated this shortening by dislocating at the elbow.

FIG 7–31.
Normal wrist. **A,** the posterior cortices of the radius *(white arrow)* and ulna *(black arrow)* are parallel and have a smooth gentle curve. Notice the straight line relationship between the axis of the radial shaft, the proximal row of carpal bones *(1 = lunate)*, the distal row of carpal bones *(2 = capitate)*, and the medial four metacarpals *(3)* *(4 = greater multangular bone)*. **B,** continuous arches are formed by the margins of the carpal bones.

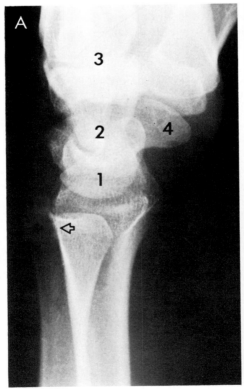

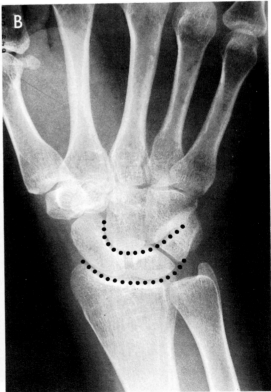

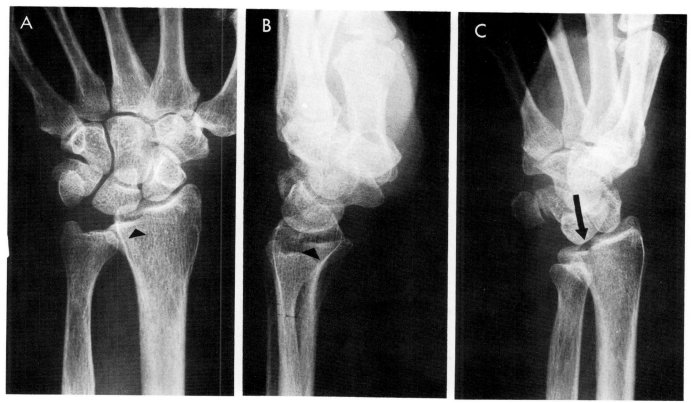

FIG 7–32.
Axial fracture of the distal radius. Although it is visible on the PA and lateral views **(A** and **B)**, this fracture is best demonstrated on a reverse oblique view **(C)**.

FIG 7–33.
A, fracture of the carpal navicular bone. The special navicular view best demonstrates the fracture **(B)**.

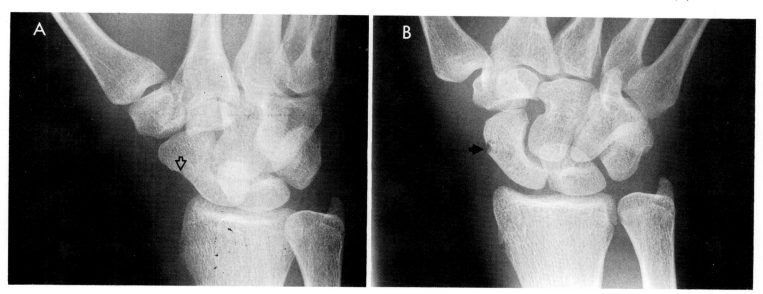

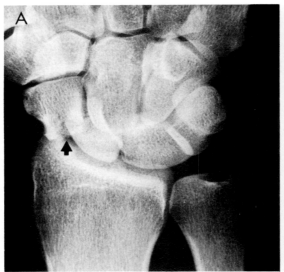

FIG 7–34.
Perilunate dislocation with fracture of the navicular *(arrow).* **A,** in the frontal projection, there is disruption of the arch configuration of the distal portions of the proximal row of carpal bones and overlapping of the distal row. **B,** in the lateral projection, the lunate retains its normal relationship to the radius, but the capitate *(2)* is dislocated posteriorly from its usual articulation in the concavity of the lunate *(1).*

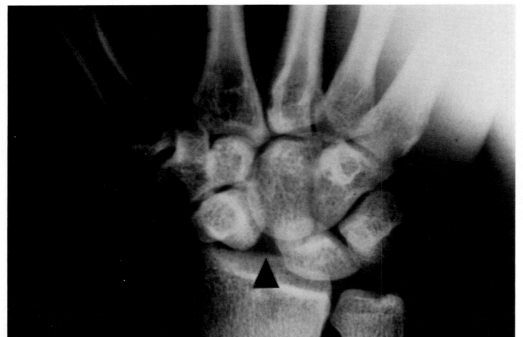

FIG 7–35.
Rotary dislocation of the carpal navicular bone. In the frontal projection there is an abnormally wide space between the lunate and the navicular.

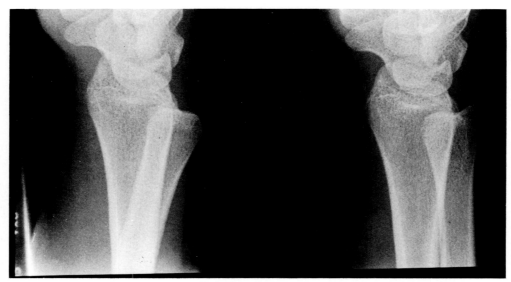

FIG 7–36.
Spurious dislocation of the distal ulna. Lateral view made by pronating the hand from the frontal projection. Accurate lateral view shows no dislocation.

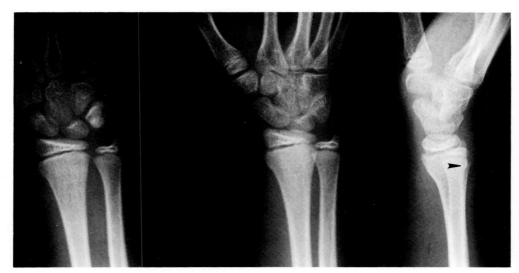

FIG 7–37.
Fracture of the distal radius. Note that the fracture is seen only on the true lateral view. Accurate positioning is therefore critical in diagnosing this injury.

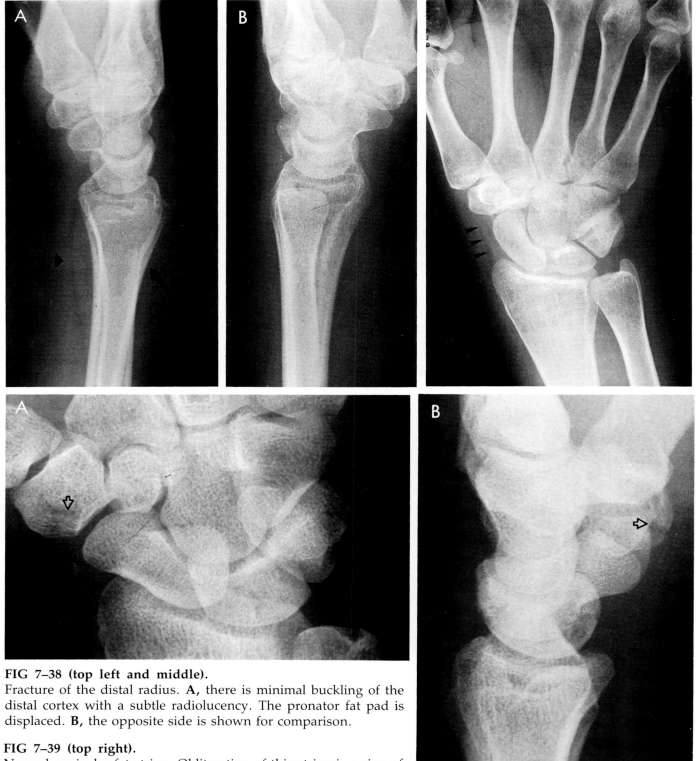

FIG 7–38 (top left and middle).
Fracture of the distal radius. **A,** there is minimal buckling of the distal cortex with a subtle radiolucency. The pronator fat pad is displaced. **B,** the opposite side is shown for comparison.

FIG 7–39 (top right).
Normal navicular fat stripe. Obliteration of this stripe is a sign of navicular fracture.

FIG 7–40 (bottom left and right).
A and **B,** fracture of the greater multangular bone.

Radiography

Routine wrist examination involves frontal, lateral, and oblique projections. The latter is made with the palm down and the hand supinated 45 degrees. These projections may be supplemented by a view with the palm up and the hand pronated 45 degrees (Fig 7–32). A special view of the carpal navicular is most helpful in diagnosing suspected fractures of that bone. This view is obtained in the PA projection with the hand in ulnar deviation and the tube angled toward the elbow (Fig 7–33).

Dislocations

Knowledge of the above-described relationships of the wrist bones is basic to the diagnosis of dislocations. Perilunate dislocation of the wrist occurs most frequently. Characteristically the lunate retains it normal relationship to the radius, and the capitate is displaced posteriorly from its usual position within the concavity of the lunate. There is almost always an associated fracture of the navicular bone. The medial navicular fragment remains attached to the lunate, and the lateral fragment remains attached to the adjacent carpal bones which are displaced (Fig 7–34). More rarely, the lunate or the navicular bone alone may be dislocated (Fig 7–35).

Spurious dislocation of the distal end of the ulna may be produced in the lateral view by pronating the hand rather than by moving the entire forearm (Fig 7–36). This undesirable expedient produces frontal and lateral views of the radius, but only frontal views of the ulna.

Fractures

Fractures of the distal radius and ulna are the most frequent fractures of the wrist. The classic Colle's fracture is an impacted fracture of the distal radius with dorsal angulation of the distal fragments, producing the "silver fork" deformity. It is associated with avulsion of the ulnar styloid. Frequently, however, radial fractures will be seen only as a minimal alteration in the contour of the cortex of the distal radius (Fig 7–37).

The pronator fat pad sign is useful in detecting minimal injuries. When the fat pad sign is positive, the fat stripe normally visible over the pronator muscle is displaced from the radius by hemorrhage or other swelling (Fig 7–38).

Next most frequent in occurrence is fracture of the navicular bone. This fracture is quite rare in children. Obliteration of the normally visible navicular fat stripe (Fig 7–39) is a sign of navicular fracture. The special navicular view may be necessary to establish the diagnosis of subtle fractures (see Fig 7–33).

Fracture of the greater multangular (trapezium) bone may be identified only by noting irregular radiolucency within the bone. Interruptions of the cortex may not be visible. The bone is best seen in the lateral projection with the thumb flexed at the carpometacarpal joint (Fig 7–40).

Small avulsion fractures on the posterior aspect of the proximal row of carpal bones almost always originate in the triquetrum. Since the small fragment is lost to observation when the hand is rotated into the frontal projection, one may have to rely on clinical correlation to identify the involved bone (Fig 7–41).

Fractures of the remaining carpal bones are quite rare. They are usually the result of direct rather than transmitted trauma (Fig 7–42). Fracture of the hook (hamulus) of the hamate may be seen, particularly among participants in baseball and racket sports. The classic radiographic sign is disappearance of that structure in the frontal projection. This may be confirmed by a tangential view of the wrist (Fig 7–43).

Hand

Anatomy

In the lateral projection, the shafts of the second, third, fourth, and fifth metacarpal bones should lie on a straight line extending along the axis of the radius passing through the lunate and capitate bones. The first metacarpal bone articulates with the greater multangular bone. The epiphyses of the second through fifth metacarpals are at the distal ends, and the epiphysis for the first on the proximal end. A frequently seen variation is the appearance of an additional epiphyseal line at the distal end of the first metacarpal.

Radiography

The hand is usually examined in the frontal, lateral, and oblique projections. Although the medial four metacarpal bones are superimposed on the lateral view, valuable information may still be obtained from it (see Fig 7–7). Occasionally, the reverse oblique may supplement these projections.

Fractures

The lateral view of the hand or fingers should not be neglected. Small fractures of the articular surfaces

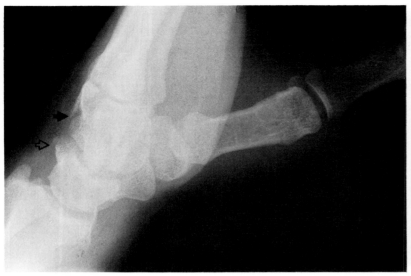

FIG 7–41.
Fractures of the triquetrum and hamate.

FIG 7–42.
Fracture of the capitate. There is also a faintly visible fracture of the greater multangular.

FIG 7–43 (bottom left).
Fracture of the hook (hamulus) of the hamate demonstrated on tangential view of the wrist.

FIG 7–44 (bottom right).
Bennett's fracture-dislocation of the first metacarpal bone. The smaller fragment has retained its normal relationship to the greater multangular, while the larger has slipped laterally and overlaps that bone.

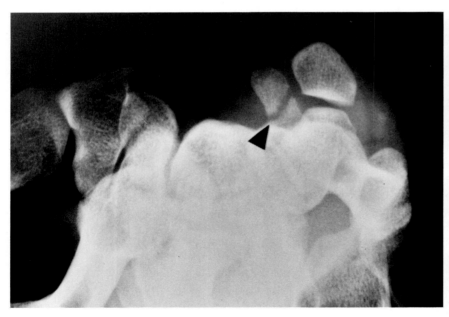

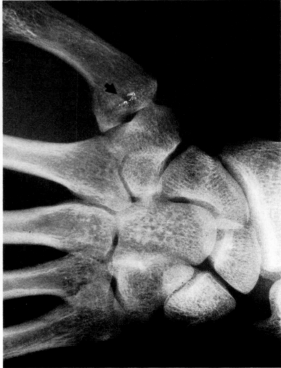

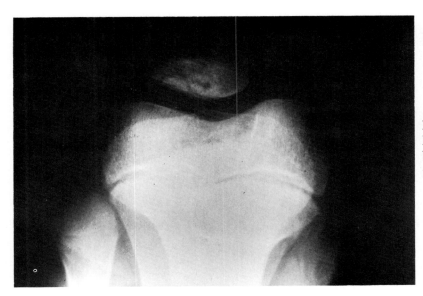

FIG 7–45.
Normal irregular ossification of the patella. The bone on the unaffected side is as irregular as the injured side.

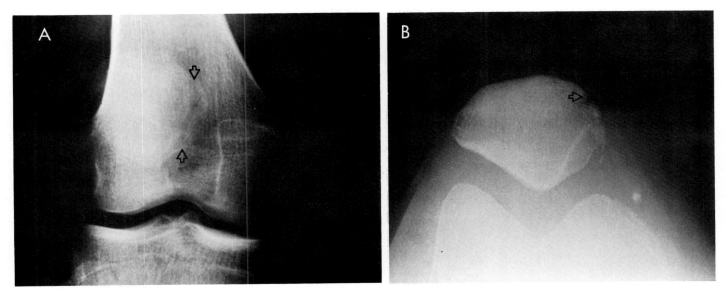

FIG 7–46.
Vertical fracture of the patella. The fracture is barely visible on the frontal view **(A)** but well seen on the "sunrise" view **(B)**.

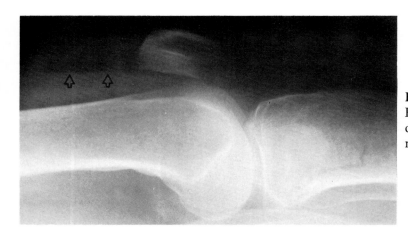

FIG 7–47.
Fat-blood level seen on horizontal-beam lateral view of the knee. Fracture causes communication between medullary canal of tibia and joint space.

FIG 7–48.
Tear of the medial collateral ligament. Stress views of the knee. **A,** on first attempt diastasis was not demonstrated, although enough force was employed to produce vacuum cleft. The edge of the medial meniscus is visible. **B,** second attempt demonstrates abnormal widening of the medial aspect of the joint.

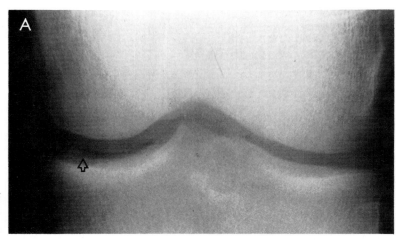

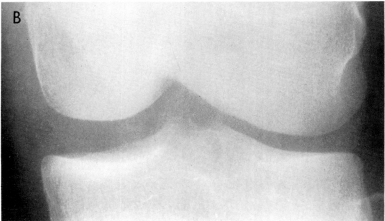

of the phalanges are frequently visible only in this projection. Occasionally, a metacarpal shaft fracture may be best seen in this view. Bennett's fracture, a fracture-dislocation of the proximal end of the first metacarpal bone, is a serious injury because muscle pull makes it difficult to maintain the position of the fragments. Therefore, one should not lightly dismiss a small cortical break at the proximal end of the first metacarpal. Failure to stabilize the fracture will cause increasing disability (Fig 7–44).

Knee

Anatomy

The patella is centered in a groove between the femoral condyles. The medial and lateral tibial plateaus should be on the same plane as, and at a right angle to, the axis of the shaft of the tibia.

Development

The epiphysis of the lower femur ossifies in the last trimester of gestation. The epiphysis of the upper tibia ossifies at birth. Identification of these centers on radiographs of the maternal abdomen was formerly employed as a marker of fetal maturity. Ossification of the center for the tibial tubercle is subject to considerable variation normally. The patella ossifies between the 2nd and 6th years. The ossification pattern in children is irregular and sometimes misleading (Fig 7–45). The patella may develop from more than one center, producing a bipartite or tripartite structure. The radiolucent cleft so formed is usually oblique across the patella, whereas fractures are usually vertical or transverse. Also, the smaller bone does not conform as closely to the contour of the apparent defect as does a fracture. Well-developed adults may have striations in the patella.

There is a cephalad extension of the knee joint capsule known as the suprapatellar bursa. This structure is sandwiched between two fat pads and is nicely demonstrated in the lateral projection when filled with fluid or blood. In the normal individual, this extension is not visible, and the fat pads coalesce to form a single radiolucency just anterior to the distal femoral shaft.

Radiography

Routine knee examinations usually include only frontal and lateral projections. We also routinely obtain an intercondylar view, which is particularly help-ful in patients with chronic difficulty, since it shows more of the knee joint space and the femoral condyles. In suspected patellar injury, a tangential ("sunrise") view of the patella is indicated. Vertical fractures of the patella are easily obscured on frontal and lateral views (Fig 7–46). A transverse patellar fracture may be invisible on the tangential view, being best seen on the routine lateral view. Oblique views of the knee are indicated when a tibial plateau fracture is suspected and the routine views are negative or only suggestive. Lateral views with horizontal beam may show blood-fat levels in the suprapatellar bursa of the knee joint (Fig 7–47). This sign indicates the presence of a fracture that has permitted fat from the marrow to enter the joint.

A stress view of the knee may be employed to assess the integrity of the ligaments of the knee (or other joint) (Fig 7–48). The attendant considerations were discussed earlier.

Fractures

The presence of hemorrhage or effusion in the knee joint space should initiate search for fracture. However, since most effusions in the knee joint result from soft tissue injury, an effusion in the knee does not have as strong an association with fracture as does a positive fat pad sign in the elbow. On the other hand, the blood-fat level in the knee is highly specific for fracture.

Fractures of the tibial plateau may be quite subtle. One should be most suspicious of any increased density in this area since such a density may be the only indication of an impacted fracture on the routine examination. A discontinuity in a portion of the cortex may be the only other sign. Oblique views can be valuable in detecting subtle plateau fractures (Fig 7–49). Tomography may establish the diagnosis in those cases in which suspicion remains.

An osteochondral fracture of one of the femoral condyles occurs when trauma drives the patella against the condyle, a fracture that can be difficult to see (Fig 7–50). Patellar fractures have been discussed in the preceding paragraphs on anatomy and technique. Pelligrini-Stieda calcification is an area of calcification or ossification overlying the medial condyle of the femur at the point of attachment of the adductor magnus muscle (Fig 7–51). This type of calcification is related to chronic stress and does not indicate a fracture. Avulsions of the quadriceps tendon and cruciate ligaments may be associated with separation of their osseous attachments (Fig 7–52).

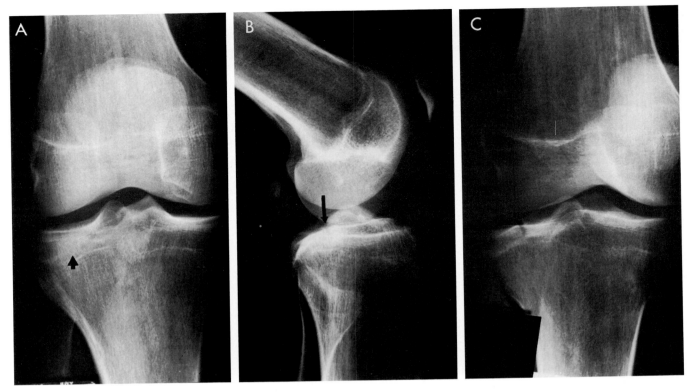

FIG 7–49.
Tibial plateau fracture. **A,** fracture is manifest by increased density in lateral aspect of proximal tibia and small cortical break. Oblique view shows fragment to be depressed and distracted **(C).**

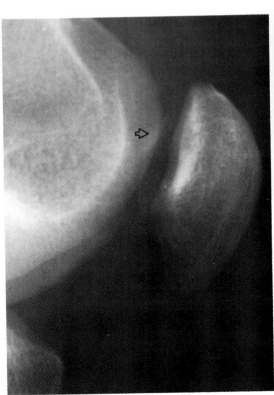

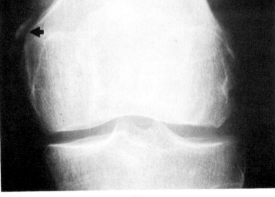

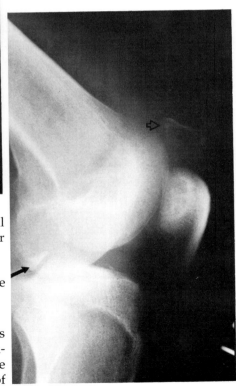

FIG 7–50 (bottom left).
Osteochondral fracture of the knee. The small fragment of the articular surface of the femur is shown.

FIG 7–51 (bottom middle).
Pelligrini-Stieda calcification adjacent to the medial condyle of the femur.

FIG 7–52 (bottom right).
Avulsion of the attachment of the quadriceps tendon *(open arrow)* and of the posterior cruciate ligament *(arrow)*. These small fracture fragments indicate a major derangement of the knee.

FIG 7-53.
Normal ankle (examined for foreign body). **A,** there are three dense centers of ossification for the tuberosity of the calcaneus *(arrow).* **B,** there is an accessory center of ossification for the medial malleolus *(arrow).*

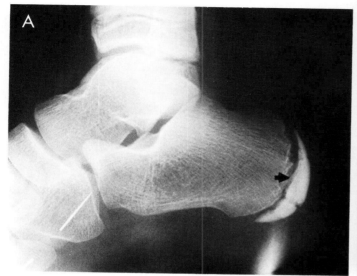

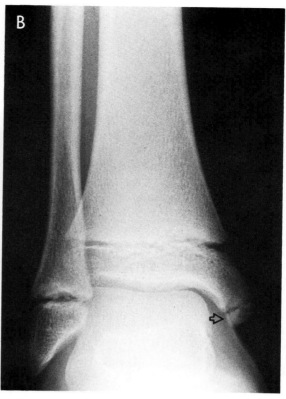

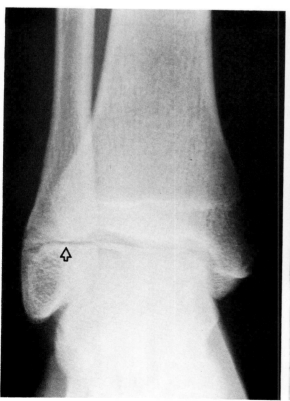

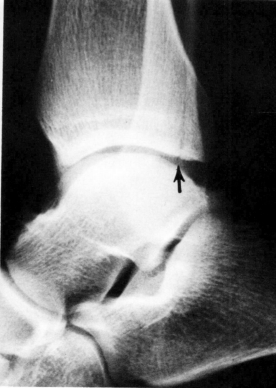

FIG 7-54 (far left).
Salter I fracture of the distal fibula. The epiphyseal line of the tibia and fibula should be the same width. There is traumatic diastasis of the fibular epiphysis.

FIG 7-55 (near left).
Undisplaced fracture of the posterior malleolus. The fracture is visible only on the lateral view.

FIG 7–56 (top right).
Fracture of the articular surface of the tibia. There is buckling of the anterior cortex.

FIG 7–57 (middle left).
Avulsion fracture of the lateral aspect of the talus.

FIG 7–58 (middle right).
Talar neck fracture.

FIG 7–59 (bottom).
Normal foot.

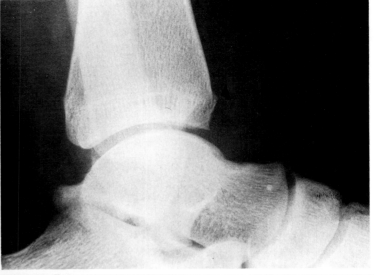

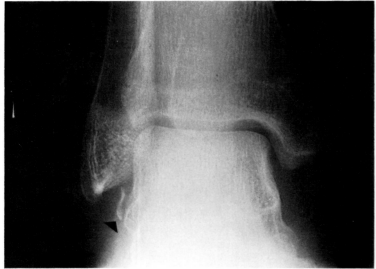

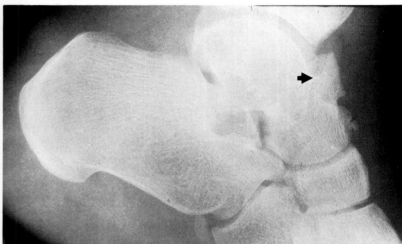

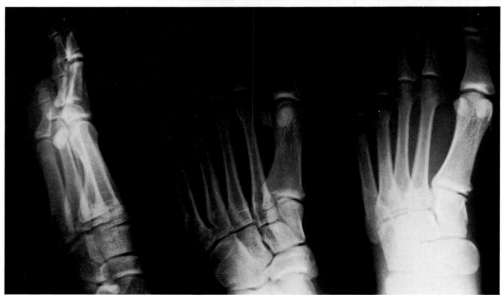

Leg

Since the knee and ankle have been discussed in other sections, only a brief discussion of the shafts of the tibia and fibula will be given.

Radiography in two projections is usually all that is required. Because the tibia and fibula are often longer than the film, their shafts are often shown with one or both ends cut off. Before accepting such an examination, one must consider that these are paired bones that are rigidly connected at both ends. Therefore, if an injury shortens or angulates one bone, there will probably be a corresponding injury to the other. If the complementary fracture is seen, the situation is clear. If not, since the compensating fracture may be at the opposite end of the other bone, its entire length should be evaluated.

Ankle

Anatomy and Development

Ossification of the lower epiphyseal centers of both the tibia and fibula begins in the 2nd year. These centers fuse at approximately the 18th year. Usually, the medial malleolus develops as a portion of the distal tibial epiphysis. It may, however, have its own center of ossification (Fig 7–53,B). The tibia and the fibula are tightly bound to each other by the intraosseous membrane. At their lower ends, a convexity on the fibula articulates with a concavity on the tibia. In the frontal projection, the notch formed by the lateral malleolus of the fibula, the medial malleolus of the tibia, and the articular surface of the tibia conforms to the top of the talus and forms the ankle mortise.

Radiography

Frontal, lateral, and oblique views should be obtained. The oblique view is made with the foot turned inward 30 to 45 degrees. The opposite oblique projection will rarely be necessary. Calcaneal fractures are not shown to advantage, if they are shown at all, on ankle (or foot) films. Stress views of the ankle may be obtained as previously discussed. Ankle arthrograms reveal tears of the ligaments and are useful in determining appropriate therapy. Arthrograms are easily obtained and are associated with low morbidity. Arthrography demonstrates ligamentous tears for only approximately 24 hours. Generally, it shows only that a tear of a given ligament exists, not the extent of the tear.

Fractures

Fracture of the distal fibula (lateral malleolus) is the most common fracture of the ankle. It may be evident on only one of three views. It is not rare for fibular fracture to be seen only on the lateral view through the tibia and the talus. Fractures of the distal fibula may be subtle, particularly during the developing years. The only sign of a fracture of the distal fibula may be that the fibular epiphysis is wider than the tibial epiphysis (Fig 7–54). These epiphyseal lines should have the same width. If the ankle mortise is widened or asymmetrical, one should consider the possibility of an occult fracture. Fracture of the medial malleolus may occur as an isolated finding, but it is usually associated with a fracture of the lateral malleolus and possibly the posterior malleolus as well (Fig 7–55). Fractures of the anterior aspect of the tibia are less common (Fig 7–56).

Fractures of the tibia and fibula are almost always readily recognized. Error may occur by failing to recognize that one of the bones in the vicinity is fractured. The same inversion injury that causes malleolar fracture may instead cause an avulsion fracture of the lateral aspect of the talus inferior to the lateral malleolus (Fig 7–57). On initial clinical examination, more serious injuries, such as calcaneal fracture and fracture of the neck of the talus, may be mistaken for ankle injuries (Fig 7–58). Therefore, careful evaluation of adjacent bones is indicated, possibly supplemented by other views. Calcaneal fracture, particularly when bilateral, may be associated with spinal fracture.

Foot

Anatomy

The anatomical relationship between the various bones of the foot is best seen on the lateral radiograph. The articular surface of the talus has a dome-shaped configuration. Anterior to the dome of the talus, the superior surface of the talus is continuous and even with the superior surfaces of the tarsal navicular, the cuneiform, and metatarsal bones. The talus has three articulations with the calcaneus. The calcaneus articulates with the cuboid, which usually protrudes laterally from the articular surface. This arrangement may simulate discontinuity. Careful scrutiny of this area will reveal where the articular surface ends. The articular surfaces of the calcaneus should coincide with the articular surface of the cuboid. A similar relationship exists with respect to the articulation between the cuboid and the fifth metatarsal bone. The proximal end of the latter clearly overhangs the articulation. In the frontal and oblique projections, a more or less continuous line joins the surfaces of the bones on the top and medial aspect of the foot. This surface is rough but level—somewhat like a cobblestone street (Fig 7–59).

Development

The primary ossification centers for the phalanges, metatarsals, calcaneus, talus, and cuboid are present at birth. Centers for the other tarsal bones together with the secondary centers for the calcaneus, the metatarsals, and phalanges appear through the 10th year.

The secondary center of ossification of the calcaneal tuberosity is of particular interest. This apophysis may be formed of more than one center. In health, it has an extremely dense appearance that should not be mistaken for aseptic necrosis (see Fig 7–53,A).

The fifth metatarsal bone has two secondary centers of ossification. In addition to one at the distal end (like the second through fifth metatarsals), there is a center for the tuberosity on the lateral aspect of the base of the fifth metatarsal. This center is formed in such a way that the radiolucency is almost parallel to the shaft and should not be confused with a fracture, which is usually transversely oriented (Fig 7–60).

Radiography

Frontal, lateral, and oblique views are the routine for examining the foot. By directing the central ray slightly posterior in the frontal projection, the articulations of the central foot are shown to better advantage. If a fracture of the calcaneus is suspected or if there are suspicious findings on other views, a special calcaneal view should be made, since calcaneal fractures may not be visible on routine views (Fig 7–61).

Dislocations

Most dislocations of the foot are dislocations of the interphalangeal or metatarsophalangeal joints. Dislocations of the central foot are usually the result of direct trauma. The Lisfranc fracture-dislocation occurs more frequently in the pediatric age group and is usually the result of a jump or fall. Careful scrutiny should be given to the continuity of the bones of the foot—particularly to the alignment between the lateral aspect of the first metatarsal and the first cuneiform bone, which should be continuous in the frontal projection (see Fig 7–59). Interruption of this alignment is often the only clue to a significant dislocation (Fig 7–62). These injuries can be difficult to define. Thus, the axial views of CT have been employed in evaluating them.

Fractures

Fractures of the phalanges and metatarsals are the most frequent fractures of the foot. With trauma to the lateral aspect of the foot, the most common injury is a fracture of the proximal end of the fifth metatarsal. The fracture line is usually oriented transversely with respect to the axis of the shaft, and only occasionally obliquely. The radiolucent line produced by the apophysis for the tubercle is parallel to the axis of the shaft. When the fracture occurs in the presence of an open apophysis, a cross-shaped radiolucent shadow results (see Fig 7–60).

The presence of many complex planes makes fracture of the tarsal bones difficult to visualize. Careful observation of the surfaces of the foot may reveal interruptions of contour produced by shifting of fragments. Referring to radiographs of a normal foot or the opposite foot can be invaluable (Fig 7–63).

Foreign Bodies

Retained foreign bodies have a substantial potential morbidity following trauma. Detection is usually easy if the foreign body is sufficiently dense to be visible on radiographs. Considerable difficulty may be encountered with a foreign body whose specific gravity is close to that of tissue and therefore provides little contrast. Obscuring by normal body structures, particularly bone, creates additional difficulty. Considerable patience and ingenuity may be required. It may be desirable to counsel the patient that all foreign bodies may not be visible radiographically, particularly those of some frequently encountered materials such as wood and glass.

The goal of the examination should be to exclude a foreign body or to demonstrate its location when detected. The location should be shown relative to the entry site, using an opaque marker if necessary to indicate its depth from the surface. While two views at right angles may accomplish this, tangential or other special projections may be required (Fig 7–64).

Xeroradiography may be employed in the search for suspected foreign bodies. The image produced by a special processor provides high detail and contrast

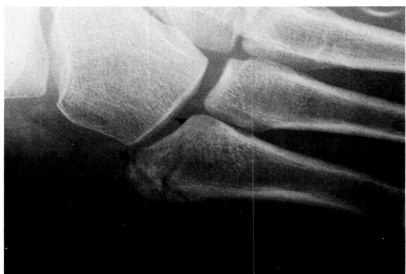

FIG 7–60 (top left).
Fracture of the fifth metatarsal *(arrowhead)* in a patient with an unfused center for the tuberosity. The latter produces a radiolucent line parallel to the axis of the bone *(arrow)*.

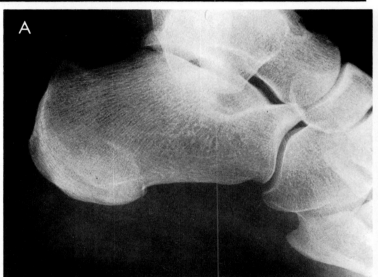

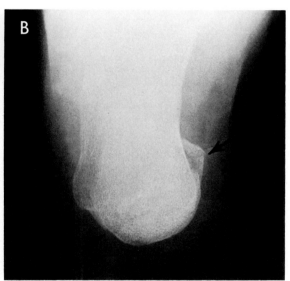

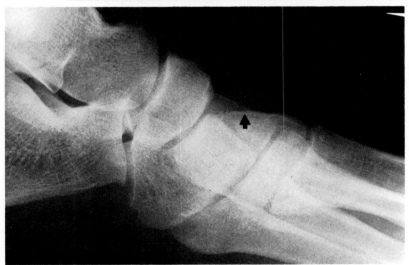

FIG 7–61 (middle left and right).
Fracture of the calcaneus. The fracture is almost invisible on the conventional foot views initially obtained **(A)**. It is clearly shown by the calcaneal view **(B)**.

FIG 7–62 (bottom left).
Dislocation of the forefoot. Notice the absence of normal alignment between the tarsals. The second cuneiform bone is markedly depressed *(arrow)*.

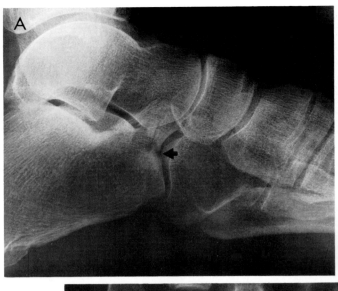 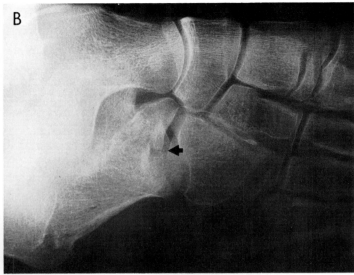

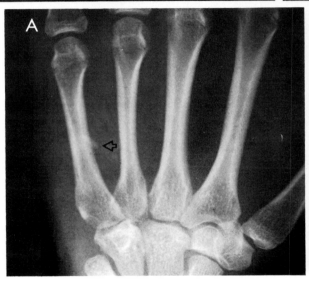 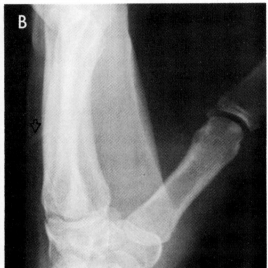

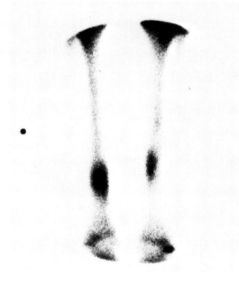

FIG 7–63 (top left and right).
Fracture of the anterior articular surface of the calcaneus.

FIG 7–64 (middle left and right).
Foreign body (pencil lead). Only on the tangential view are the size and location fully visible.

FIG 7–65 (bottom left).
Fatigue fracture of the tibias. Vivid demonstration on radionuclide scan of radiographically occult fatigue fractures.

resolution. Moreover, there is an inherent edge-enhancement effect between objects of different density. For small body parts, the radiation dose is less than for conventional radiography. For larger body parts, such as the elbow or knee, the dose becomes equal or greater. Several factors restrict the availability of this modality. Since some warm-up is required, it is not instantly ready. The equipment requires special maintenance. Many radiology departments have changed to special film-screen techniques instead of xeroradiography and no longer have xeroradiographic capability. Fortunately, anything seen on xeroradiography can usually be seen on high-contrast film examination.

A foreign body may be remote from its site of entry. Obviously high-velocity missiles may pursue a circuitous route as they dissect along body planes and are deflected by rigid structures. Vascular transmission may occur. We have even encountered migration within the spinal canal. The object may lodge in a moving structure, such as a muscle or tendon, and its position on subsequent examinations may therefore be inconstant. A deeply penetrating object may break off or carry foreign material with it.

Fatigue Fractures

Fatigue fracture results from unusual stress on a bone. The bone involved and the type of stress dictate where the fracture will occur. These fractures are most frequently seen in the feet and other portions of the lower extremity. Many fatigue fractures are radiographically invisible for a week or 10 days. The most sensitive diagnostic examination is radionuclide bone scanning (Fig 7–65). Fatigue fractures appear as areas of increased density in bone, often accompanied by local subperiosteal new bone production and occasionally by a small amount of callus formation (Fig 7–66).

Nontraumatic Conditions

At one time or another virtually every known affliction of man will be seen in an emergency department, either primarily or incidentally. Regardless of experience the physician cannot be expected to recognize all of them. When confronted with this situation, it is necessary to attend to the most pressing clinical problem(s) and have the patient return or be referred for evaluation of the incidental findings. One should be particularly attentive when unexpected radiographic findings are present. Figures 7–67 and 7–68 show such findings of significant disease that were seen incidental to trauma.

Osteomyelitis

Osteomyelitis results from hematogenous spread or direct inoculation of microorganisms. Direct inoculation may result from a puncture wound, surgery, or spread of infection from a contiguous area. Although the inoculation form of osteomyelitis may occur in any portion of the bone, hematogenous infections most frequently begin in the vascular metaphyseal area, particularly in children.

Although a week or 10 days is required before radiographic bone change will appear, soft tissue swelling may be present early. The earliest sign will be loss of the visibility of the fat lines in the tissue planes. The earliest skeletal sign is loss of bone density in the area of infection. This process progresses to frank destruction with initial loss of trabecular markings and then loss of cortex (Fig 7–69). A portion of bone may be deprived of blood supply and become separated from the adjacent bone (sequestrum). Subperiosteal new bone production will produce a fine dense line parallel to the cortex. Unchecked metaphyseal osteomyelitis can break into the adjacent joint and result in pyogenic arthritis.

If the distinction between osteomyelitis and malignant tumor is based solely on a single radiographic observation, diagnosis may be difficult. There are, however, some useful differentiating points. In acute osteomyelitis, the history and clinical examination will usually be characteristic. Bone neoplasms usually have greater localized bone destruction and larger soft tissue masses. It is rare for a tumor to cross a joint. Eosinophilic granuloma, a localized area of bone destruction, may be confused with osteomyelitis. Ewing's tumor, a malignant neoplasm, may have an appearance similar to osteomyelitis.

Arthritis

The differential radiologic diagnosis of joint disease is a very complex subject. While arthritic conditions may present in an emergency setting, the early roentgen findings are usually nonspecific. Specific findings are usually seen in patients with longstanding disease.

Acute septic arthritis may show evidence of fluid distending the joint capsule and loss of the adjacent fat lines resulting from edema of those tissues. Neglected or unsuccessfully-treated cases may progress to destruction of the articular cartilage, with loss of joint space and eventual destruction of the articular bone.

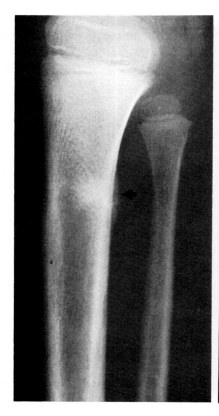

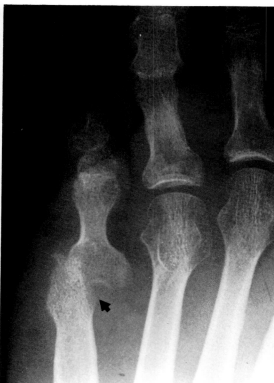

FIG 7–66 (far left).
Fatigue fracture of the tibia. Sclerotic area in the tibia with subperiosteal bone production.

FIG 7–67 (near left).
Diabetic osteoarthropathy. Extensive destruction in the region of the fifth metatarsophalangeal joint. Discovered as an incidental finding in a patient who had traumatized foot.

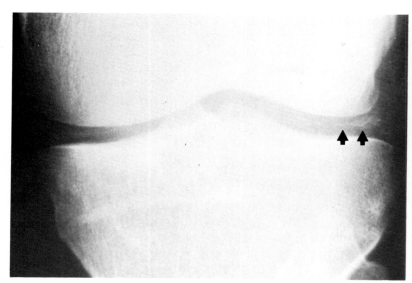

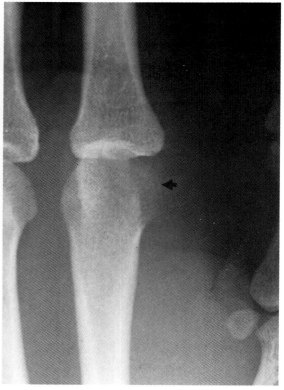

FIG 7–68 (left).
Chondrocalcinosis as part of calcium pyrophosphate deposition disease, detected as incidental finding in knee trauma.

FIG 7–69 (right).
Osteomyelitis of the head of the second metacarpal. There is destruction of the trabeculae, with a break in the cortex.

FIG 7–70 (near right).
Gouty arthritis. Notice that there are randomly distributed destructive lesions adjacent to the joints. A partially calcified soft tissue lesion at the wrist represents a tophus.

FIG 7–71 (far right).
Rheumatoid arthritis. Notice the symmetric distribution of the swelling at the proximal interphalangeal joints. A single erosion is present at the distal end of the proximal phalanx of the second finger.

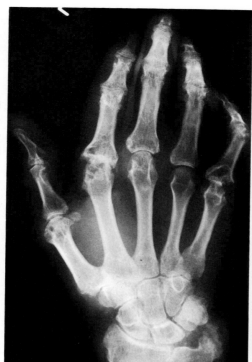
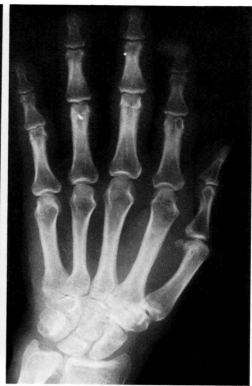

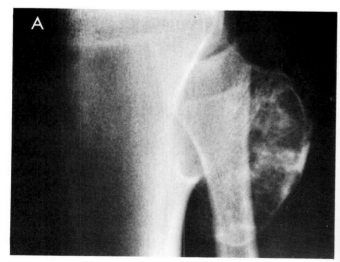
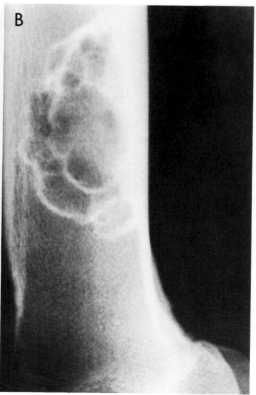

FIG 7–72.
Benign tumors. **A,** osteochondroma. **B,** nonossifying fibroma of the femur.

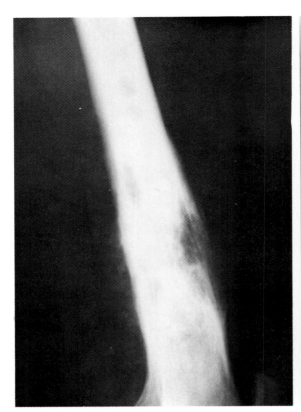

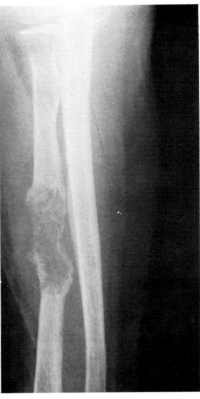

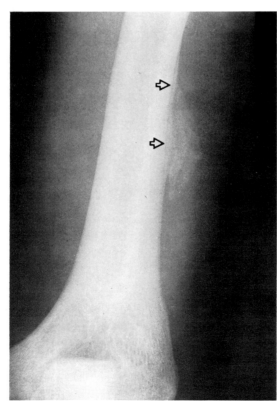

FIG 7–73 (top left).
Osteosarcoma of the femur. Notice the lamellar subperiosteal bone production and calcified soft tissue mass posteriorly.

FIG 7–74 (top right).
Metastatic renal carcinoma to the radius. Note the poorly-defined zone of transition from tumor to normal bone.

FIG 7–75 (left).
Myositis ossificans. There is a pyramidal area of bone production. This lesion is at times confused with osteosarcoma. Notice that there is a characteristic radiolucency between the lesion and the bone *(arrows)*. This separation differentiates myositis ossificans from sarcoma.

Just as in clinical diagnosis, general factors, such as the age and sex of the patient and the distribution of the processes, are considerations in radiologic diagnosis of arthritic disorders. Whether a process is random or bilaterally symmetric is an important clue. For example, the distribution of lesions would help differentiate gout from rheumatoid arthritis. One should look at the radiograph from a distance to appreciate the general appearance. This may reveal a helpful pattern of soft tissue swelling or demineralization (Figs 7–70 and 7–71).

Neoplasms

Bone neoplasms may be seen as incidental findings in an acute setting. However, a neoplasm may be the underlying abnormality in a pathologic fracture. Metastatic deposits are particularly liable to this complication. In the emergency setting, the critical issue is the realization that the patient's symptoms or his fracture are due to an underlying bone neoplasm. Once the neoplasm is discovered, the physician should decide whether the lesion represents a threat to the strength of the host bone and whether to protect the extremity until appropriate diagnosis and therapy can be carried out.

In general, benign bone neoplasms are characterized by well-defined sclerotic margins with intact overlying cortex and the absence of soft tissue mass (Fig 7–72). Malignant neoplasms tend to infiltrate bone, breach the cortex, and invade adjacent soft tissues. Periosteal bone production in the absence of fracture suggests malignancy (Figs 7–73 and 7–74).

There is a group of entities, including myositis ossificans (Fig 7–75), whose radiologic findings may be mistaken for those of neoplasm. For the most part, confusion arises in the misinterpretation of normal growth phenomena or normal variations. This subject is dealt with in the next section.

Suggested Reading

1. Edeiken J: *Roentgen Diagnosis of Diseases of Bone,* Vols 1 and 2, ed 3. Baltimore, Williams & Wilkins Co, 1981.
2. Harris JH Jr, Harris WH: *The Radiology of Emergency Medicine,* ed 2. Baltimore, Williams & Wilkins Co, 1981.
3. Keats TE: *Atlas of Normal Roentgen Variants That May Simulate Disease,* ed 4. Chicago, Year Book Medical Publishers, 1988.
4. Rogers LF: *Radiology of Skeletal Trauma,* vols 1 and 2. New York, Churchill Livingstone, 1982.

Normal Variants

Theodore E. Keats, M.D.

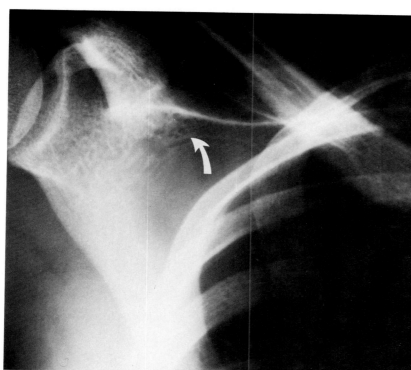

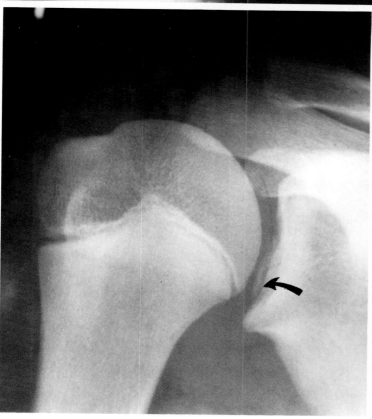

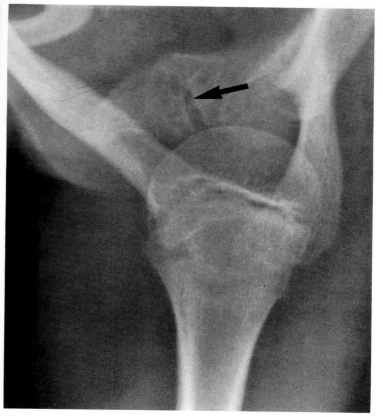

FIG 7–76 (top left).
The vascular channel *(arrow)* of the nutrient artery of the scapula, which should not be mistaken for a fracture.

FIG 7–77 (bottom left).
Secondary ossification center of the glenoid fossa *(arrow)*, which should not be mistaken for fracture.

FIG 7–78 (bottom right).
Axial projection of the shoulder. The coracoid process develops as a separate center *(arrow)* which may persist until 18 to 20 years of age and should not be mistaken for fracture.

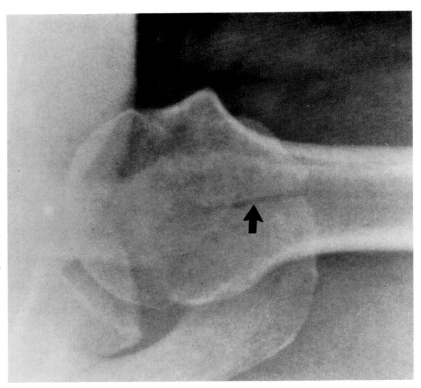

FIG 7–79 (top right).
Axial projection of the shoulder, showing the os acromiale *(arrow)*. This secondary center persists into adult life as a separate bone and may be mistaken for a fracture of the acromion process. It is usually, but not invariably, bilateral.

FIG 7–80 (bottom left and right).
The normal physeal lines *(arrow)* of the proximal portion of the humerus in a 17-year-old boy. **A,** external rotation. **B,** internal rotation. The physeal line in this view sometimes is mistaken for a fracture.

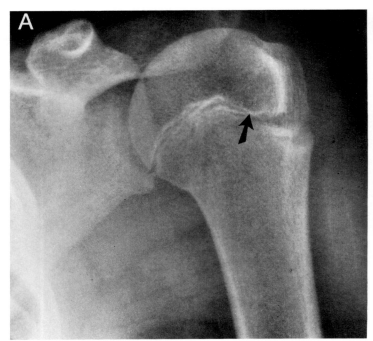

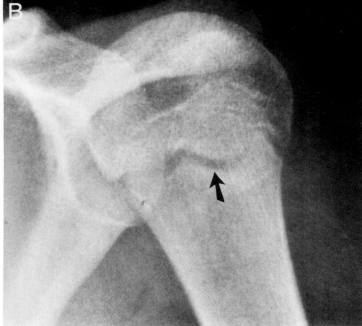

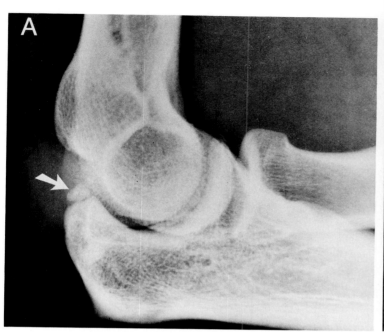

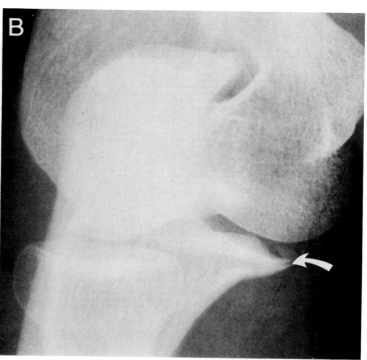

FIG 7–81 (top left and right).
A, ununited separate nucleus of ossification for the olecranon process *(arrow)* which may be mistaken for a fracture. **B,** persistent ossification center of the coronoid process *(arrow)* which simulates a fracture.

FIG 7–82 (bottom left).
Accessory ossification center at the distal end of the first metacarpal *(arrow)*, with a developmental epiphyseal spur at its medial margin *(notched arrow)*.

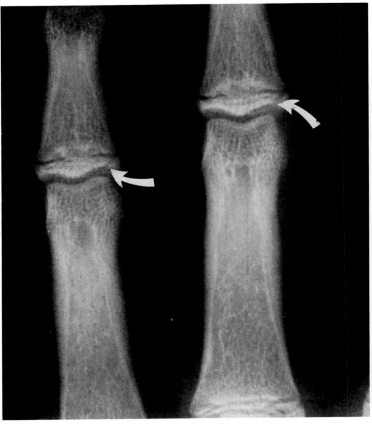

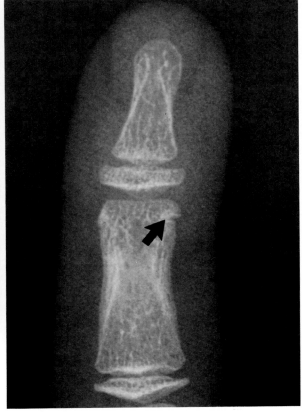

FIG 7–83 (top left).
Normal lucent fissures *(arrow)* in the epiphyses of an adolescent, which may be mistaken for fractures.

FIG 7–84 (top right).
Attempt to form an accessory ossification center *(arrow)* at the distal end of a middle phalanx in a 10-year-old boy. This may be mistaken for an incomplete fracture.

FIG 7–85 (bottom right).
Normal irregular mineralization of the ossification center of one femoral head. This appearance in a single center in a young infant does not necessarily indicate disease. (Ref: Caffey J: *Pediatric X-Ray Diagnosis,* ed. 8. Chicago, Year Book Medical Publishers, 1985, p 787.)

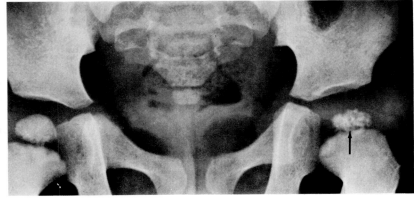

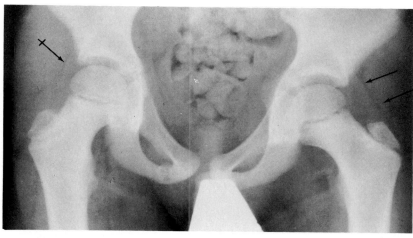

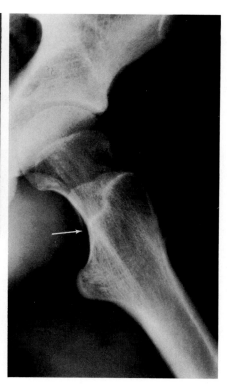

FIG 7–86 (top left).
Apparent bulging of the hip "capsule" suggesting synovitis or hemarthrosis may be produced by filming the hip in abduction and external rotation as in this 6-year-old boy *(arrow)*. Note normal fat lines on opposite side *(notched arrow)*. (Ref: Brown I: A study of the "capsular" shadow in disorders of the hip in children. *J Bone Joint Surg* 1975; 57B:175.)

FIG 7–87 (top right).
Simulated periostitis of the femoral neck produced by overlapping shadow of the greater trochanter.

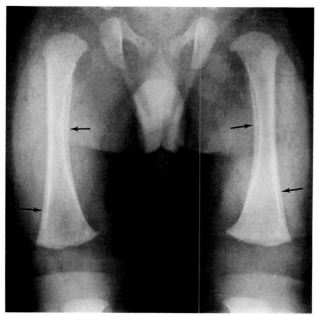

FIG 7–88 (bottom left).
Physiologic "periostitis" of the newborn. This is not seen before the age of 1 month and is symmetric in distribution, although not necessarily concentric, and may be seen in only one view. (Ref: Shopfner CE: Periosteal bone growth in normal infants: A preliminary report. *Am J Roentgenol* 1966; 97:154.)

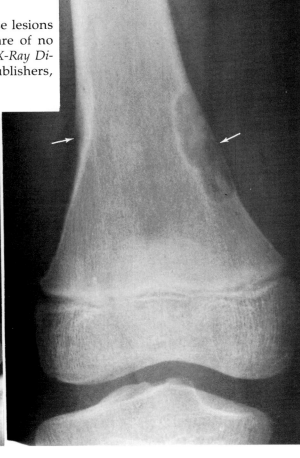

FIG 7–89.
Typical juvenile benign cortical defects. These lesions are very common in the distal femur and are of no clinical significance. (Ref: Caffey J: *Pediatric X-Ray Diagnosis,* ed 8. Chicago, Year Book Medical Publishers, 1985, p 460.)

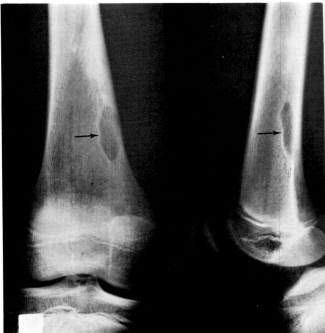

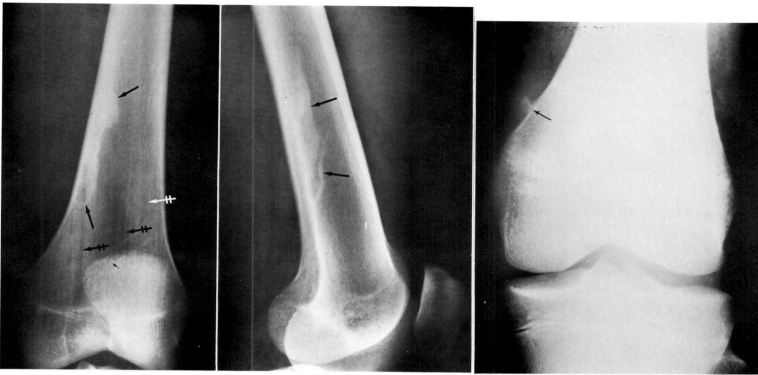

FIG 7–90 (top left and middle).
Sclerosis of a healed juvenile benign cortical defect in a 17-year-old boy *(arrows)*. Note also longitudinal striations in the metaphysis, a common finding in young people *(notched arrows)*.

FIG 7–91 (top right).
"Tug" lesion of distal portion of the medial aspect of the distal portion of the femur in an adolescent, representing bone formation in the insertion of the adductor magnus muscle. (Ref: Barnes GR Jr, Gwinn JL: Distal irregularities of the femur simulating malignancy. *Am J Roentgenol* 1974; 122:180.)

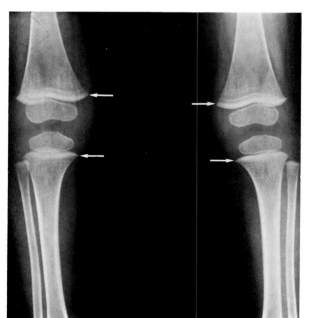

FIG 7–92 (bottom left).
Dense zones of provisional calcification are often mistaken for the lines of heavy metal poisoning. These zones vary considerably in thickness in healthy children and in the same child at different ages. They tend to be proportionately thicker during the second to fifth years. (Ref: Caffey J: *Pediatric X-Ray Diagnosis*, ed 8. Chicago: Year Book Medical Publishers, 1985, p 781.)

FIG 7–93.
Irregular defect in the cortex of the medial posterior aspect of the distal femur is a common finding between the ages of 12 and 16 years. This is a normal growth phenomenon, which often demonstrates fine perpendicular spiculation of bone **(B)**, and is often mistaken for a malignant bone tumor. It appears to be developmental in origin and disappears with advancing age. (Refs: Brower AC, et al: The histological nature of the cortical irregularity of the medial posterior distal femoral metaphysis in children. *Radiology* 1971; 99:389; and Barnes GR Jr, Gwinn JL: Distal irregularities of the femur simulating malignancy. *Am J Roentgenol* 1974; 122:180.)

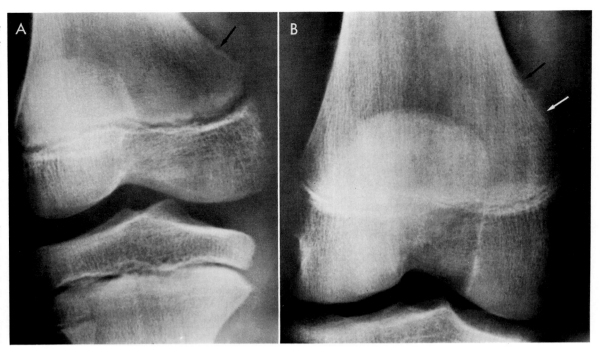

FIG 7–94 (bottom left and middle).
Two examples of normal irregularity in ossification of the posterior aspect of the distal femur in 2-year-old infants.

FIG 7–95 (bottom right).
Irregularity of the posterior aspect of the distal femur in adolescents is a common finding often mistaken for the new bone formation of a neoplasm. It has been suggested that it may be related to an avulsive injury, but it is probably the same phenomenon described in Figure 7–93. (Ref: Bufkin WJ: The avulsive cortical irregularity. *Am J Roentgenol* 1971; 112:487.)

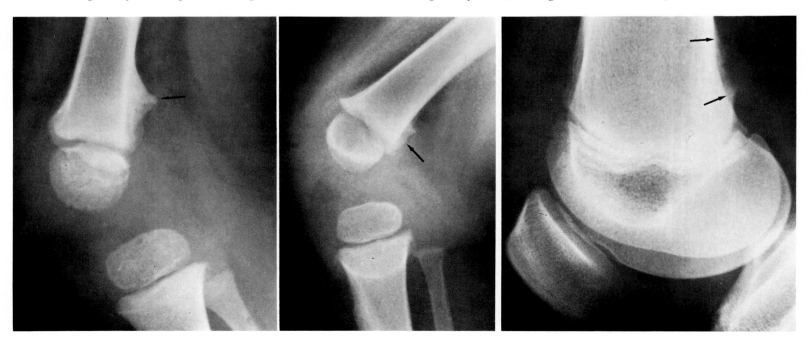

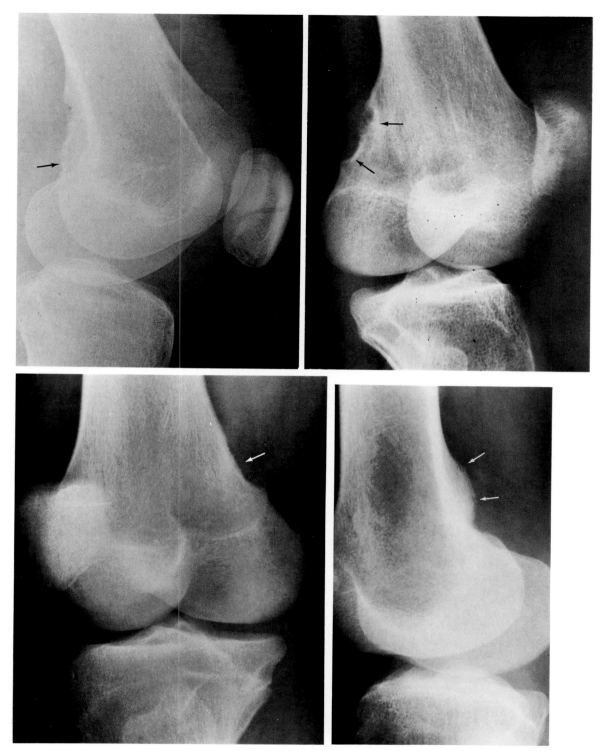

FIG 7–96.
Four examples of cortical irregularities in the posterior cortex of the distal femur that have persisted into adult life, presumably the end product of the process shown in Figure 7–95. These defects are important only that they not be mistaken for significant lesions.

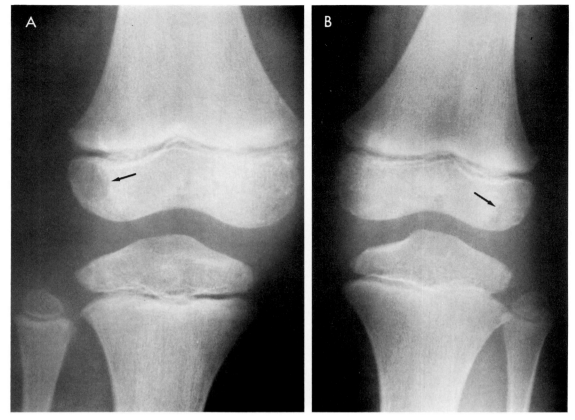

FIG 7–97.
A, normal developmental lucency of the lateral aspects of the distal femoral epiphyses, simulating a destructive lesion in a 6-year-old boy. **B,** similar, but less marked, changes are present in the opposite limb.

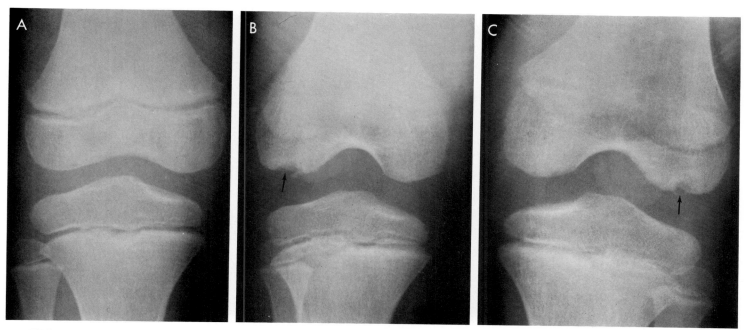

FIG 7–98.

Normal irregularity of the lateral condyles of the femur in a 7-year-old boy. These irregularities are posteriorly located and are seen in the tunnel views of both knees **(B and C)** but not in the conventional anteroposterior projection **(A)**. Such irregularities should not be mistaken for osteochondrosis dessicans. (Ref: Caffey J, et al: Ossification of the distal femoral epiphysis. *J Bone Joint Surg* 1958; 40A:647.)

FIG 7–99.

An excellent example of the normal irregularity of the distal femoral epiphyses in an 8-year-old girl that explains the misleading shadows seen in the frontal projections of the knees of children of this age.

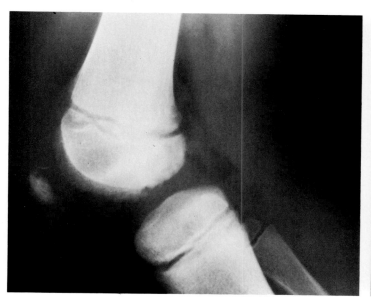 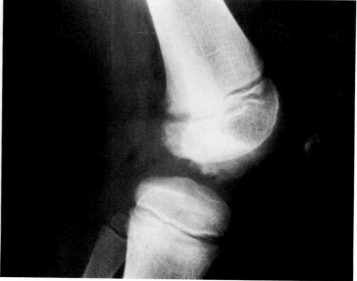

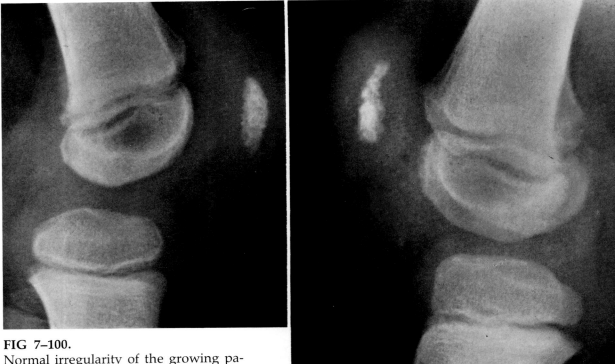

FIG 7–100.
Normal irregularity of the growing patellae in a 7-year-old boy.

FIG 7–101.
Normal asymmetric development of accessory ossification centers in a 9-year-old. Note apparent fragmentation of the lower pole of the patella in **B.**

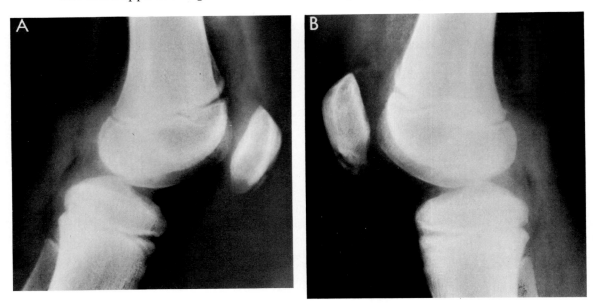

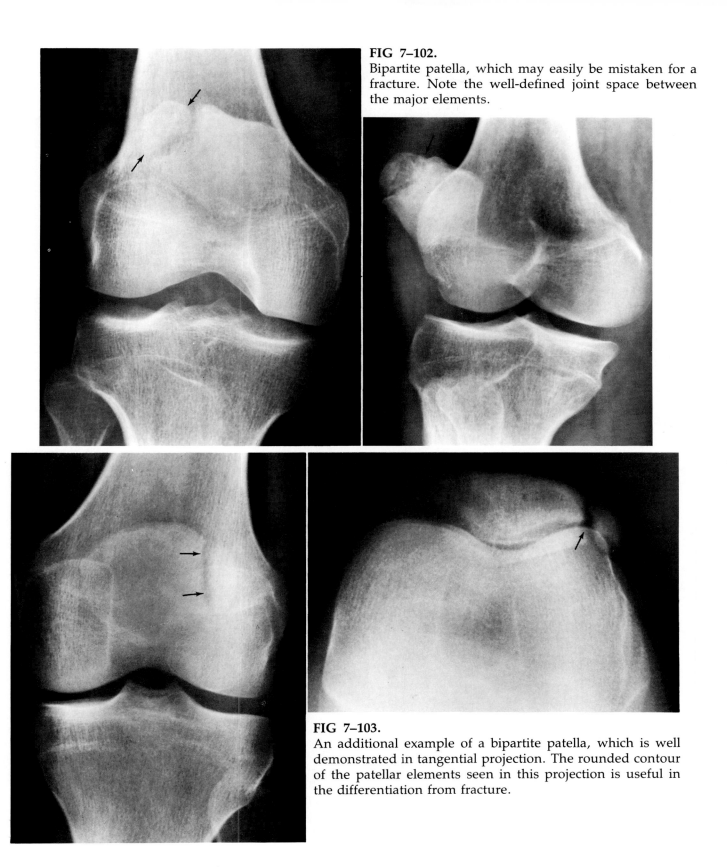

FIG 7–102.
Bipartite patella, which may easily be mistaken for a fracture. Note the well-defined joint space between the major elements.

FIG 7–103.
An additional example of a bipartite patella, which is well demonstrated in tangential projection. The rounded contour of the patellar elements seen in this projection is useful in the differentiation from fracture.

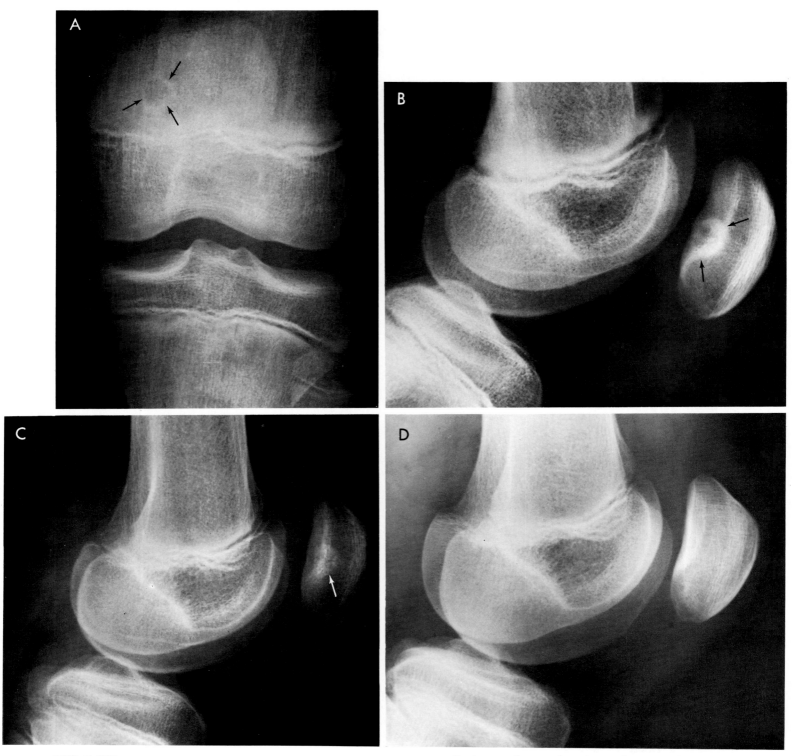

FIG 7–104.
A and **B** are cortical lucencies of the patella in a 13-year-old boy which represent a normal variation in growth of the patella. These are of no clinical signifi-cance. **C,** 1 year later, showing sclerosis of healing. **D,** 2 years later, showing complete resolution. (Ref: Haswell DM, et al: The dorsal defect of the patella. *Pediatr Radiol* 1976; 4:238.)

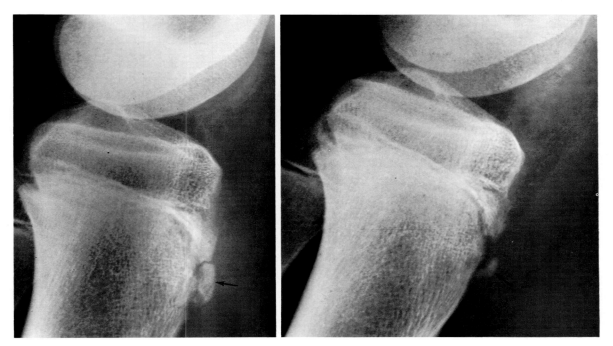

FIG 7–105.
Normal variations in appearance of the ossification center of the tibial tubercle in adolescence, which might be mistaken for osteochondrosis or traumatic avulsion.

FIG 7–106.
Spurs at metaphysis of the proximal fibula, not to be mistaken for an osteochondroma. These result from pull of the soleus muscle.

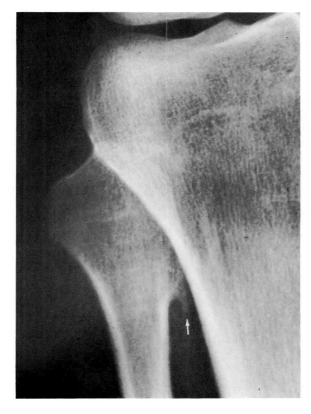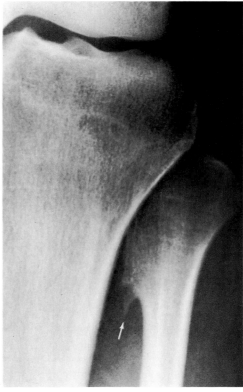

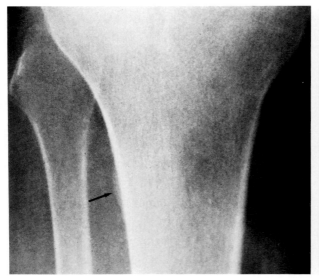

FIG 7–107.
Two examples of pseudoperiostitis, simulated by the tibial tuberosity *(arrow)*. (Ref: Kohler A, et al: *Border-lands of the Normal and Early Pathologic in Skeletal Roent-genology,* ed 3. Philadelphia, Grune & Stratton, 1968, p 442.)

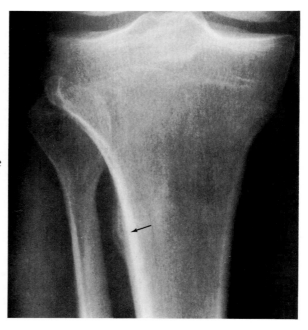

FIG 7–108.
Laminated appearance of the tibial tubercle, not to be confused with periosteal new bone formation.

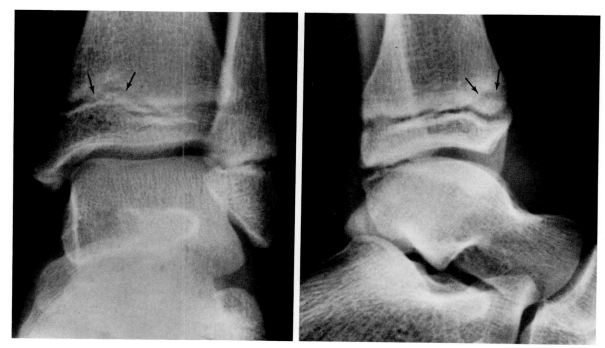

FIG 7–109.
Normal localized angulation of the distal epiphyseal plate of the tibia in an 11-year-old boy.

FIG 7–110.
The fibular ossicle, a scale-like ossification center in the epiphyseal line, simulating a fracture.

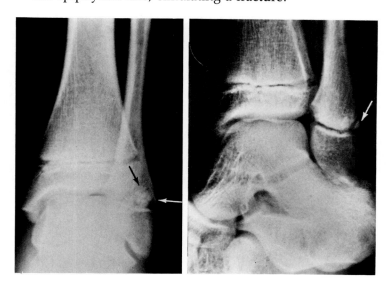

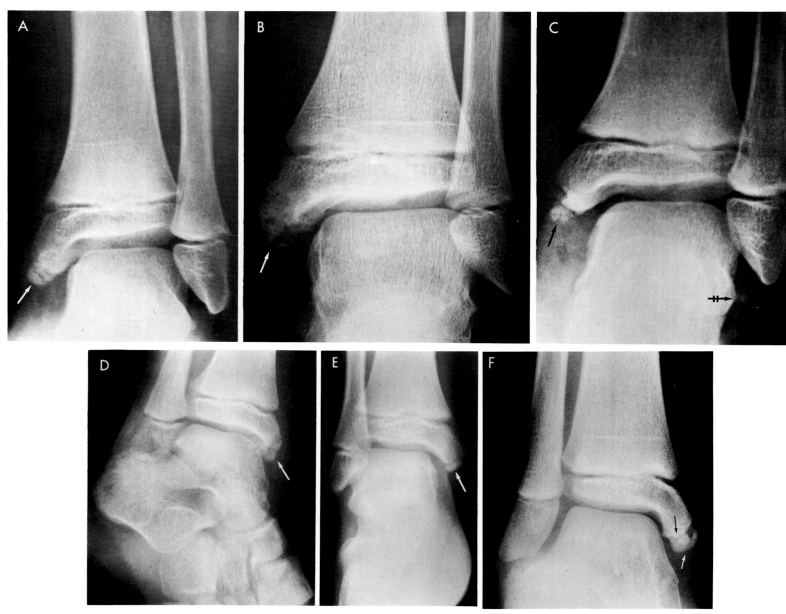

FIG 7–111.
Normal irregular ossification of the tip of the medial malleolus in adolescent children. In **C,** an ossicle is seen between the calcaneus and the lateral malleolus, which represents the os trochleae calcanei *(notched arrow).*

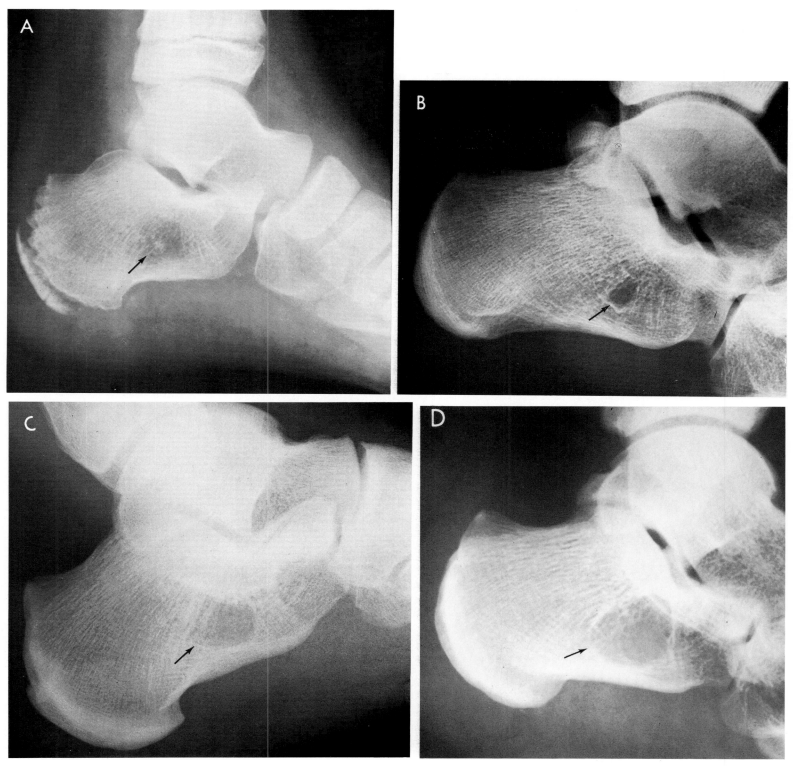

FIG 7–121.
Four examples of simulated calcaneal cysts due to the normal arrangement of the trabecular pattern in this area. The presence of the nutrient channel within the cyst, as in **A,** is useful in identifying the area of radiolucency as a pseudocyst. This variant is confused with true cysts of the calcaneus. (Ref: Kohler A, et al: *Borderlands of the Normal and Early Pathologic in Skeletal Roentgenology,* ed 3. Philadelphia, Grune & Stratton, 1968, p 482.)

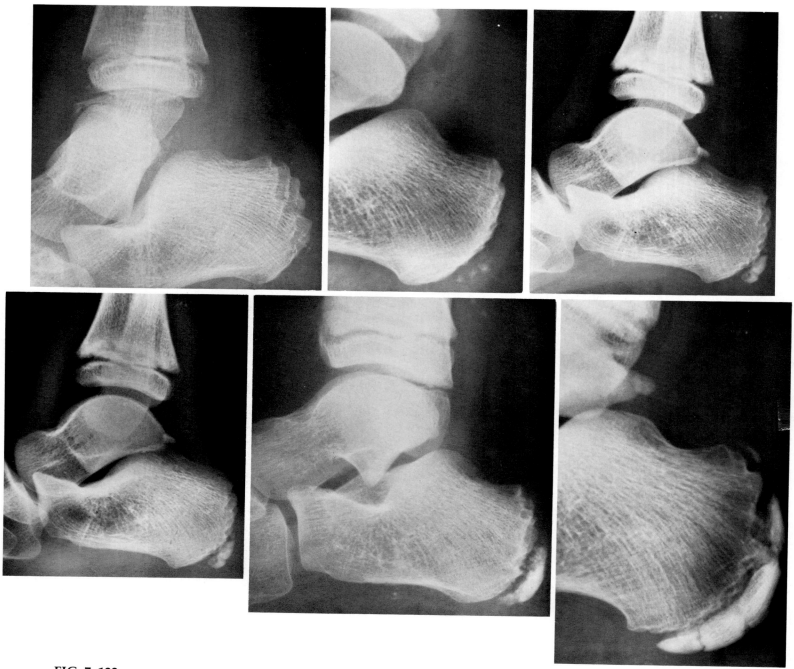

FIG 7–122.
Normal variations in appearance of the growing calcaneus in adolescence. The irregularity of the calcaneal tuberosity before fusion of the secondary ossification center, as well as the density and fragmentation of the secondary ossification center, is a normal manifestation of growth.

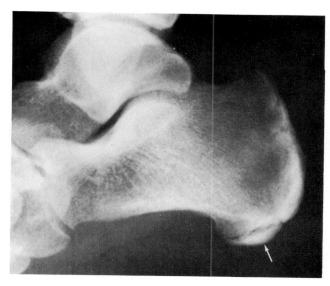

FIG 7–123.
Incomplete closure of the distal portion of the calcaneal apophysis in a 15-year-old boy.

FIG 7–124.
Normal ossification of the navicular from multiple centers in an 8-year-old boy. This appearance may be confused with osteochondrosis or a fracture.

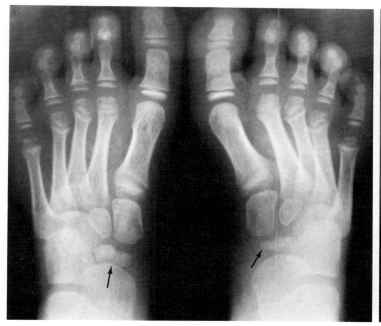 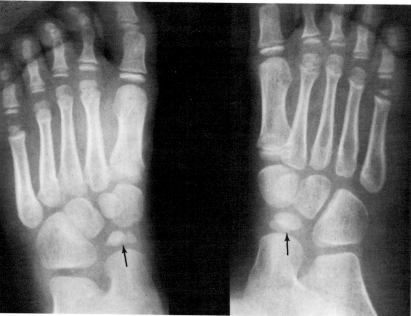

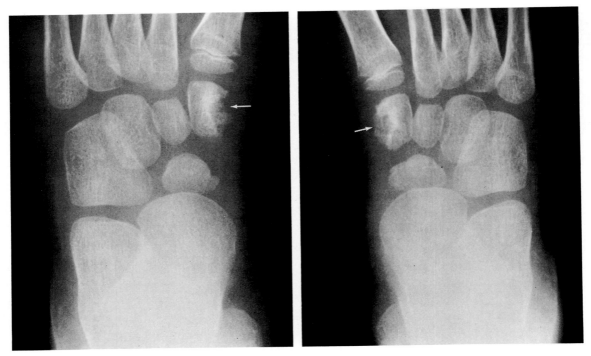

FIG 7–125.
Irregular mineralization of the first cuneiforms in a 6-year-old boy.

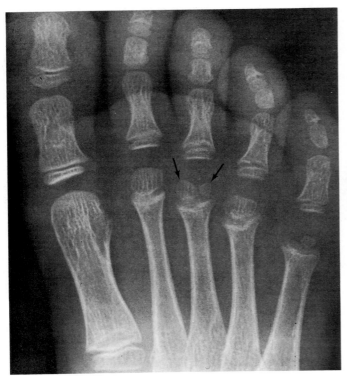

FIG 7–126.
Duplication of the ossification center of the head of the third metatarsal, not a fracture.

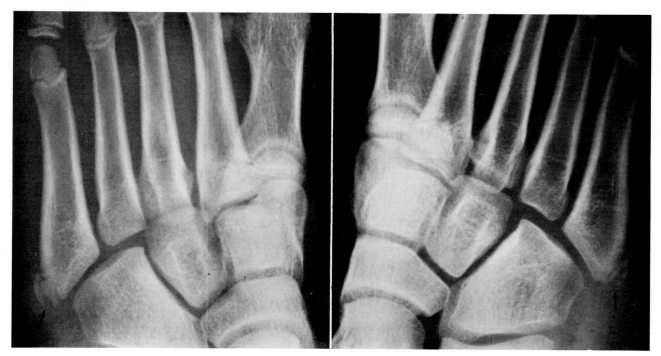

FIG 7–127.
Multicentric ossification centers of the tuberosity of the fifth metatarsals in a 12-year-old girl, simulating fractures.

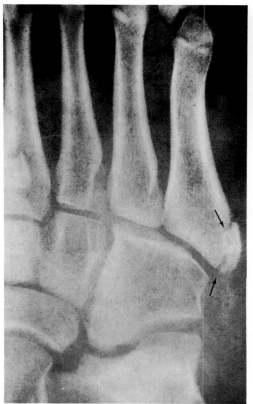

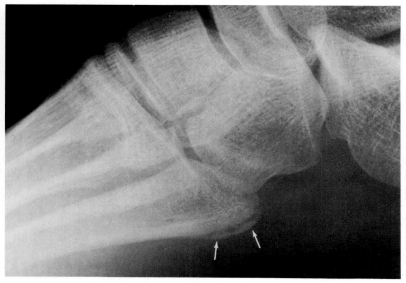

FIG 7–128.
The normal apophysis of the tuberosity of the base of the fifth metatarsal, which resembles a fracture. Most fractures of this area are horizontal rather than vertical.

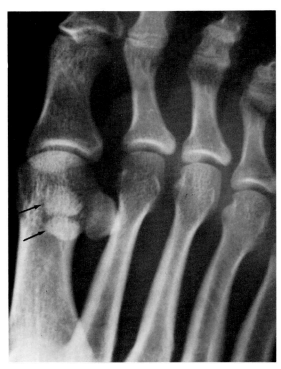

FIG 7–129.
Symmetric oval bipartite sesamoids of the first toe.

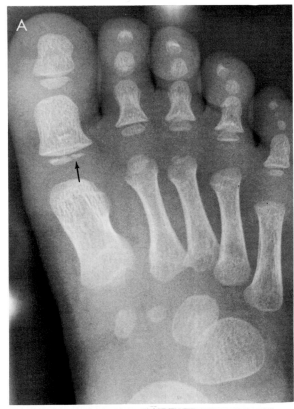

FIG 7–130.
Divided epiphysis at the base of the proximal phalanx of the first toe, not a fracture. **A,** a 3-year-old boy; **B,** an 11-year-old boy; **C,** a 13-year-old boy.

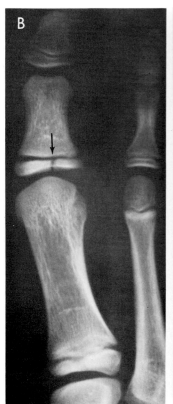

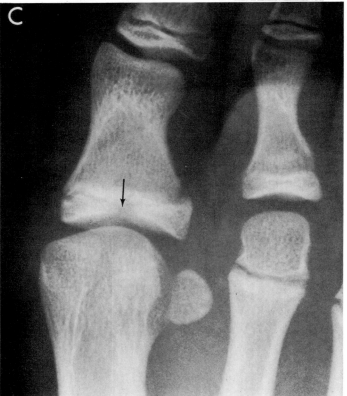

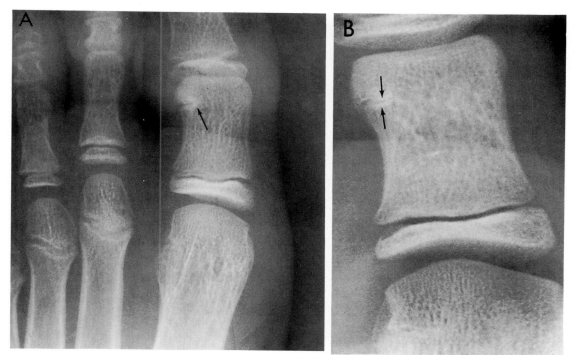

FIG 7–131.
Incomplete developmental fissures through the proximal phalanx of the first toe. **A,** 10-year-old boy; **B,** 12-year-old boy.

8

The Pediatric Patient

W. Gray Mason, Jr., M.D.

"Children are not just little adults."

Although this statement is a cliché, children's emergencies and their radiographic findings are indeed different from their adult counterparts. Different diseases affect the child's body, different structural characteristics result in different reactions to trauma, and child abuse is often evaluated first in an emergency department.

In many ways, radiographs serve as an extension of the physical examination in these patients, pinpointing an abnormality in a young patient who is unable to describe his or her symptoms. These studies may also reassure concerned adults that a child's nonverbal complaint, such as a persistent limp or intractable crying, does not represent a danger to life or health.

The best use of radiological examinations in pediatrics involves studies at clinical "branch points" of the decision tree. The physician seeing a febrile, coughing child with few physical findings faces a branch point: should this child receive antibiotics? A chest film may be normal, suggesting that symptomatic treatment is sufficient. Or it may show a consolidating pneumonia, indicating that antibiotics are necessary.

On the other hand, the situation at the conclusion of two weeks of antibiotics is a less significant branch point. The follow-up chest film in the same child, without fever or other symptoms, would be less likely to alter therapy: a normal film would be expected, but residual findings of pneumonia may reflect the slowness of resolution rather than a new disease requiring additional treatment.

Technical Problems

The actual process of radiographing children is often difficult. The structures are small, the bones incompletely ossified, and the child often uncooperative.

The most difficult children are the toddlers, from 12 to 36 months of age. Younger infants are not usually a problem since they are compliant and can often be soothed by feeding or a pacifier. Older children can usually be persuaded to cooperate. In my experience, copious praise ("What a big boy! I can't believe how well you're holding still!") works better than criticism or commands.

Toddlers, however, are old enough to have an independent opinion ("I'm not going to do this!") and too young to be influenced by anything the emergency or radiology staff says. The term "terrible two's" certainly applies to pediatric radiology.

Sometimes parents can help, although the presence of a sympathetic parent may make the problem worse since the child expects the parent to extricate him from his unpleasant situation. If the child is uncontrollable in the presence of the parent, we ask mom or dad to wait outside. The reunion with the reassuring parent is the child's reward for a successfully completed study.

Even the most experienced pediatric radiology departments have to resort to physical restraint with some toddlers. Although "brat boards" with Velcro straps are available commercially, a bedsheet wrapped tightly around a toddler's arms and torso, papoose-style, will usually provide adequate restraint.

Selecting the proper films for each examination is also important. The routine views should adequately visualize the area studied. But we try to combine thoroughness with the lowest reasonable radiation dose.

Although the radiation risk from modern diagnostic radiology is exceedingly low, the adverse effects of radiation exposure are most prominent in children. Carcinogenesis is a late effect of radiation, occurring 10 to 15 years after exposure. Radiation-induced cancer is therefore of greater concern in a young child with 70 or 80 years of remaining life expectancy than in an elderly patient. Likewise, genetic effects, which are passed on as mutations to subsequent generations, are of more concern in children exposed to radiation, since the reproductive portion of their lives will carry the burden of their radiation dose.

To balance these considerations, the Wolfson Children's Hospital uses the standard radiographic views listed in Table 8–1. Some of the studies include fewer views than similar adult examinations. However, our radiologists and emergency physicians are encouraged to supplement the basic examination with additional views when these may be helpful. For instance, a skull series in a patient with a suspected scalp foreign body would include the standard views, but might be supplemented with a tangential soft tissue view of the suspicious area of the scalp to check for radiopaque debris.

TABLE 8–1.
Standard Radiographic Views

Skull	AP*/PA*, lateral, Townes
Sinuses/facial bones	Upright Waters (under 5 years); Waters, PA, and lateral, all upright (5 years and older)
Cervical spine	Lateral (upright), AP, odontoid
Soft tissue neck	Lateral and AP, both upright
Chest	PA and lateral, upright if possible
Abdomen	Upright AP, supine AP, optional PA chest
Pelvis	AP
Hips	AP of pelvis to include both hips, frogleg lateral of symptomatic hip
Femur	AP and lateral
Knee	AP, lateral, tunnel view
Lower leg	AP and lateral
Ankle	AP, mortise, and lateral
Foot	AP and lateral (under 2 years)
	AP, lateral, and oblique (2 years and older)
Clavicle	AP, AP angled 20° caudad
Shoulder	AP internal rotation, AP external rotation, lateral scapular view
Scapula	AP through chest, lateral
Humerus	AP and lateral, include both ends of bone
Elbow	Lateral, AP, and oblique AP
Forearm	AP and lateral
Wrist	AP and lateral (under 5 years); AP, lateral, and angled navicular (5 years and older)
Hand, finger	AP, oblique, lateral of affected part

*AP = anteroposterior; PA = posteroanterior.

Because the soft tissues of children contain a great deal of useful information, our views of extremities and skull are exposed somewhat lighter than similar films on adults. A bright viewing light is often helpful in studying the soft tissue areas of these films, especially if they are conventionally exposed.

Skull

Sutures make radiographs of the pediatric skull challenging. They mimic fractures, and one must take care not to mistake a normal variant for a fracture or vice versa. In addition, it is often difficult to tell if the sutures are normal in width. There are no reliable measurements. The examples of normal variants in this book certainly help decide what is and is not a fracture. A reference book of normal anatomy is also useful.

Normal Skull

In babies the sutures are widely patent, and the anterior fontanelle is open for the first 18 months of life.

In addition to the major sutures (sagittal, coronal, lambdoid, and temporalis), accessory sutures may also be present in normal infants. The metopic suture between the frontal bones, accessory sutures in the parietal bones, and the mendosal sutures (as well as others) in the occipital bone are all potentially misleading.

The sutures usually appear to interdigitate by 12 months of age. The sagittal suture fuses at about 6 years, and the coronal and lambdoid sutures by 10 and 14 years, respectively.

Spread Sutures

The child's skull is more compliant to changes in intracranial volume than the adult's. Before the sutures fuse, an intracranial mass or any increase in intracranial volume may cause sutures to spread.

A rapid increase in intracranial volume anywhere in the brain affects all the open sutures. In a child with open sutures, a posterior fossa mass will affect the coronal as well as the sagittal and lambdoid sutures.

Figure 8–1 shows a skull with spread sutures. Unfortunately there is no reliable measurement of suture width. Experience and normal "controls" are the best criteria. Age must be taken into account as well. A normal suture width in a newborn would represent profound diastasis in a three-year-old child.

Fractures

Linear skull fractures resemble vascular grooves and sutures. Some hints for distinguishing these lucencies are listed in Table 8–2.[1]

TABLE 8–2.
Fracture vs Vascular Groove vs Suture

Finding	Fracture	Vessel	Suture
Soft tissue swelling	Yes	No	No
Symmetrical	No	Probably	Yes
Branching	Maybe	Yes	No
Dense margin	No	Yes	No

Some skull fractures are more complex than the linear fractures. Severe head trauma may produce "shattered globe" fractures with several bones involved (Fig 8–2).

Spine

Spinal lesions are similar in children and adults. The chief pitfalls usually involve unrecognized normal variants.

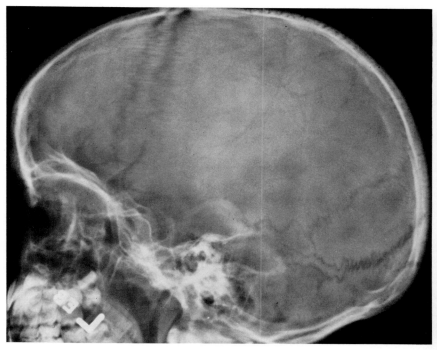

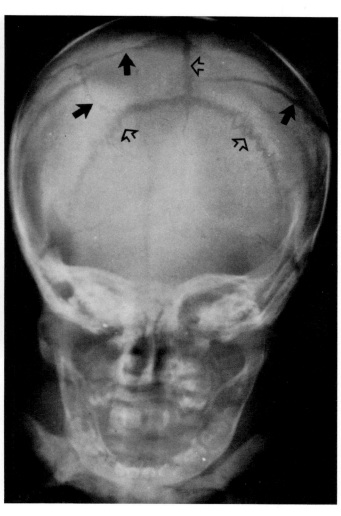

FIG 8–1 (left).
Spread sutures. The sutures are spread in this 4-year-old boy with ataxia and morning vomiting. Note the wide coronal sutures extending vertically from the top of the skull down towards the orbits. The lambdoid sutures are wide posteriorly as well. A CT scan showed a large posterior fossa cerebellar astrocytoma, demonstrating that an intracranial mass will cause diffuse suture spreading, not just spreading of the adjacent sutures.

FIG 8–2 (right).
Skull fractures and sutures. The fractures (*solid arrows*) are different from the sutures (*open arrows*) in this three-year-old who was hit by a car. The sutures occupy predictable locations and show interdigitations, especially in the lambdoid suture on the patient's left. The fractures are straighter, show branching, and are not in typical locations for sutures.

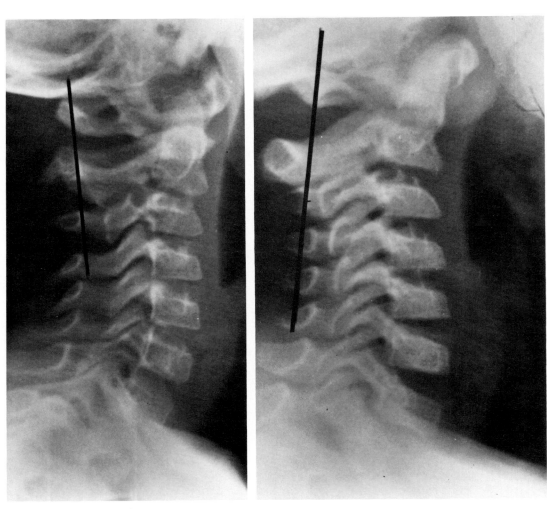

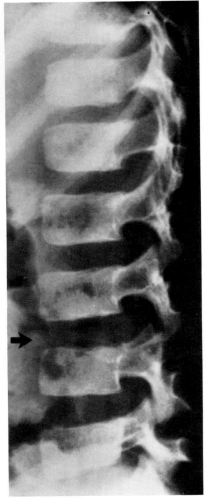

FIG 8–3 (left).
Pseudosubluxation of C2–3. Although C-2 appears tilted forward on C-3, the line connecting the posterior arches of C-1 and C-3 passes through the arch of C-2; this is a normal finding and does not represent fracture.

FIG 8–4 (middle).
Cervical fracture with positive posterior spinal line. This three-year-old has a sub-luxed upper cervical spine, but the posterior spinal line misses the posterior arch of C-2 by more than a millimeter. The fractured odontoid allowed C-1 to sublux anteriorly, and the posterior spinal line confirms the disruption of the cervical anatomy.

FIG 8–5 (right).
"Lap belt" spinal fracture. The acute flexion injury to the lumbar spine has disrupted the posterior ligaments of the lumbar spine, allowing distraction of the posterior elements at L3–4 *(arrow)*. Notice that the disk space is wider posteriorly, and the holes of the neural foramina are larger. (Courtesy of Dr. George Taylor, Department of Radiology, Children's Hospital National Medical Center, Washington, DC)

Two subjects deserve special mention, however. The pediatric cervical spine may be difficult to evaluate. And, with the advent of laws requiring the use of seat belts and car seats in children, injuries from these restraints are becoming more common.

Cervical Spine

The most useful views of the cervical spine in childhood are the lateral, anteroposterior, and odontoid views. As with adult patients, all seven cervical vertebrae should be radiographed although accomplishing this is sometimes quite difficult, and the technologist may have to use special views. The "swimmer's" view, centered on the cervicothoracic junction with one arm extended overhead and the other reaching toward the feet, is useful in demonstrating the upper thoracic and lower cervical spine. Occasionally, computed tomography (CT) may be needed.

An important normal variant occurs at C2–3. When a child flexes his neck forward, C-2 may appear to tilt out of alignment with C-3. Fortunately, the posterior elements of the spine remain in alignment, and these serve as a reassuring guide. If the line connecting the C-1 and C-3 vertebral bodies passes through the anterior cortex of the dorsal spinous process of C-2, the neck is in normal alignment as shown in Fig 8–3.

With a cervical spine fracture disrupting the upper spinal ring or allowing vertebral subluxation, the C-2 dorsal spinal surface will fall behind the line (Fig 8–4).

A word of warning: in children, the dorsal spinal line only applies when the neck is "pseudo-subluxed" during flexion. When the vertebral bodies line up properly, the posterior spinal line will not always be intact.[2]

Lap Belt Injuries

All states now have laws requiring the use of car seats and seat belts by children. During the sudden deceleration when one car crashes into another car or an immovable object, the seat belt may injure the child. (If the child was wearing no seat belt, worse injuries would undoubtedly occur.)

Typically, this is a lumbar flexion injury. The anterior component consists of a compression fracture of the anterior vertebral bodies. Posteriorly, ligamentous injury allows facet dislocation and distraction of the posterior elements of the vertebrae. Radiographic findings may be subtle (Fig 8–5). The anterior compression fractures may be difficult to see, but the widening of the foramina on the lateral view is evidence of injury.

Airway

Airway diseases are ubiquitous in childhood. Usually these diseases are self-limited and benign, with cough and mild fever as the most common symptoms. But epiglottitis, which may have similar symptoms, is potentially life threatening.

The clinical presentation of epiglottitis is somewhat different from croup (Table 8–3), but the differences are not always as clear in real life as they are in the textbooks. To make matters worse, physical examination of children with epiglottitis may worsen the airway obstruction. As a result, radiographs of the soft tissues of the neck are crucial to the evaluation of upper airway diseases.[3]

TABLE 8–3.
Diseases of the Airway

	Epiglottitis	Croup
Age (peak)	3 to 4 years	1 to 2 years
Onset	Rapid	Gradual
Position of child	Upright	Supine
Drooling	Yes	No
Fever	High	Lower
Cough	Not prominent	Barking
Voice	Soft, muffled	Hoarse

Although the anatomy of the hypopharynx is straightforward and the findings of epiglottitis are usually unequivocal, many emergency physicians and even some radiologists are uncomfortable interpreting these examinations.

Radiographic Technique

For our routine soft tissue neck study, we obtain lateral and anteroposterior views of the neck. If the patient has great respiratory distress, a lateral view alone is usually adequate to detect or exclude epiglottitis. Ideally, the patient should be upright with the neck in extension. Although the films should be taken during inspiration while the patient is not swallowing, precise timing of the exposure is often difficult. If soft tissue density obscures the air spaces on the lateral view, that view should be repeated.

Normal Anatomy

To read a soft tissue neck film, first identify the important anatomic structures (Fig 8–6). On the lateral

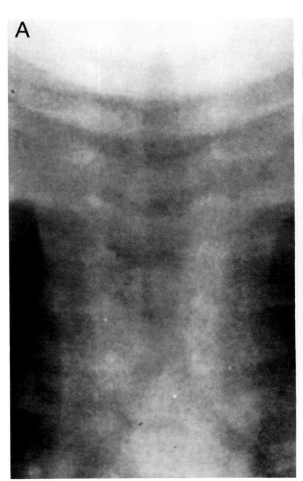

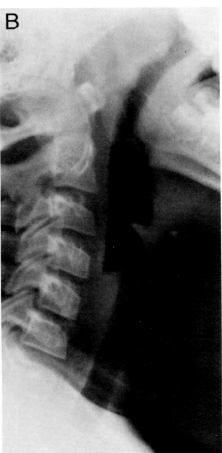

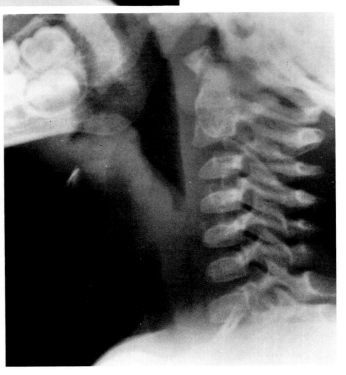

FIG 8–6 (top).

Normal airway. The upper airway has shoulders and tapers abruptly (**A** and Fig 8–8). On the lateral view (**B**) the epiglottis is located just posterior to the transverse segment of the hyoid bone. Air outlines the epiglottis's posterior surface. The delicate aryepiglottic folds extend down and posteriorly from the tip of the epiglottis to the arytenoid cartilages.

FIG 8–7 (right).

Epiglottitis. This radiograph of a 2½-year-old girl with fever and respiratory distress shows the two hallmarks of epiglottitis. First, the airway above the vocal cords appears completely blocked by the swollen aryepiglottic folds. Epiglottitis involves supraglottic structures, and the swelling of these folds is responsible for the airway obstruction. Second, the epiglottis itself is enlarged. No air column is visible within the shadow of the epiglottis, a finding that distinguishes epiglottitis from the "omega-shaped" epiglottis.

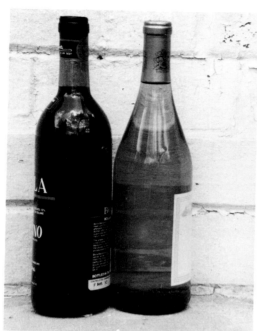

FIG 8–8 (top left).
Shape of tracheal shadows. These two wine bottles illustrate the configuration of the trachea in normal patients and in croup. The red wine bottle on the *left* has shoulders, similar to the normal appearance of the trachea. The white wine bottle on the *right* tapers like the airway in laryngotracheobronchitis (croup). (Photo by A. Gardner.)

FIG 8–9 (bottom).
Croup. The supraglottic portion of the airway is normal in this 13-month-old girl with croup. Note the slender epiglottis posterior to the transverse segment of the hyoid bone. The normal aryepiglottic folds extend from the epiglottis inferiorly and posteriorly to the arytenoid cartilages at the rear of the larynx.

Croup is visible on the lateral film as the density just below the dark shadow of the laryngeal ventricle. In the normal patient, the airway should be visible up to the larynx. In this patient, the airway is nearly obliterated by the tracheal inflammation.

The lateral film shows the tapering of the upper trachea, similar to the profile of the chablis bottle in Figure 8–8.

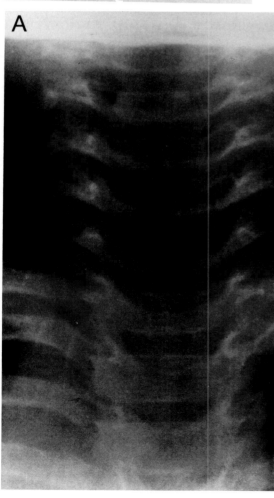

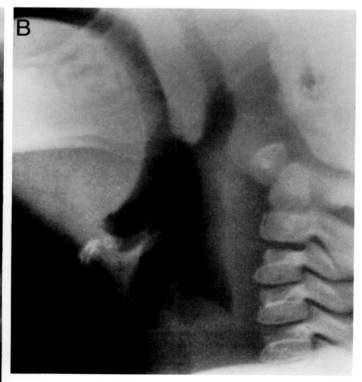

view, the hyoid bone in the anterior neck is usually easy to find. The airspace posterior and superior to the hyoid bone is the vallecula. The superior and anterior border of the vallecula is the base of the tongue. The posterior border of the vallecula is the epiglottis. The epiglottis is usually blade-shaped with the upper portion slightly narrower than the base. There is considerable variation, however, and the top portion of the epiglottis, although still flat, may expand in its lateral dimension so that it is shaped like the Greek letter omega. These side lobes may sometimes mimic enlargement. The normal epiglottis, outlined by the air in the vallecula and in the supraglottic region, is thin, whether or not "omega flaps" are present.

The appearance of aryepiglottic folds is critical in the diagnosis of epiglottitis. The folds extend from the upper posterior epiglottis inferiorly and posteriorly to the arytenoid cartilages. The vocal cord area and laryngeal ventricle are present below the aryepiglottic folds at the top of the tracheal air column. Higher up, the uvula, adenoids, and retropharyngeal soft tissues are visible.

The anteroposterior film shows the shape of the upper airway. The air column in the trachea should taper sharply inward at the true vocal cords in the normal patient.

Epiglottitis

Usually the result of *hemophilus influenza* infection in the soft tissues above the glottis, epiglottitis is named for the bright red, inflamed epiglottis that is visible laryngoscopically. In fact, the life-threatening airway obstruction is also due to edema in the aryepiglottic folds that flank the glottic opening. Some authorities call the condition "supraglottitis."

There are two important radiographic findings to look for in patients with epiglottitis (Fig 8–7). Aryepiglottic fold swelling is the most reliable radiographic finding. This soft-tissue density bridges the airway above the glottis. Although normal folds are thin, veil-like structures, swollen aryepiglottic folds may be several millimeters thick.

The second finding is swelling of the epiglottis itself. The swollen epiglottis is round like a finger tip. The supraglottic air column is not visible within the silhouette of the epiglottis. Sometimes the swollen epiglottis will obliterate the vallecula.

"Ballooning" of the hypopharynx may also be seen in these patients, but this sign is not specific and may vary with the phase of inspiration.

Beware of relying solely on the size of the epiglottis without looking for aryepiglottic folds. The omega epiglottis described above may mimic swelling. If it is really epiglottitis, the air column within the silhouette of an inflamed epiglottis will be obliterated by the edema, and the aryepiglottic folds should appear as a density across the air column above the glottis.

Patients with epiglottitis usually need intubation and antibiotic therapy.

Croup

The most common airway disease causing cough and upper airway obstruction is viral laryngotracheobronchitis or croup. Patients with croup often have a characteristic cough, tend to be younger than epiglottitis patients, and seldom require intensive treatment.

In croup, narrowing of the subglottic portion of the airway by edematous tracheal mucosa causes the airway symptoms. This narrowing is visible radiographically on the anteroposterior view as a tapering of the upper tracheal airway. The croupy airway resembles the tapered neck of a chablis wine bottle. In contrast, the normal airway resembles the shouldered neck of a Bordeaux bottle (Fig 8–8).

On the lateral film, using the laryngeal ventricle as a landmark, the subglottic narrowing appears as a soft tissue density that gradually becomes more lucent as the airway widens (Fig 8–9). Distension of the hypopharynx with air may also be seen, especially in severe cases.

The radiographic findings of croup are not as reliable as those of epiglottitis. Patients with symptoms of croup often have few radiographic findings, and an occasional asymptomatic patient may have a subglottic configuration that looks like croup.

Usually symptomatic treatment is all that is needed in patients with laryngotracheobronchitis, but an occasional patient may have more severe respiratory embarrassment and require intubation.

Chest

Chest films are the most common radiographs in children. Yet these studies are a constant technical challenge. Immobilization of children is difficult, and the automatic exposure controls on some x-ray machines have difficulty with the short exposure times and small radiation doses that pediatric chest radiography demands.

Unless special equipment is available, most x-ray installations use supine and recumbent radiography for the frontal and lateral radiographs of children too small or too wiggly to stand for conventional "adult" views. Often the parent may hold the child in position for the exposures, with sandbags to immobilize thrashing arms and legs.

The radiographic examination of the chest should include a lateral view, which is especially helpful in assessing the diaphragms and lower lobes and in locating pathology visible on the frontal view.

Ideally, both chest views should be taken during full inspiration. Expiratory films may mimic pneumonia (Fig 8–10).

Normal Anatomy

A child's chest is certainly smaller than an adult's, but there are other differences as well.

The most spectacular difference is often the thymus. A normal thymus in a child is proportionately larger than it is in an adult. In children below the age of 2 years, the thymus can be so big it obliterates the cardiac shadow. It may even be visible in older children. The thymus is an anterior structure and does not cause tracheal displacement. A soft and compliant organ, the thymus can sometimes extend along pulmonary fissures, especially the minor fissure on the right, resulting in oddly-shaped mediastinal and paramediastinal densities. The wavy edge of the thymus where it interdigitates with the intercostal muscles is a common marker helpful in identifying this benign "mass" (see Fig 8–12).

Another difference between babies and adults is the more lordotic position of the chest on frontal films. The clavicles are typically projected above the lung fields. In addition, the heart may appear proportionately larger in a child than in an adult.

The diaphragms are a good indicator of aeration in children. In a child with normally-inflated lungs, the diaphragms are curved. The heart appears to rest in the diaphragm silhouette and resembles a softball lying in a soft pillow.

The trachea is a flexible structure in childhood. Respiration, crying, or squirming may all contribute to remarkable tracheal tortuosity on either the frontal or the lateral view. Even right angle turns of the trachea are usually normal in children below the age of 3. Repeat films in a different position should show the tracheal flexibility.

Bronchiolitis and "Viral Pneumonia"

Lower respiratory viral infection is by far the most common pulmonary illness encountered in a general pediatric setting. These infections tend to be seasonal, worse in the fall and winter. Children under the age of 2 are especially susceptible because of the small size of the bronchioles, the relatively greater production of mucus, and the greater reactivity of the airways.

Clinically, these children are sick. They have fever, cough, and tachypnea. They and their parents have probably had little sleep for several nights because of the coughing.

Radiographically, these patients have variable findings, but usually demonstrate a combination of air trapping, atelectasis, hilar adenopathy, and pulmonary interstitial prominence (Fig 8–11).

The air trapping and atelectasis are actually two aspects of the same pathological process. The bronchioles are small in children. When the mucosa lining these passages thickens with edema, the airway narrows, causing greater resistance to air flow on expiration than on inspiration. The obstruction to expiration causes air trapping. As the disease progresses, the edematous mucosa blocks the bronchioles, or they become plugged with mucus, and the blocked segment of lung becomes atelectatic.

Radiographically, the diaphragm shadow is one of the best indicators of air trapping. While the normal diaphragm is curved, in air trapping the diaphragms are depressed and straighter. With over-inflated lungs, the heart appears to sit on top of a mountain, rather than in the normal pillow.

The atelectasis in these patients appears as a streaky density with varying orientations (Fig 8–12). Most atelectases will arise in the hila and extend peripherally. Usually these are fleeting findings, arising abruptly and resolving just as quickly. Occasionally, a whole lobe may become atelectatic.

A lower respiratory viral infection characterized by prominent air trapping is called bronchiolitis and is frequently caused by respiratory syncytial virus.

Interstitial infiltrates in children with lower respiratory viral infections are most often perihilar. Both the pulmonary interstitium and the bronchial walls are involved, and the resulting appearance looks shaggy. Hila and heart border may be indistinct.

Adenopathy is another common finding in these patients, with the hila occasionally becoming quite large. Although adenopathy is also a sign in tuberculosis, lymphoma, histiocytosis X, and sarcoid, the common viral syndromes are a far more common cause.

Typically children with viral pneumonias do not have pulmonary consolidation. Pulmonary densities in patients with the typical viral clinical picture usually represent collapsed lung. Atelectasis should be distinguished from pulmonary consolidation, which

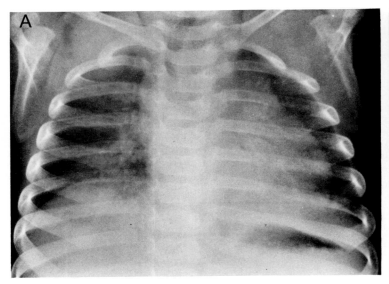
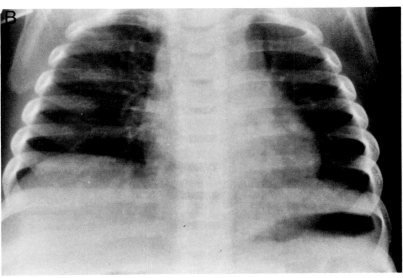

FIG 8–10.
Inspiratory and expiratory chest radiographs. These two chest films taken only minutes apart, show the vast difference between an expiratory film **(A)** and an inspiratory film **(B).** The expiratory film suggests pneumonia, and the heart appears large. The repeat film, during inspiration, shows normal lungs and heart size.

FIG 8–11.
Viral lower airway disease. This 9-month-old girl had a mild fever, a runny nose, and a bad cough. The chest x-ray shows flattening of the diaphragms bilaterally. Both pulmonary hila are large, with the right side more prominent. The lung fields appear less clear when compared to a normal chest (see Fig 8–10,B).

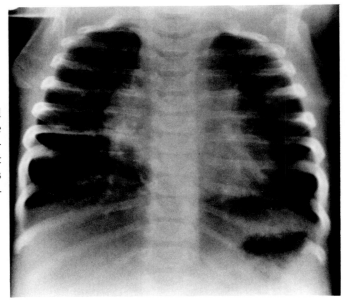

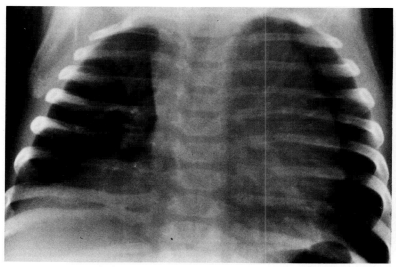

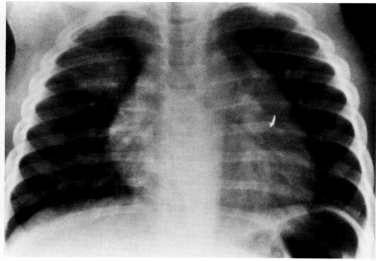

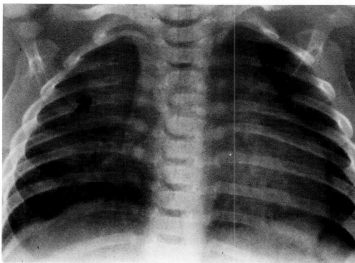

FIG 8–12 (top left).
Bronchiolitis with right upper lobe and left lower lobe atelectasis. This 4-month-old infant with tachypnea and cough has x-ray findings typical of viral lower airway disease. Besides diaphragmatic flattening, there are two areas of atelectasis. A wedge of density is present in the medial aspect of the right upper lobe representing collapse of the medial portion of that lobe. More subtle is a linear lucency behind the cardiac silhouette in the left lower lobe. Both of these findings resolved on a follow-up film.

Two incidental findings are also present. The eighth and ninth ribs on the right are fused, and the thymus is especially prominent in the left chest.

FIG 8–13 (top right).
Round pneumonia. The spherical density in the right upper lobe is a round pneumonia, usually caused by pneumococcus *(Streptococcus pneumoniae)*. The white streak in the left hilum is an artifact.

FIG 8–14 (bottom left).
Tumor masquerading as round pneumonia. The subtle round density in the right upper lobe *(arrow)* resembles the pneumonia in Figure 8–13. Closer inspection reveals distortion of the second and third ribs on the right. This round density was a ganglioneuroblastoma. Because of the occasional mass which mimics a round pneumonia, a follow-up radiograph to document clearing of the round density is reassuring.

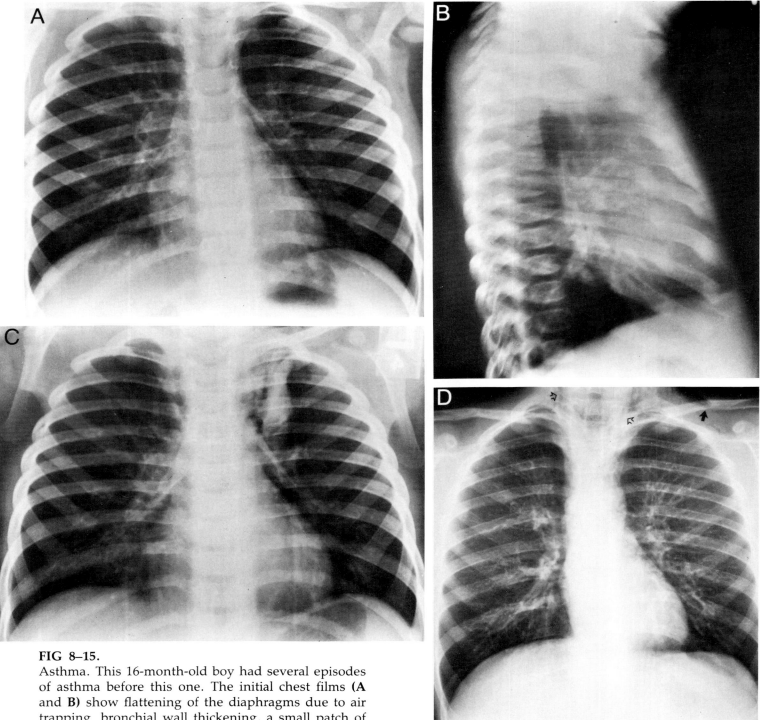

FIG 8–15.

Asthma. This 16-month-old boy had several episodes of asthma before this one. The initial chest films **(A and B)** show flattening of the diaphragms due to air trapping, bronchial wall thickening, a small patch of atelectasis in the right base, and a small pneumomediastinum in the left pulmonary hilum. A repeat film **(C)** the next day shows how quickly the atelectasis may change. The small patch in the right base has resolved, but a larger wedge of atelectasis is visible in the left upper lobe. **D,** an older patient with asthma shows dissection of air into the mediastinum and neck *(open arrows)* and subcutaneous tissues *(solid arrows)* during an episode of bronchospasm.

represents a portion of lung distended by inflammatory fluid.

Round Pneumonia

Most often caused by *Streptococcus pneumoniae*, these pneumonia are spherical air space densities (Fig 8–13).

Children with a round pneumonia have less severe symptoms, but a higher fever, than children with lower respiratory viral infections. There may be no physical findings. A round pneumonia has clinical implications identical to those of a lobar consolidation.

These are important lesions since they should be recognized as bacterial infections requiring antibiotic treatment. In addition, these patients should have a follow-up film to document resolution of the pneumonia. What appears to be a round pneumonia may turn out to be a mass (Fig 8–14)!

Asthma

Asthma is a common problem in children. It is a disease of bronchospasm induced by a variety of substances and circumstances.

Radiographically, bilateral air trapping is the most common feature of an acute asthma attack. Similar to bronchiolitis in younger patients, asthma results in flattened diaphragms and dark lung fields. The heart looks like it is on top of a mountain instead of resting in a cushion (Fig 8–15).

Mucus plugging of bronchi and bronchioles is a frequent feature of asthma, and linear or plate-like atelectasis is the result. This atelectasis appears streaky and often arises from the pulmonary hilum. It is a fleeting phenomenon that resolves rapidly and reappears just as rapidly elsewhere in the chest. These streaks of density do not represent pneumonia (see Fig 8–15).

During an asthma attack, air can leak out of the air spaces and into the mediastinum by way of the pulmonary interstitium. Pneumomediastinum is usually visible as a thin stripe of pleura along the mediastinal surface of the lung on the anteroposterior view. Occasionally, the pneumomediastinum may leak out into the soft tissues of the neck (see Fig 8–15) or into the abdomen. Usually these air leaks are not clinically significant.

Probably the most useful task a chest film accomplishes in a patient undergoing an asthma attack is to exclude a consolidating pneumonia. Bacterial pneumonia may trigger an asthma attack in a susceptible individual. The presence of consolidation superimposed on the asthma is an indication for antibiotics as well as the bronchodilators the bronchospasm requires.

There is a lot of similarity in the radiographs of babies and toddlers with bronchiolitis and older children with asthma. Both diseases are characterized by interstitial pulmonary density, bilateral air trapping, bronchial wall thickening, and atelectasis. Both may accompany a lower respiratory viral infection. But bronchiolitis in babies and toddlers does not respond as well as asthma to beta adrenergic drugs. Bronchiolitis usually has a viral etiology, while asthma's triggers are protean. A bronchiolitis in an infant or toddler does not mean that the child will be asthmatic later in life. Because of the overlap between the two diseases, many pulmonologists do not make the diagnosis of asthma before the age of two.

Foreign Bodies in the Airway

Aspirated foreign bodies are a common occurrence in children. Usually the aspirated object is not radiopaque. Peanuts are the most common offender.

Often the presenting clinical story mentions the sudden onset of coughing or a paroxysm of choking. A specific history of swallowing something the wrong way occasionally steers the clinician in the right direction.

If the foreign body is radiopaque, it is easy to see. More typically, it is lucent, and the secondary pulmonary effects provide the clues. Radiographically, bronchial foreign bodies can have several appearances.

An endobronchial foreign body may demonstrate ipsilateral air trapping (Fig 8–16). This occurs because the bronchi expand slightly during inspiration due to the negative pressure in the chest. Some air may squeeze by the object. On exhalation, the bronchi are not expanded, and the trapped air cannot easily escape from the air spaces. This is called a "ball-valve" or "check-valve" effect.

The hyperexpanded side may show flattening of the diaphragm, spreading of the pulmonary vessels, and shift of the mediastinum toward the normal side. Different levels of the two diaphragmatic surfaces on the lateral film is a helpful clue. Sometimes these findings are prominent enough on the regular chest films to suggest the diagnosis.

Usually, however, additional radiologic studies will make the diagnosis with greater certainty. If fluoroscopic equipment is available, the "check valve" effect is easy to see on the television screen. The affected diaphragm does not move as briskly as the normal side. The mediastinum will move paradoxically toward the affected side during inspiration (as the healthy lung expands) and toward the healthy side during expiration (as the healthy lung empties out).

If fluoroscopic equipment (or a radiologist) is not available, lateral decubitus films of the chest may help. A lateral decubitus film is an anteroposterior or posteroanterior film taken with the patient lying on his side and the x-ray beam horizontal. This technique works because, in the normal patient, the heart and mediastinum are heavy enough to compress the dependent lung. When a foreign body is present, the healthy side is compressible, but the hyperexpanded side remains inflated. A comparison of the two sides usually shows the difference.

Abdomen

There is a poem that radiology residents recite when faced with an abdominal film. It is an exhortation to look at the abdomen in a systematic manner.

Bones, stones,
Mass, gas.
Study the corners,
And cover your . . . rear end.

It certainly is not iambic pentameter, but a systematic approach to pediatric abdomen films can increase the likelihood of recognizing abnormalities.

"Bones," although always present, are easy to overlook. In patients with trauma, pelvic and lumbar fractures are sometimes incidental findings on abdomen films. "Stones" can represent gall bladder disease (especially in children with hemoglobinopathies), kidney stones, or coproliths due to appendicitis. "Masses" in children may be full hollow organs (stomach, urinary bladder), neoplasms (Wilm's tumor, neuroblastoma, hepatic or ovarian masses), or pathologic obstructions (intussusception, ureteropelvic junction obstruction). And the gas pattern may give a clue to the presence of bowel obstruction, perforation, or paralytic ileus.

The conditions covered in this section are more frequently encountered in children than in adults.

Intussusception

The classical patient with intussusception is between 6 and 30 months of age, has a history of a recent viral syndrome, and an immediate history of vomiting, abdominal pain, and bloody stools. The stools are often described as "currant jelly" in appearance, dark red and gelatinous. The classical patient will also have a midabdominal mass and an empty right lower quadrant.

Pathologically, the intussusception usually involves the ileocolic region as the lead point. A minority of intussusceptions are ileoileal (and these tend to be post-operative) or ileoileocolic.

Radiographically, an intussusception can have almost any appearance, and the lack of specific findings should not dissuade anyone from further studies if the clinical presentation warrants (Fig 8–17).

In patients with a "tight" intussusception, a small bowel obstructive pattern may be seen. "Looser" intussusceptions may show no evidence of obstruction. Paradoxically, sometimes the patients with symptoms of the longest duration have the loosest intussusception; perhaps children with the most obstructive intussusceptions become sicker more quickly.

In rare cases, the intussusceptum may be visible on plain films.

When an intussusception is suspected clinically or radiographically, a contrast enema is required. The standard in this country is a barium enema, although some pediatric radiologists now prefer water-soluble contrast because of the infrequent, but potentially devastating, complication of perforation. Recently, some centers borrowed a technique from the Republic of China that uses air or carbon dioxide as contrast.

The goals of the enema are both diagnostic and therapeutic. The intussusceptum is visible as a rounded density in the colon, outlined by the contrast. As the study continues, the hydrostatic (or aerostatic) pressure of the contrast pushes the intussusceptum proximally. In about two thirds of the cases, the ileocolic intussusception can be completely reduced by this method; reports in the literature range from 40% to 85%.

Although patients who have their intussusceptions reduced by enema do not need surgery, a small percentage of patients will experience bowel perforation during the procedure, usually in an area of bowel necrosis. Therefore, it is prudent to notify the surgery service that a patient may require surgery.

Foreign Bodies

Children put all sorts of things in their mouths—coins, jacks, batteries, safety pins, small toys, razor blades. Anything small has found its way into some child's mouth. These foreign bodies are often swallowed.

The clinical presentation usually has the parent reporting the ingestion, but some children will present with a sudden onset of drooling and dysphagia.

The radiographic approach is straightforward. A frontal film of both the chest and abdomen are re-

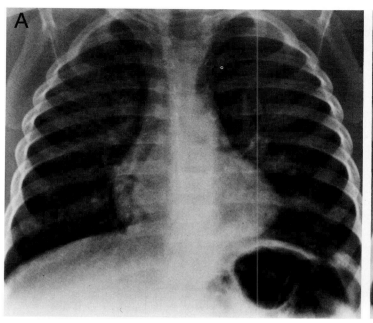

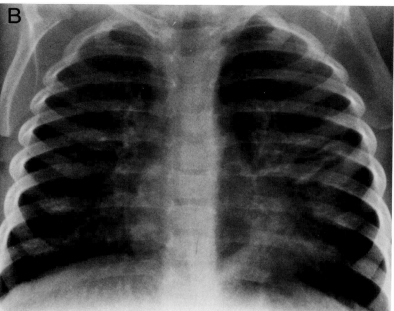

FIG 8–16.
Endobronchial foreign body. This toddler suddenly began coughing. The initial chest film **(A)** showed left lower lobe pneumonia. Although not noticed on the original film, the left lung appears darker than the right. The child returned to the emergency depart-ment 36 hours later with no improvement. The second chest film again showed the hyperlucent left lung with more extensive infiltrate and atelectasis in the left lower lobe. Fluoroscopy showed paradoxical motion, and subsequent bronchoscopy removed a peanut from the left mainstem bronchus.

FIG 8–17.
Intussusception. Although an abdominal film may suggest intussusception with dilated small bowel loops reflecting obstruction **(A),** a contrast enema diagnoses intussusception **(B)** and, in many cases, will reduce it.

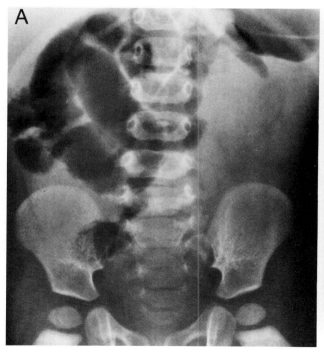

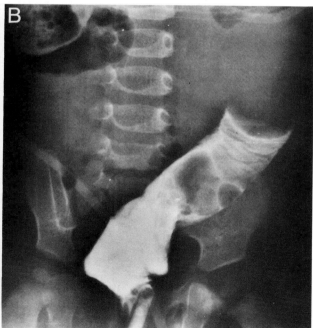

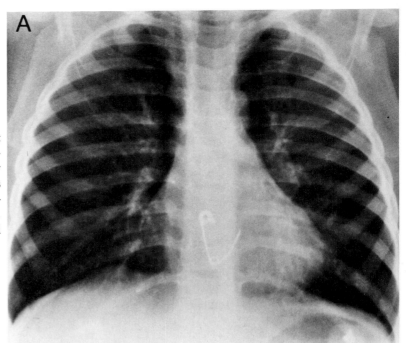

FIG 8–18.
Passage of a foreign body. This open safety pin is first seen at the esophagogastric junction **(A).** Surgical removal was planned, but a few hours later, the safety pin had passed into the stomach **(B).** Since objects that reach the stomach are almost always passed rectally, the child was watched. Forty-eight hours later, the open safety pin had been uneventfully expelled **(C).**

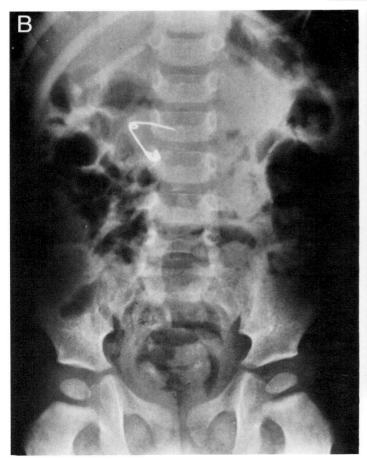

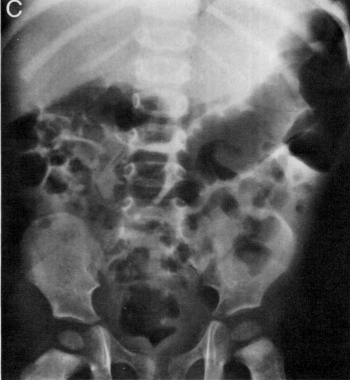

quired. If no foreign body is visible, a lateral neck film (if the neck is not visible on the other views) excludes a pharyngeal foreign body.

When a foreign body is present, the response is based on its location. The esophagogastric junction is the "isthmus" of the alimentary tract (Fig 8–18). Foreign bodies that pass this point and enter the stomach are almost always passed rectally. Although open safety pins and razor blades usually pass without incident, we usually obtain repeat films to document passage of the foreign body. Repeat films are also warranted if any foreign body is not seen in the child's stool within a week. Occasionally, oddly shaped objects that become impacted in the alimentary tract may require surgical removal.

On the other hand, esophageal foreign bodies that do not pass into the stomach remain in the esophagus until removed (Fig 8–19). Radiopaque objects like coins are easy to see; lucent objects (buttons, pull rings from soft drink cans) may require barium to visualize. The three most common sites for impaction in the esophagus are the upper esophagus just below the cricopharyngeus muscle, the region immediately above the aortic arch, and the esophageal vestibule above the esophagogastric junction. Swallowed coins are the most common esophageal foreign bodies.

Objects lodged in the esophagus can usually be removed under fluoroscopic control with a Foley catheter. After immobilizing the child, a deflated Foley catheter is inserted in the mouth, NOT the nose, of the patient. We find it helpful to use a tongue depressor wrapped in a cotton 4 by 4 padding to ensure that the mouth stays open. The catheter is passed beyond the foreign body and inflated with air. As the catheter is withdrawn, the inflated balloon catches the coin and pulls it up and out. The child's body is rolled to the side as the catheter is withdrawn to allow the coin to fall out of the mouth.

Coins lodged in the lower esophagus are sometimes more easily pushed into the stomach, an acceptable alternative since foreign bodies which reach the stomach are usually passed rectally.

Vomiting in the Neonate

Newborn babies have poorly-developed gastroesophageal sphincters. Some babies regurgitate after every feeding. One pediatrician has a "buttermilk clinic" for his vomiting babies because that is what their clothes smell like.

But vomiting, especially vomiting of recent origin, may signify more serious disease. In babies not born with intestinal obstructions, the most common causes are hypertrophic pyloric stenosis, midgut volvulus, and hernias.

Pyloric stenosis typically occurs in babies 4 to 12 weeks of age. It is uncommon in premature babies. The male/female ratio is 4 to 1. A baby with pyloric stenosis has intractable vomiting and is very hungry. The physical examination will show the "olive" or pyloric mass, but even experienced physicians may have difficulty eliciting this sign.

Abdominal films may show gastric distention, even when the baby has been vomiting (Fig 8–20). In addition, the more distal bowel loops often contain little gas. Although these signs are far from foolproof, they are useful in guiding further work-up. When the abdominal films suggest pyloric stenosis, the child receives a careful physical examination by a pediatric surgeon, with confirmation of the diagnosis by ultrasound in cases where the olive is difficult to feel. Ultrasound shows the pyloric tumor well and avoids the administration of barium in a patient who is likely to need surgery. On the other hand, if the abdominal films do not suggest obstruction (no gastric distension, plenty of bowel gas in small and large bowel loops), an upper gastrointestinal series with barium is appropriate since gastroesophageal reflux is more likely.

Midgut volvulus is a less common obstruction. When the obstruction is jejunal or ileal, the plain film findings may be nonspecific. Small bowel obstruction is the most common appearance. When the obstruction is more proximal, abdominal films are more likely to show gastric distension. Further work-up may include a barium upper gastrointestinal series or a barium enema. Needless to say, volvulus can be a surgical emergency when accompanied by bowel necrosis.

Finally, hernias may result in obstruction. The abdominal study typically shows a small bowel obstructive pattern, but as the poem above suggests, "Look at the corners . . ." so the little gas bubble in the inguinal hernia sac does not escape notice.

Pelvis and Hips

The relatively common hip diseases affecting children include transient synovitis (sometimes called "toxic synovitis"), septic arthritis, Perthes disease (also called Legg-Perthes or Legg-Calve-Perthes disease), and slipped capital femoral epiphysis.

A hip is the only joint which requires a comparison view for routine evaluation. Even if only one hip is painful, the AP view should include the whole pelvis and contralateral hip. This procedure allows evaluation of the ossification of the two femoral heads, com-

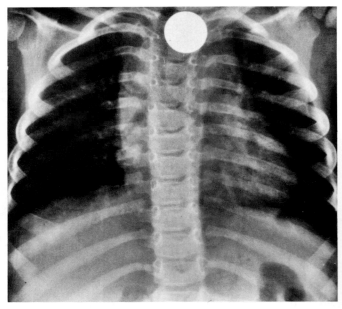

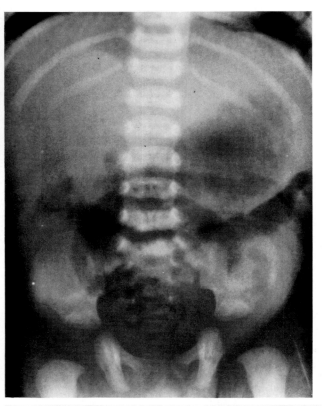

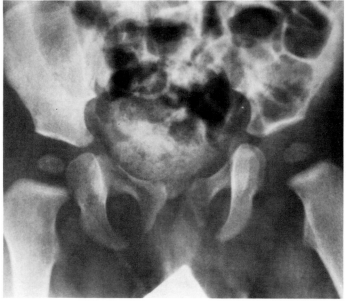

FIG 8–19 (top left).
Esophageal foreign body. This toddler was drooling and could not swallow food after swallowing this coin. Esophageal foreign bodies often do not pass into the stomach and must be removed, either endoscopically or by means of Foley catheter.

FIG 8–20 (top right).
Pyloric stenosis. The abdominal film on this 5-week-old boy with severe vomiting shows the typical plain film findings of pyloric stenosis. The stomach is distended in the left upper quadrant, and the bowel gas in the small intestine and colon is sparse. These findings may be confirmed with physical examination (by feeling the olive), ultrasound of the pyloric tumor, or barium swallow to show the contour of the gastric obstruction.

FIG 8–21 (bottom right).
Transient synovitis. This 15-month-old boy refused to walk on his left leg. Physical examination suggested that his hip was tender, and the hip films confirm the lateral displacement of the left femoral head. Comparison with the right femoral head is helpful.

parison of the acetabular configuration, and use of the asymptomatic side as a control in measuring the joint space width.

To measure the width of the joint, use a film marking pencil or crayon marker to mark the edge of the epiphysis medially and the acetabular wall. Make a similar measurement from the top of the epiphysis to the acetabular roof. The measurements should be within a millimeter of each other in patients with two normal hips. Although a helpful sign when present, hip effusion and pyarthrosis may be present with minimal hip joint widening.

Normal Anatomy

The femoral heads are not normally ossified in newborns. Hips become visible at three to six months of age. By 18 months, the femoral head ossification centers conform to the shape of the cartilaginous femoral head.

In the normal patient, the acetabulum should cover the femoral head. The center of the head should be clearly medial to the lateral edge of the acetabulum. A more lateral position of the femoral head indicates ligamentous laxity (which may be seen in neuromuscular diseases affecting the hips) or a dislocated hip. In addition, Shinton's arc is a useful index of alignment. The arc of the medial femoral neck should be continued superiorly and medially. This extension of the arc should coincide with the inferior edge of the superior ramus of the pubic bone. When the arc is disrupted, the location of the hip in the acetabulum is abnormal.

Transient Synovitis

Sometimes called "toxic synovitis," this is an extremely common cause of painful hip in children under 10 years of age. This synovitis is probably caused by a virus and is painful enough to interfere with ambulation. Onset is rapid, and its course benign. Typically, it is self-limiting, requiring only symptomatic treatment. Radiographically, the only finding is widening of the affected joint space, present in about half the cases (Fig 8–21).

Transient synovitis must be distinguished from more ominous diseases. Septic arthritis also presents with a painful hip and evidence of joint space widening. Fever and elevation of the white blood cell count are usually present as well. Because of the damage to the joint by septic arthritis, a painful hip accompanied by clinical findings suspicious for infection should be aspirated.

Perthes Disease

The etiology of this aseptic necrosis of the femoral head is unknown. Boys are affected six times more often than girls. Peak ages are 6 to 8, although the disease does occur in younger and older children. Clinically, it presents with a painful limp, usually of a few weeks duration.

The earliest radiographic sign of Perthes disease is hip effusion. This first stage may last up to 2 weeks, and, during this time, the condition is radiographically indistinguishable from transient synovitis.

Early signs of aseptic necrosis in the hip provide the first evidence of Perthes disease (Fig 8–22). Increased density of the affected femoral head with respect to the normal one indicates devascularization. Presumably, there is mild demineralization of the skeleton, but the unperfused head is unaffected.

Subchondral infraction, a line of lucency paralleling the joint space in the femoral head, is a later sign of avascular necrosis. If the child continues to walk on the hip, fragmentation and flattening of the femoral head may occur.

Some patients present with the earliest findings, but some are not brought to medical attention until severe femoral head deformity is present.

Slipped Capital Femoral Epiphysis

Occurring during the early teens, slipped epiphysis is three times more common in boys than in girls and is often bilateral. It may cause avascular necrosis of the femoral head, articular cartilage narrowing, decreased range of motion, and eventual degenerative joint disease in the hip.

Slipped capital epiphyses may be difficult to detect. Often the slip is more visible on a lateral view of the hip (Fig 8–23). Differences between the hips on AP views may hint at the slippage. Subtle alteration of the epiphysis or the position of the head on the neck are often only appreciated in comparison with the normal side.

Skeletal Emergencies in Children

The child's skeleton is very different from an adult's. The relative strength of the various components of the child's skeleton are different from those of the adult. The skeleton is still growing, structurally weak cartilage plates occupy ends of compliant long bones. The ligaments are the strongest part of the skeleton in children. An epiphyseal fracture or an avulsion is more likely than a ligament tear. Hence, an injury that produces a sprained ankle in a 23-year-

FIG 8–22 (top right).
Perthes disease. The right femoral head of this 8-year-old boy is more dense than the left, and a crescent of lucency (subchondral infraction) is visible just below the cortex. These are classic signs of idiopathic femoral head aseptic necrosis or Perthes disease.

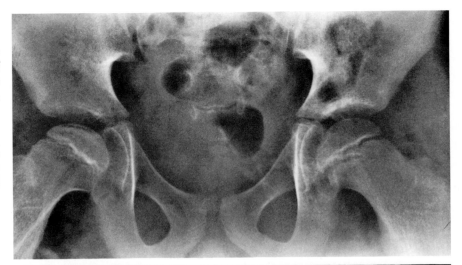

FIG 8–23 (middle right).
Slipped capital femoral epiphysis. The left femoral head is displaced medially and inferiorly in this 14-year-old boy with hip pain. Often, the frog leg lateral position is best for detecting this abnormality.

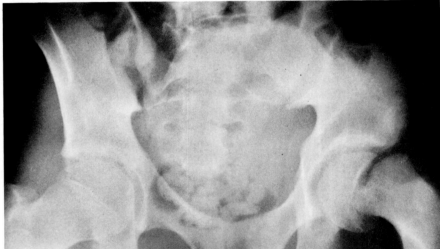

FIG 8–24 (bottom left).
Elbow effusion. This lateral view of a child's elbow shows fat pads both anteriorly and posteriorly. The posterior fat pad should never be seen normally; it is usually hidden in the olecranon notch. The anterior fat pad usually rests against the distal humerus. When it is billowed outward, as in this patient, it also indicates joint fluid. In a trauma patient, a positive fat pad sign is a fracture until proven otherwise.

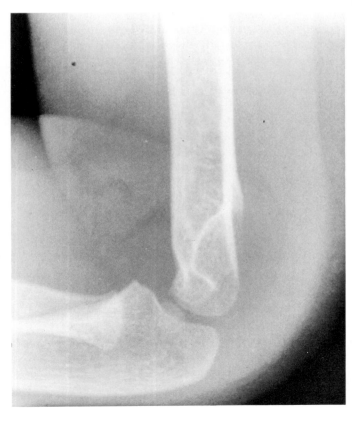

old would probably cause an epiphyseal fracture in a 12-year-old.

Technical Factors

Soft tissues are important in the radiographic diagnosis of skeletal injuries in children. In the elbow, knee, and ankle, joint effusion may provide an important clue to injury (Fig 8–24). Some nondisplaced fractures may exhibit soft tissue swelling as the only evidence of injury.

Because the soft tissues are so important, the x-ray exposure should be light enough for the soft tissues to be visible. When viewing skeletal films, a bright light is often helpful, although one has to be careful since the heat from the lamp may wrinkle the film.

Proper attention to technique is important in positioning as well. In the elbow, for instance, the lateral positioning must be precise. An oblique view may mask the presence of an effusion.

Because the pediatric skeleton is replete with normal lucencies which may mask fractures, a normal examination should be followed by a repeat film in 10 to 14 days if the patient's symptoms persist. Sometimes even the most experienced observers will miss fractures that only become visible when the healing process becomes visible. A delayed film of an occult fracture may show periosteal reaction, sclerosis through the fracture site, and osteoporosis of the remainder of the bone.

Finally, there is controversy about the role of comparison films. The availability of a handy "baseline" must be balanced against the additional expense and the extra radiation burden to a healthy part of the body. Certainly some parts of the body require comparison. The AP view of a painful hip must include the contralateral hip since the difference in joint width is the criterion for joint effusion. Generally, however, routine comparison views are not necessary. A book of normal anatomy replaces most comparison views in our department,[4] and we rarely obtain a comparison unless the films of the affected body part are confusing.

Epiphyseal Fractures

The Salter-Harris classification of epiphyseal fractures (Fig 8–25) describes the spectrum of these injuries. Fractures with higher classifications generally have a greater chance of poor outcome, with limb shortening and fracture site deformities the most likely complications.

Type 1 fractures traverse the epiphyseal plate. If these fractures are not displaced, the only radiographic sign may be soft tissue swelling.

Type 2 fractures are the most common. A fragment of metaphysis remains attached to the epiphyseal plate. The epiphysis and the metaphyseal fragment are displaced.

In type 3 fractures, the fracture plane extends through the epiphysis. The metaphysis remains intact, and a portion of the epiphysis and growth plate remain attached to the metaphysis. The fracture fragment consists of the displaced portion of the epiphysis.

The type 4 fracture extends across the epiphyseal plate, with both metaphyseal and epiphyseal components to the fracture.

Type 5 is a crush injury, with obliteration of all or part of the growth plate by the longitudinal impact. This type fracture commonly results in growth arrest or, if only part of the plate is damaged, angled growth with subsequent deformity.

Greenstick, Torus, and Plastic Fractures

Children's bones are much less brittle than adults' bones. As a result, a child's long bone is less likely to shatter. The term "greenstick" graphically describes the pliability of the pediatric skeleton (Fig 8–26). A diaphyseal fracture in a child often shows fracture of the convex cortical surface and bending of the concave surface. Just like its namesake, it looks like a broken green stick.

A similar fracture may occur at the metaphysis of a long bone. Because of a compressive force, the metaphyseal surface may buckle out. This type of buckle fracture is called a "torus" fracture. In Greek architecture a torus is the bump at the base of a column (Fig 8–27) and this type of buckle fracture resembles that bump (Fig 8–28).

A third type of fracture which demonstrates the pliability of the pediatric skeleton is a bowing fracture. When the force deforming the bone is great enough to cause bending but not sufficient to snap the bone, the bone may be bowed (Fig 8–29). This type fracture is common in the radius, ulna, and tibia. Normal curves of these bones may be confusing; a comparison view may help determine if a confusing curve in an injured bone represents bowing. When a long bone is bowed, it is treated like a fracture. If the deformity is severe enough, it may need to be straightened.

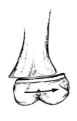 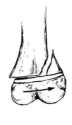 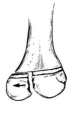

TYPE I TYPE II TYPE III

FIG 8–25 (top right).
The Salter-Harris classification of epiphyseal fractures. A type I epiphyseal fracture involves avulsion of the entire epiphysis. If nondisplaced, a type I fracture may be difficult to detect. Type II fractures extend through the epiphysis, but carry a fragment of metaphysis. This is the most common epiphyseal fracture. A type III fracture involves the epiphysis itself, with the fracture line extending through the growth plate. In the type IV injury, the fracture line involves both the metaphysis and the epiphysis. A type V fracture is a crushing injury to the growth plate.

In general, the prognosis worsens as the numbers get bigger. Type V epiphyseal fractures have a high likelihood of residual deformity, either growth arrest or angled growth.

FIG 8–26 (near right).
Greenstick fracture.

FIG 8–27 (far right).
"Torus" in Greek architecture.

TYPE IV TYPE V

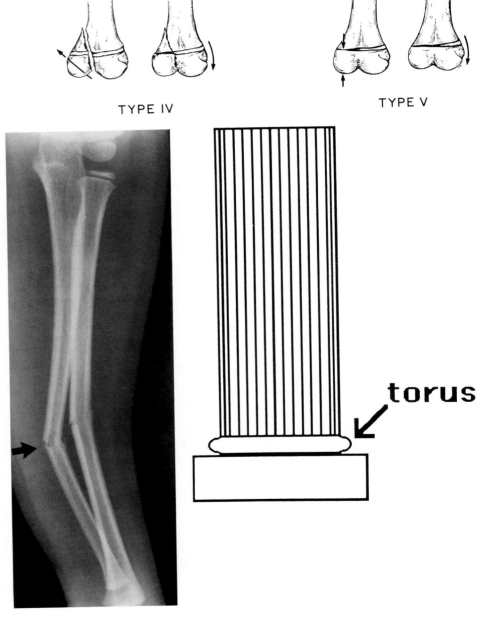

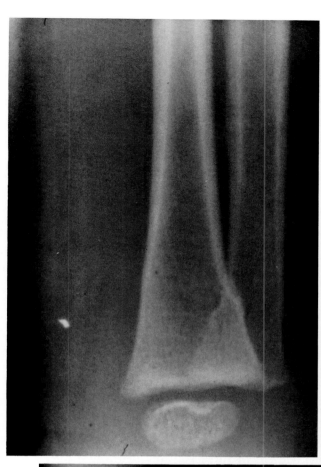

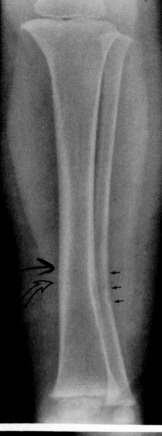

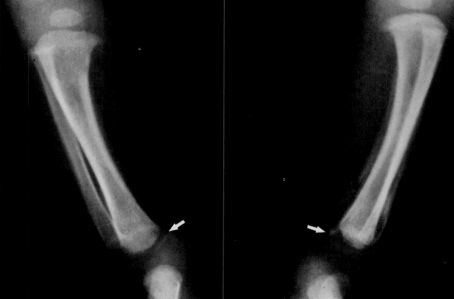

FIG 8–28 (top far left).
Torus fracture.

FIG 8–29 (top near left).
Plastic bowing fracture. The *small arrows* show the bent fibula, a plastic deformity resulting from many microfractures. In addition, the tibia is fractured (*open, curved arrow*) transversely. The *large black arrow* does not point to anything.

FIG 8–30 (bottom left).
Bucket handle fractures of child abuse. Note the rim of density at the distal ends of the tibias. These resemble the wire handles of buckets (the metaphysis is the bucket). These fractures are strong indicators of child abuse. In addition, periosteal reaction cloaks the left tibia, indicating that some of the trauma occurred a week or more prior to the radiograph.

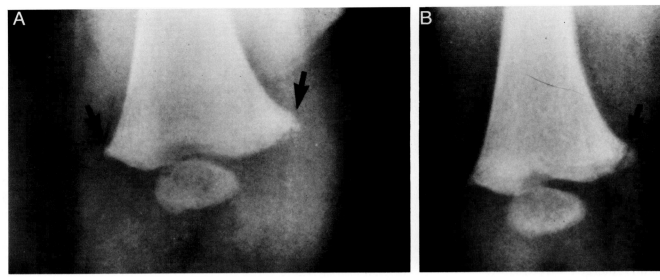

FIG 8–31.
Corner fractures of child abuse. This infant's distal femur shows corner fractures. In the AP projection, both metaphyseal corners are involved (*arrows* in **A**), while only the posterior corner is fractured on the lateral view (*arrow* in **B**). Actually, these corner fractures are a single fracture fragment extending around the periphery of the metaphysis. Corner fractures are pathologically identical to bucket handle fractures.

FIG 8–32.
Rib fractures in child abuse. Posterior rib fractures *(solid arrows)* strongly suggest abuse. They are often subtle, but the callus around the lower right fractures helps to make them more visible. The more lateral rib fractures are not as specific for abuse, but should be regarded as suspicious.

FIG 8–33.
Subdural hematoma from shaking. This CT scan on an abused infant shows increased density around the falx posteriorly. Acute bleeding appears dense on the CT scan. The interhemispheric location is typical for subdurals caused by shaking the baby violently back and forth in a sagittal plane. The decreased density anterior to the frontal lobes at the top of the picture represents older hematomas.

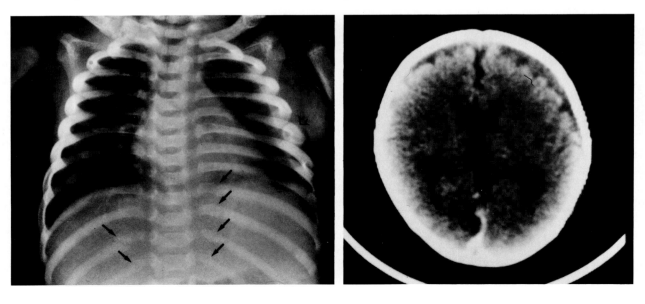

Child Abuse

For this discussion, child abuse is physical harm to a child committed by the child's parents or guardians. Although the problem of child abuse is certainly not a new one, its medical history is relatively short. An article by John Caffey in 1946 first brought attention to children with characteristic fractures and subdural hematomas.[5] A landmark article by Kempe and colleagues in 1962 coined the term "battered-child syndrome" and brought new attention to this disturbing subject.[6]

Although the incidence of child abuse is difficult to determine, there were about 1 million reports of child abuse to child protection authorities in 1983, and that figure certainly seriously underestimates the actual incidence of the problem.

In an emergency setting, there are radiographic findings that strongly suggest child abuse.

Skeletal Abuse

Fractures occur in a minority of cases of child abuse, but are more common in children under 3 years of age. Certainly any injury can be due to abuse. But some fractures occur in child abuse almost exclusively, and the presence of these fractures usually indicates a "battered-child" (Table 8–4).

TABLE 8–4.

Skeletal Trauma in Child Abuse

---

1. *Fractures indicating child abuse*
   "Bucket-handle" or corner metaphyseal fractures
   Posterior rib fractures
   Scapular fractures

2. *Fractures suspicious for child abuse*
   Multiple fractures of different ages
   Fractured fingers and toes
   Complex skull fractures

3. *Fractures common in child abuse but not specific for abuse*
   Clavicular fractures
   Diaphyseal fractures
   Linear skull fractures

Metaphyseal lesions, specifically corner fractures and "bucket-handle" fractures, are, according to Kleinman, "virtually pathognomonic of infant abuse."[7] These lesions are two different appearances of the same injury. The fracture represents a plane of separation between the metaphysis and the epiphyseal plate of the developing bone. The distal fracture fragment—the epiphysis and cartilaginous growth plate—has a dense peripheral margin. When this peripheral margin is viewed obliquely, it resembles the wire handle of a bucket (Fig 8–30). When the same lesion is viewed from the side, only the portion of the fracture peripheral to the metaphysis is visible, and it looks like a corner (Fig 8–31). Often, corner fractures are visible in both AP and lateral views, indicating that the corners are affected in all planes.

These fractures are different from Salter fractures. With these metaphyseal fractures, the periosteum is intact, and there is little displacement. The mechanism of injury is the torsion and traction applied to the limbs while the infant is shaken. The femur and humerus are most commonly involved, but the tibia and radius are often involved as well.

Posterior rib fractures also suggest child abuse (Fig 8–32). Babies seldom suffer rib fractures in the absence of nonaccidental trauma. In infants, these fractures are usually the result of thoracic compression during shaking, although in older children rib fractures may be due to direct blows to the chest or to the impact of being thrown against a wall or other solid object.

Rib fractures are often difficult to see immediately after they occur. After callus formation, however, they may be more visible. Oblique chest views may demonstrate them better than conventional views.

Lateral rib fractures are less common than posterior fractures and are less specific for abuse. The presence of unexplained lateral rib fractures warrants careful study of the posterior ribs and awareness of the possibility of child abuse. Incidentally, resuscitation seldom results in rib fractures in children.

The scapula is another fracture site strongly suggesting abuse. These fractures are unusual and often difficult to see, but a scapular fracture in the absence of a severe direct blow almost certainly represents nonaccidental trauma. Scapular fractures probably result from traction on tendons and ligaments as the child is vigorously shaken. When present, these fractures are often seen with typical child abuse fractures elsewhere.

Other features of fractures suggest abuse, but without the specificity of the three types of fractures noted above. Fractures of different ages suggest an ongoing pattern of injury to the child. Without a history of accidental injury, fractures in different stages of healing should raise a red flag. Bilateral fractures suggest abuse as well, since accidental injuries are usually unilateral. Fractures of the hands, feet, vertebrae, and complex skull fractures are also suspicious, particularly when the history does not match the pattern of injury.

CNS Injuries Due to Abuse

When an infant is shaken by the arms or torso, the head moves rapidly to and fro with the neck as a pivot point. The rotational acceleration and deceleration may disrupt bridging veins between the surface of the brain and the dura, resulting in subdural hematomas. Although the initial report by Caffey included the presence of subdural hematomas, conventional skull radiography is often normal in patients with extensive bleeding. Sutural widening is the most common abnormality, but it may be difficult to detect, especially in young infants. The availability of CT has been a major advance in detecting this type of injury.

On a CT scan, an acute collection of blood appears white, clearly different from brain density. As the clot ages, it becomes progressively less dense. After 3 or 4 days, the clot may be the same density as brain. After 1 or 2 weeks, it will be less dense.

One of the most common appearances of an acute subdural hematoma in a shaken baby is a bright interhemispheric stripe that represents an acute subdural hematoma along the falx (Fig 8–33). In normal babies, the falx is more dense than brain, but real subdural hematomas may be distinguished from a normal falx by patchiness of the density, extension over the tentorium or over the surface of one hemisphere, or asymmetry with respect to the falx.

Small subdural hematomas over the convexity of the brain are harder to see because the proximity of the dense bone of the skull may mask the abnormal density. CT slices through the top of the vertex may show these better than lower slices, and effacement of the sulci on the affected side may provide a useful clue.

Magnetic resonance imaging has advantages over CT in imaging small subdural and subacute hematomas and may clarify confusing CT findings.

When the CT scan shows both acute and subacute subdural hematomas, the findings are highly suspicious for child abuse. When the hematoma appears to result from a single insult, the findings must be weighed with clinical history. In infants, birth trauma may cause subdural bleeding, making the presence of subdural hematoma less specific in the first few weeks of life.

Recommendations When Abuse Is Suspected

Obviously the diagnosis of child abuse should not be taken lightly. On the one hand, the welfare of the child may be at stake, but on the other hand, an unwarranted accusation of child abuse will have serious repercussions with the parents and caretakers of the child.

In the initial stage of work-up, a skeletal survey is the first radiographic step. Skeletal films are the usual first step, but nuclear medicine skeletal surveys are preferred at some institutions. If retinal hemorrhages, suspicious fractures, or central nervous system signs are present, an unenhanced CT scan is indicated.

References and Suggested Reading

1. Steiner GM: *Essential Pediatric Radiology.* London, Blackwell Scientific Publishers, 1983.
2. Swischuk LE: *Emergency Radiology of the Acutely Ill or Injured Child.* Baltimore, Williams & Wilkins Co, 1986, p 536.
3. Battaglia JA: Severe croup: The child with fever and upper airway obstruction. *Pediatrics in Review* 1986; 7:227–233.
4. Keats TE, Smith T: *An Atlas of Normal Developmental Roentgen Anatomy,* ed 2. Chicago, Year Book Medical Publishers, 1988.
5. Caffey J: Multiple fractures in the long bones of infants suffering from chronic subdural hematoma. *AJR* 1946; 56:163–173.
6. Kempe CH, Silverman FN, Steele BF, et al: The battered-child syndrome. *JAMA* 1962; 181:105–112.
7. Kleinman P: *Diagnostic Imaging of Child Abuse.* Baltimore, Williams & Wilkins Co, 1987, p 10.

Index

A

Abdomen
  acute
    decision tree, 296
    routine films, 249–250
  adynamic ileus, 256–258, 260
  anatomical approach, 244–249
  ascites, 212, 287
  barium vs. water-soluble contrast, 260–262
  blunt trauma, 309–329
    angiography, 319–320
    bladder complications, 320–325
    blood in peritoneal cavity, 311–313
    duodenal injury, 317, 319
    intrahepatic hematoma, 310
    magnetic resonance imaging, 319–320
    nuclear medicine for, 319–320
    radiographic technique, 312
    rectus sheath hematoma, 310
    renal injuries, 325–329
    ruptured diaphragm, 318, 319
    ruptured spleen, 313–317
    ultrasonography, 319–320
    urethral complications, 320–325
    viscus perforation, 317
  calcific densities, 244, 245
  cholecystitis, acute, 277–281
  distal colon obstruction vs. adynamic ileus, 257, 259, 260
  diverticulitis, 285, 286
  flank pain, 296–305
  gallstone ileus, 284–286
  inflammatory lesions, recognizing, 293
  interposition, 272, 274, 277, 348
  intussusception, 268–270
  masses, 249, 267, 268
    simulation of, 270, 350
  mechanical obstruction, 253–257
  mesenteric ischemia, 294–296, 297
  nonspecific, 251–253
  normal variants, 330–336
    abdominal mass simulation, 350, 351
    bladder, 363
    bladder simulation, 364
    calcifications, 352, 354–356, 360
    distention of infantile stomach, 353
    emphysematous cystitis simulation, 363
    fissured biliary calculus simulation, 353
    gallstone simulation, 351
    kidneys, 356–357, 360
    neoplasm simulation, 352, 358, 364
    pneumoperitoneum simulation, 347, 348
    psoas shadow, 356
    renal calculus simulation, 351
    retrocaval ureter, 361
    soft tissue shadows, 354
    ureters, 361–362
  pancreatitis, acute, 277–281
  pediatric
    foreign bodies in, 492, 494, 495
    intussusception, 492, 493
  penetrating trauma
    foreign bodies, 328, 336
    gunshot wounds, 327, 329
    stab wound, 328
  perception of disease, 243
  peritoneum, free air in, 268, 271–273
  peritonitis, 285–287
  pregnancy, radiation exposure during, 301, 306–309
  strangulation obstruction, 263–266
  testicular torsion, 301, 306
  ureteral colic, 296, 301, 304, 305
Abdominal aortic aneurysm: calcified, 338
Abortion: septic, 309
Abscesses
  appendiceal, 275–277
  intra-abdominal, 285–288
  lung, 187, 188
Acetabular rim, 396
Acetabulum: ossification centers, 399, 400
Acromioclavicular separation, 415
Adrenal gland: calcified, 338
Adult respiratory distress syndrome, 184, 194, 196
Adynamic ileus, 251, 256–258
Air: in biliary tree, 284–285
Air bronchogram, 162, 163
Airway
  foreign bodies in, 491–493
  normal pediatric, 483, 484, 486
  obstruction, 206–209
Alveolar fractures, 48, 51
Aneurysm
  abdominal aortic, calcified, 338
  descending aorta, 200
  thoracic aortic, 198–199
Angiography
  blunt abdominal trauma, 319–320
  pulmonary, 205, 206, 208
  renal, 329
Ankle
  anatomy and development, 433, 435
  fractures, 433–435
  radiology, 435
Ankylosing spondylitis, 92, 120, 394
Ankylosis, 120
Aorta
  abdominal, calcified, 339
  aneurysm, 198–200, 297–301
  rupture, 179, 183, 184, 186
Aortography, 199, 200
Apendicitis, 275–277
Appendiceal abscess, 275–277

Appendicitis: gangrenous, 257
Appendicolith, 275–277
Appendix: perforated, 272, 276, 277
"Apple core" configuration, 293
Arcuate foramina, 129
Arnold-Chiari malformation: hydrocephalus, 17
Arteriography: abdominal, 320
Arthritis, 439, 441, 443
Arthrography, 406
Ascaris, 340
Ascites, 212, 287
Aseptic necrosis, 389
Asthma, 209, 490, 491
Atelectasis, 161, 166–169, 199, 209
Atherosclerotic aneurysm, 197
Atlas
  anterior arch, inferior accessory ossicles, 137
  cleft in neural arch, 129
  pseudonotch, 136
Azygos fissure, 152, 153

B

"Bamboo" spine, 120
Barium vs. water-soluble contrast, 260–262
Bennett's fracture-dislocation of metacarpal bone, 428, 431
"Bent-finger sign," 249, 252, 256, 343
Bipartite patella, 459
"Bird's beak" configuration, 293
Bladder, urinary
  complications from abdominal blunt trauma, 320–325
  normal anatomy, 246, 247
  normal distention, 363
  rupture, 321–323
  simulation of, 364
Bladder stones: calcified, 339
Bleeding: intraperitoneal, 246. *see also* Hemorrhage
Bone neoplasms, 441–443
Bowel. *see also* Large bowel; Small bowel
  ischemic disease, 297
  obstruction, terminology, 250–251
Breast carcinoma
  pelvis and hips metastases, 387
  skull metastases, 16, 19
  spinal metastases, 123, 124
Bronchial asthma, 207
Bronchial obstruction: pneumonia from, 187, 191
Bronchiectasis, 191
Bronchioles: viral infections, 190, 192
Bronchiolitis, 190, 193, 487–489, 491
Bronchopneumonia, 164, 190

Bronchus
    fractured, 182
    viral infections, 190, 192

C

Calcaneus
    apophysis, incomplete closure, 471
    cysts, simulated, 469
    fracture, 437, 438
    normal variants, 470
Calcifications
    abdominal, 244, 245, 336–344, 354–356
    choroid plexus glomus, 29–30
    pancreatic, 337
    Pelligrini-Stieda, 431, 432
    pineal, 14
    skull, 28–30
Calculus: renal, 296
Caldwell view: of orbital blow-out fracture,
        63, 67
Calvarium
    normal, 26
    prominent digital markings, 24
    thickened, 17, 19, 27
Capitate fracture, 428
Cardiomegaly, 198
Cardiomyopathy, 172
Carpal navicular bone
    dislocation, 424
    fracture, 423–424
Cavitation
    diagnosis, 165, 186
    in pneumonia, 187
Cecal volvulus, 292, 293
Central nervous system: injuries from child
        abuse, 502, 504
Cervical spine
    anatomy, 95, 96
    anterior subluxation and unilateral
            locked facet, 102
    compression, 103
    degenerative disease, 119, 121, 124
    diagnostic approach, 94
    dislocations, "corner clues," 19
    flexion injuries, 98
    fractures, 100, 104, 105
        classification, 95, 98
        "corner clues," 19
        hangman's, 103, 118
        lamina, 108
        odontoid, 106
        old healed, 101
    hyperflexion injuries
        compressive, 98, 103
        distractive, 98, 102
    hyperostosis, 119
    injury, 102
    normal anatomy, 138

normal variants
    cervical pedicle, congenital absence,
        141
    fracture simulation, 139, 140, 142
    pseudosubluxation, 139–140
    superimpositions, 138
    transverse processes, 144
pathology, 95, 97–111
pediatric, 482, 483
pseudosubluxation, 107
soft tissue swelling, 95, 98
stable injuries, 98
suspected injury, technique for, 91–95
swimmer's view, 111
unstable injuries, 98
ununited ossification centers, 142
vertebral bodies, normal wedge shape,
        142
widening between odontoid and anterior
        arch, 18
Chest
    adult respiratory distress syndrome, 195
    circulatory disorders, 195
    computed tomography, 156–159
    diaphragm, 177–178
    infections, 191–195
    infections, adult vs. pediatric, 193, 195
    inhalation of noxious gases and smoke,
        195–208
    interpretation of radiological findings,
        163–177
        air-space filling, 161–163
        lobar collapse, 166
        pulmonary consolidation and collapse,
            164–165, 167
        pulmonary edema, 162, 163, 167
        shadows, 168–171
    intrathoracic manifestations of abdominal
        disease, 211–212
    mediastinum, 178–181
    normal anatomy, 156, 157
    normal variants, 216–239
        air in esophagus, 219, 230
        arytenoid cartilage, calcification, 218,
            219
        azygos lobes, 225
        breast, dense juvenile, 220
        costal cartilage, calcified, 222
        diaphragm, 238–239
        epipericardial fat shadows, 233
        extrapleural fat deposits, 223
        infant expiration, 227
        inferior vena cava radiolucencies, 235
        lung apex in lateral projection, 219
        paramediastinal stripe, 229
        paravertebral stripe displacement, 228
        parenchymal abnormalities, simulation
            of, 226
        patent ductus arteriosus, 233

pleural thickening simulation, 221
pneumomediastinum simulation, 230
pneumothorax simulation, 220, 221
prevertebral fat stripe, cervical, 217
pseudotumors, mediastinal, 224, 228
retropharyngeal soft tissues, 216
ribs, anomalous articulations of, 221
right atrial size in infants, 230
scapular spine, radiographic
        innominate lines, 222
size variation in pulmonary artery, 234
soft tissue mass simulation, 224
soft tissues of neck, physiologic
        calcification, 219
straight back syndrome, 232
stylohyoid ligaments, calcified,
        217–218
superior cornua of thyroid cartilage,
        calcification, 218
supraclavicular fossa, 220
thymus, 235–237
trachea, lateral deviation, 227
vertical fissure line, 226
partial volume artifact, 158, 159
pediatric
    asthma, 490, 491
    bronchiolitis and viral pneumonia,
        487–489, 491
    foreign bodies in airway, 491–492, 493
    normal anatomy, 486–488
plain radiographs
    abnormal, 159–163
    azygos lobe fissure, 152, 153
    bilateral paravertebral swelling, 113
    categorizing abnormalities, 151
    decubitus views, 156
    expiration effects, 155
    expiration views, 156
    lordotic views, 156
    rib views, 156
    routine views, 151, 152, 153
    shadow detection, 153, 154
    technical evaluation, 155, 156
    thymic shadow, normal, 152
pleura
    pneumothorax, 176, 177, 179
    thickening, 176, 177
pleural effusion, 170, 171–177
pneumonia, 168, 186–191
pulmonary edema, 195
rib disease, 153
streak artifact, 159
window widths and centers, 158, 159
Chest trauma
    aortic rupture, 183, 184, 186
    chest wall emphysema, 184
    fat embolism, 184
    lung contusion and laceration, 180, 181,
        182

pleural and chest wall abnormalities, 181, 182, 184
  rib fracture, 181
  tracheobronchial tear, 184
Chilaiditi's syndrome, 272, 274, 277
Child abuse, 502–504
"Choke urethrogram," 321
Cholecystitis, 277–281, 341
Chondrocalcinosis, 440
Choroid plexus: glomus calcification, 29–30
Chronic obstructive pulmonary disease, 209, 211
Clavicle
  dislocations and subluxations, 413, 416
  fracture, 415
Cleidocranial dysostosis, 26
Coccyx
  injuries, 369
  normal anterior angulation, 148
"Coffee bean sign," 265, 291
Colon
  distal obstruction vs. adynamic ileus, 257, 259, 260
  fecal accumulation, 341
  interposition, 272, 274, 277, 348
  "thumbprinting" configuration, 297
  volvulus, 291–293
Colon carcinoma
  obstructive, 264, 290
  perforated, 272
Computed tomography
  aortic dissection, 199, 200
  aortic rupture, 186
  ascites, 287
  cervical spine degenerative disease, 121
  chest
    basic technical factors, 156–159
    indications, 156
    intrathoracic manifestations of abdominal disease, 212
    normal, 156, 157
  epidural hematoma, 13
  extremities, 409
  facial trauma, 73, 76–80
  head trauma, 3–4
  hip fracture, 389
  intrahepatic hematoma, 310
  intraventricular hemorrhage, 14
  kidney trauma, 327
  lung contusion and laceration, 181
  mediastinum, 178
  pelvic hematoma, perivesical, 323
  pelvic trauma, 369, 370
  pericardial effusion, 197, 198
  pleural effusion signs, 174–177
  pneumothorax, 182, 184
  psoas abscess, 288
  pubic ramus fracture, 376
  ruptured spleen, 315, 316

sacral fracture, 375, 376
skull fracture, 6, 9–10, 15
spinal fracture, 112
subdural fluid collection, 13
subdural hematoma, 502, 504
Congenital defects
  airway obstruction from extrinsic compression, 209
  parietal foramina, 34
Contusion: pulmonary, 180
Coprolith, 275–277
"Corner clues," 17-19, 109, 111
Corner fractures of child abuse, 502, 503
Coronal suture: simulation of skull fracture, 42
Coronoid process fracture, 55, 57
Cor pulmonale, 206, 208
Costal cartilage: calcification, 360
Croup, 207, 485, 486
Cuneiforms: irregular mineralization, 472
Cystitis: simulation of, 363

D

Dens: pseudofracture, 134
Deprivational syndrome, 19
Diabetic osteoarthropathy, 440
Diaphragm
  localized eventration, 238
  normal, 151, 177–178
  ruptured, 183, 184, 318, 319
  scalloping, 238
Dilantin therapy: secondary skull signs, 17, 19
Diploic vascular pattern: prominent, 24
Diplopia, 63
Discoid atelectasis, 199
Diverticular abscess, 285
Diverticulitis, 285, 286
"Dog ear" sign, 273, 311, 312
Drowning, near, 194, 196, 198
Duodenal bulb: fluid-filled, 350, 359
Duodenum
  injury, 317, 319
  perforated ulcer, 272

E

Echocardiography, 198
Ectopic pregnancy, 281–284, 286
Edema, pulmonary, 193
Elbow
  anatomy, 416, 418
  dislocations, 417, 418
  effusion, 498, 499
  fracture, 420, 421
  normal, 404
  posterior humeral fat pad sign, 418, 419
  radiography, 416, 418

Emphysema
  centrilobular, 209, 211
  chest wall, 184
  orbital, 63, 67
  pneumonia and, 185, 186
  severe, 210
  signs, 206
Emphysematous cystitis: simulated by perivesical fat, 363
Empyema, 173, 176, 187
Enophthalmos, 63
Enterocolitis: necrotizing, 342
Eosinophilic granuloma, 120, 124
Epidural hematoma, 6
Epiglottis: acute, 206
Epiglottitis, 484, 486
Epiphyseal fractures: Salter-Harris classification, 405, 406, 499, 500
Epiphyses: normal lucent fissures, 450
Esophagus
  air, 230
  compression, 119
  foreign body in, 210, 211, 496
  rupture, 210, 211
Excretory urogram, 325, 326
Extremities. see also specific extremity
  anatomical considerations, 403, 404
  general considerations, 409–410
  nontraumatic conditions, 439, 440. see also specific conditions
  normal variants, 447–475
  patterns of bone injury, 403, 405
  patterns of bone repair, 406, 407
  radiographic technique, 406–409

F

Face
  fractures
    classification, 47
    Le Fort, 68–73
    in lower third of face, 47–55
    in middle third of face, 55–73
    orbital blow-out fractures, 63, 66–68
    in upper third of face, 73–75
    zygomatic arch, 61, 62
    zygomaticomaxillary complex, 62–68
  normal variants
    air shadows, 86
    fracture simulation, 83, 84
    hypoplasia of antrum, 83–84
    mental foramina, 87
    nasal bone, 87
    neoplasm simulation, 88
    polyps simulation, 85
    soft tissues of mouth and oropharynx, 88
    superimpositions, 85, 86

Face (cont.)
  trauma, computed tomography, 73,
      76–80
Fallopian tubes: calcified, 339, 356
Falx cerebri: calcification, 28
Fat
  emphysematous cystitis simulation,
      363
  pneumoperitoneum simulation, 347
Fatigue fracture, 438, 439
Fecal impaction, 269
Fecolith: calcified, 275–277
Femoral head subluxation, 371
Femur
  juvenile benign cortical defects, 452
  nonossifying fibroma, 441
  normal variants, 454–457
  ossification center, irregular
      mineralization, 450
  osteosarcoma, 442
  simulated periostitis, 451
  "tug" lesion, 453
Fetus: lobulation of kidneys, 357
Fibroma, 441
Fibula
  fracture, 407, 433
  normal variants, 461
  ossicle, 463
Flank pain, 296–305
Flank stripes: normal anatomy, 246,
      248
Fluoroscopy, 209
Fontanel bone: anterior, 25, 26
Foot
  anatomy, 434–436
  development, 433, 436
  dislocation, 434, 436, 437
  fractures, 436, 437, 438
  normal variants, 472–475
  radiology, 434, 436
  simulated calcaneal cysts, 469
  talar beak, 468
Foramen magnum, 39
Forearm
  anatomy, 421, 422
  development, 421
  fractures, 421, 422
  radiography, 421
Foreign bodies
  abdominal, 492, 494, 495
  in airway, 491–492, 493
  bronchial, 207–209
  in extremities, 436, 438, 439
  pharyngeal and upper esophageal, 210,
      211
Frontal area: localized focal dural
      calcifications, 28
Frontal sinus, fractures, 7, 73, 75, 76

G

Gallbladder: calcium in, 337
Gallstone ileus, 284–286
Gallstones, 336
  simulation of, 351
Gangrene: appendiceal, 277
Gas
  accumulation mechanism in adynamic
      ileus, 256–258
  bilary tree, 284–285
  gallblader, 341
  outside bowel, 249, 250
  retroperitoneal dissection, 342
  small-bowel, 251, 252, 265
  stomach, 239, 246
Gastric antrum: fluid-filled, 351
Gastric distention, 341
Gastroenteritis, 266
Glenoid fossa: secondary ossification
      center, 447
Granuloma: eosinophilic, 120, 124
Greenstick fractures, 499, 500
"Gull-wing" configuration, 249, 284
Gunshot wound: to abdomen, 327, 329

H

Hair arrangement: as normal skull film
      variant, 23
Hamate fracture, 428
Hampton's hump, 201, 203
Hand
  anatomy, 427
  fractures, 427, 428, 431
  radiography, 427
Hangman's fracture, 103, 111, 118
Haustrations, 246, 248, 249
Head trauma
  computed tomography, 3–4
  management strategy, 4
  primary diagnostic tests, 3
Hematomas
  epidural, 6
  intrahepatic, 310
  perivesical retroperitoneal, 324
  pulmonary, 180
  rectus sheath, 310
  subdural, 17, 502, 504
Hemidiaphragm. see Diaphragm
Hemopneumothorax, 184
Hemorrhage
  pelvic, 325, 367
  perirenal, 329
Hemothorax, 181
Hernias, 268
Hip. see Pelvis and hips
Hirschsprung's disease, 260

Histoplasmosis, 188
"Horse collar sign", 265, 292
Human chorionic gonadotropin test
      (HCG), 281
Humerus
  fractures, 408, 416, 420
  normal physeal lines, 448
Hydrocarbon pneumomia, 195
Hydrocephalus, 17
Hyperinflation, 193, 195
Hyperostosis: cranial, 27
Hypertension: pulmonary, 205
Hypoplasia
  mandibular antrum, 83
  maxillary antrum, 83, 84

I

Ileocolic intussusception, 268–270
Ileus
  adynamic, 256, 257, 258
  gallstone, 284–286
Iliac arteries: calcified, 339
Iliac fossae: normal lucency, 394
Iliac spine, 396
Ilium: grooves for nutrient arteries, 393
Inca bone, 37
Inferior vena cava: radiolucencies, 235
Inguinal hernia
  repair, tantalum mesh for, 343
  strangulated, 263
Inhalation of toxic gases, 195–196
Interparietal bones, 37, 38
Intersphenoidal synchondrosis, 43
Interstitial pulmonary edema: septal lines,
      193, 196
Intestinal perforation, 261, 273
Intracranial injury, 14, 15, 19
Intrahepatic hematoma, 310
Intraparietal suture: unilateral, 33
Intraperitoneal bleeding, 246
Intraventricular air, 16
Intussusception
  abdominal, 492, 493
  ileocolic, 268–270
Ischia: irregularities of ossification, 398
Ischiopubic synchondrosis, 397
Ischium fracture, 372

J

Jefferson bursting fracture, 104, 105, 111
Judet views, 367

K

Kehr's sign, 313
Kerley's lines, 168, 169, 187, 195

Kidney
  dromedary, 358
  fetal lobulation, 357
  injuries from blunt abdominal trauma,
    325–329
  low-lying, 356
  multicystic, calcified, 337
  pelvic, 360
Knee
  anatomy, 431
  development, 429, 431
  fractures, 430, 431, 432
  radiography, 429–431

L

Large bowel
  characteristics, 246, 248, 249
  fecal content, 246, 250
Le Fort fractures, 68, 70, 71
  classification, 69
  combinations, 72, 73
  computed tomography, 76–78
Leg, 435
Legg-Calve'-Perthes disease, 387, 495, 497,
    498
Legionella pneumophilia, 191
Legionnaire's disease, 191
Levator ani muscles: shadows of, 354
Limbus vertebra, 146
Liver: anatomy, 244, 246
Lobar atelectasis, 186
Lumbar spine
  normal, 112
  spondylolysis and spondylolisthesis, 110
Lung
  abscess, 187, 188
  contusion and laceration, 180, 181, 182
  nodules, 187, 188
  radionuclide scanning, 202–205

M

Mach bands, 134, 230
Magnetic resonance imaging
  blunt abdominal trauma, 319–320
  cervical spine trauma, 95
  extremities, 409
  head trauma, 4
Malleolus: normal irregular ossification, 464
Mandible
  condyle fracture, 110
  fracture, 109
    anteroposterior view, 48, 49, 51, 53
    condyle fractures, 55, 58
    "cross-table" lateral view, 48, 50
    lateral oblique view, 47–48, 49
    panoramic view, 48, 50, 51, 52
    ramus fractures, 55, 56

subcondylar, 55, 57
    Towne view, 48, 50
Maxilla: anterior nasal spine fracture,
    61, 62
Maxillary antrum: air-fluid levels, 13
Maxillary sinus
  air-fluid level, 14, 18
  fracture, 18
Medial collateral ligament: tear, 430
Mediastinum
  mass, normal, 237
  normal anatomy, 157
  widening, 178, 179, 228
Mendosal sutures, 35
Meningioma: differential diagnosis, 31
Mesenteric ischemia, 294–296, 297
Mesothelioma, 176
Metacarpals
  accessory ossification center, 449
  Bennett's fracture-dislocation, 428
  fracture, 403, 404, 407
Metatarsal
  fracture, 437
  normal variants, 472, 473
Metopic suture, 39
Miliary tuberculosis, 187, 188, 192
Monteggia's fracture, 422
Multiangular bone: fracture, 426
Multiple myeloma, 16, 19
Muscle spasm: cervical spine, 95
Mycoplasmal pneumonia, 192
Myositis ossificans, 442

N

Nasal region
  axial view, 55, 59, 60
  base view, 61
  fractures, 55–62
  lateral view, 55, 59, 60
  Waters view, 55, 59, 60
Nasofrontal suture, 30, 31
Navicular bone
  fat strip, 426
  normal ossification, 471
Near drowning, 194, 196, 198
Necrosis, aseptic, 389
Neoplasms. see specific neoplasms
Nephrocalcinosis, 296, 338
Neuroblastoma, 19
Nuclear bone scan: of spondylolysis, 118
Nuclear medicine: for blunt abdominal
    trauma, 319–320

O

Obesity
  displacement of paravertebral stripe, 228
  mediastinal widening, 228

Occipital bone
  thinning, 41
  venous sinuses, 41
Occipital fissure, 35
Occipital venous lakes, 40
Occipitomastoid suture, 39
Odontoid
  developmental clefts, 135
  fracture, 17
  Jefferson bursting fracture, 104, 105, 111
Olecranon process: ossification center, 449
Opacities: abdominal, 336–344
Orbital blow-out fractures, 63, 66–68, 80
Orbital rim, superior: fracture of, 73, 74
Orbit floor: fracture, 79
Os acetabuli marginalis, 400
Os acromiale, 448
Os intermetatarseum, 467
Os odontideum, 107
Os peroneum, 467
Os subfibulare, 465
Os supranaviculare, 466
Os supratalare, 466
Osteochondroma, 441
Osteochondrosis, 397
Osteogenesis imperfecta, 26
Osteomyelitis, 439, 440
Osteoporosis: postmenopausal, 35
Osteosarcoma, 442
Os tibiale externum, 467
Os trigonum, 465
Ovarian dermoid, 340

P

Pacchionian depressions, 25
Paget's disease, 123, 124, 389
Pancreas: calcification, 337
Pancreatitis: acute, 277–278, 281
Paraglenoidal sulcus, 395
Paranasal sinuses
  secondary signs of trauma, 6, 14, 19
  skull fracture communicating with, 19
Paravertebral soft tissue swelling, 113
Parietal fissure, 32, 33, 35
Parietal foramina, 34
Parietal skull fracture: pediatric, 109
Patella
  fracture, 408, 429
  irregular ossification, 429
  normal variants, 458–460
  ossification pattern, 429, 431
Patent ductus arteriosus, 233
Pediatric patients
  abdomen
    distention of infantile stomach, 353
    foreign bodies in, 492, 494, 495
    intussusception, 492, 493

Pediatric patients (*cont.*)
vomiting, neonatal, 495, 496
airway
croup, 485, 486
diseases, 483
epiglottitis, 484, 486
normal anatomy, 483, 484, 486
radiographic technique, 483
bladder, normal distention, 363
cervical spine, 482, 483
normal variants, 141, 144
vertebral bodies, normal wedge shape, 142
chest
asthma, 490, 491
bronchiolitis and viral pneumonia, 487–489, 491
foreign bodies in airway, 491–492, 493
normal anatomy, 486–489
normal variants, 152, 216, 220, 227–230, 234
child abuse, 502–504
elbow, posterior humeral fat pad sign, 418, 419
extremities, normal variants, 450–465, 470–475
mouth and oropharynx, normal configurations, 88
parietal fissures, 32, 33
parietal foramina, 34
pelvis and hips, 495, 497
normal anatomy, 368, 497
normal variants, 394, 396, 398–400
slipped capital femoral epiphysis, 497, 498
transient synovitis, 496, 497
Perthes disease, 497, 498
pneumatoceles, 165
pneumonia, 190
radiographic views, standard, 480
skeletal emergencies, 497–499
epiphyseal fractures, 499, 500
greenstick, torus and plastic fractures, 499–501
technical factors, 499
skull
fractures, 109, 480, 481
normal anatomy, 480
normal variants, 35–38, 43
spread sutures, 480, 481
small-bowel gas, 265
spine
"lap belt" fracture, 482, 483
normal variants, 129, 131, 139–140
synchondrosis, 43
technical problems, 479–480
Pelligrini-Stieda calcification, 431, 432
Pelvic arteries: calcified, 338
Pelvic inflammatory disease, 281, 283

Pelvis and hips
anatomy, 368, 369
hemorrhage, 325, 367
injury, radiographic work-up, 388
mass simulation, 355
normal
adult, 368
pediatric, 368
normal variants, 393–400
pediatric, 451
pain evaluation, 389
pathology, 369–389
acetabulum fracture, 373, 383
avulsion of ischial tuberosity, 374
breast cancer metastases, 387
comminution of trochanteric region, 370
compression fracture of T-12, 378
degenerative disease, 382
femoral head subluxation, 371
femoral neck fracture, 379, 383
fracture of superior pubic ramus, 368
fractures, 321, 322, 325
hematoma, 322, 323
hip dislocation, 383, 384
hip fractures, 381, 389
hip infection, 384
iliac spine fracture, 373, 374
ilium fracture, 373
infection, 386
intertrochanteric fracture, 378, 380, 382
ischemic necrosis, 387
ischium fractures, 372
Legg-Calve'-Perthes disease, 387
Paget's disease, 388
pelvic fractures, 369
postsurgical changes, 384–385
prostatic carcinoma metastases, 388
pubic ramus fracture, 371, 376
pubis fractures, 372
rami fracture, 380
sacral fracture, 375, 376
sacroiliac joint dislocation, 372
sacroiliitis, 387
skin fold artifacts, 380
slipped capital femoral epiphysis, 386
stress fracture, 378
postoperative evaluation, of total hip replacement, 389
slipped capital femoral epiphysis, pediatric, 497, 498
technique, 367
trauma, computed tomography for, 367
Pericardial effusion, 194, 197, 198
Pericardium: normal, 197
Periostitis: simulated, 451
Peritoneal cavity: blood in, 311–313
Peritoneum: free air in, 268, 271–273
Peritonitis, 285–287

Perthes disease, 387, 495, 497, 498
Pessary: vaginal, 341
Phalanx: normal variants, 474–475
Pharyngeal tonsils, 215
Pharynx
foreign bodies in, 210, 211
pseudomasses, 215
Phenytoin therapy: thickened calivarium from, 17, 19
"Physiologic pseudosubluxation of C-2", 107, 111
Pills, enteric-coated: in abdomen, 343
Pineal gland, 6, 14
Plastic bowing fractures, 499, 501
Pleura
capping, 178
thickening, 176, 177
simulation of, 223
Pleural effusion, 170, 171, 172
computed tomography, 171, 174–177
lamellar, 193, 196
loculated, 160, 173, 174
ultrasonography, 176, 177
Pleuropulmonary scars, 168, 169
Pneumatoceles, 165, 167, 181, 182
Pneumatosis, 342
Pneumocephalus, 16, 19
Pneumococcal pneumonia, 191
Pneumoconiosis, 170
Pneumomediastinum, 178, 180, 182, 184, 209
simulated, 230
Pneumonia
bacterial, 164
anaerobic, 191
gram-negative, 191–192
consolidation of lungs, 189
fungal, 192
hydrocarbon, 195
interstitial, 190
mycoplasma, 188
plain chest radiographs, 154, 161
pneumococcal, 185, 191
radiographic features, generalizations, 187
secondary adynamic ileus, 258
spherical, 165, 167, 187
staphylococcal, 165
upper-lobe, 185
viral, 190, 487–489, 491
Pneumonitis: postobstructive, 191
Pneumoperitoneum, 212
simulated, 347, 348
Pneumothorax
computed tomography, 182
radiographic interpretation, 176, 177, 179
simulation of, 179, 220
traumatic, 181, 184
Preauricular sulcus, 395

Pregnancy
  early, 307
  ectopic, 281–284, 286
  motion unsharpness, 308
  radiation exposure during, references, 309
  septic abortion, 308
Prevertebral fat stripe: cervical, 217
Prostatic carcinoma: metastatic, 123, 124, 388
Pseudoperiostitis, 462
Pseudosubluxation: of cervical spine, 482, 483
Pseudotumors
  abdominal, 358, 359
  right upper quadrant, 351
Psoas abscess, 288
Psoas shadows: normal anatomy, 246, 248
Pterygoid plates: involvement in Le Fort fractures, 68, 70, 72
Pubic rami fractures, 371, 376
Pubis fractures, 372
Pulmonary artery: size variation with age, 234
Pulmonary collapse: mechanisms, 174
Pulmonary disease: diffuse, 171
Pulmonary edema
  alveolar, 162, 163, 167
  "bat's wing" pattern, 162
  "butterfly" pattern, 162
  noncardiogenic, 194, 196
Pulmonary embolism, 199, 203, 204, 205
Pulmonary fibrosis: diffuse interstitial, 170
Pulmonary infarct, 201
Pulmonary infiltrates, 161–163
Pulmonary venous pressure: raised, 194–196
Pyloric stenosis, 268, 270, 495, 496

R

Radiation dose to fetus: calculation of, 306, 309
Radionuclide scanning
  extremities, 409
  lung, 202–205
Radius
  dislocated head, 417
  fractures, 423, 425, 426
Ramus fractures, 55, 56
Rectus femoris muscle: "tug" lesion at insertion, 396
Rectus sheath hematomas, 310
Renal calculus: simulation of, 351
Renal carcinoma: metastatic, 442
Respiratory tract, lower: viral infections, 190, 192
Reticulonodular patterns, 169, 170
Retrocaval ureter, 361

Retrograde cystourethrography, 321
Retrograde urethrography: technique, 372
Ribs
  disease, soft tissue swelling and, 153, 154
  fractured, 181
    in child abuse, 502, 503

S

Sachs-Hill deformity, 413
Sacral fracture, 375, 376
Sacroiliac joint
  dislocation, 372
  sclerosis and irregularity, 394
Sacroiliitis, 387
Sacrospinal ligaments: calcification, 354
Sacrotuberous ligaments: calcification, 355
Sacrum fractures, 369
Sagittal suture: simulation of skull fracture, 42
Salter-Harris classification of epiphyseal fractures, 405, 406, 499, 500
Scalp laceration, 15
Scapula
  fractures, 413, 414, 503
  radiography, 413
  vascular grooves, 404, 447
Sclerosis: of nasofrontal suture, 31
"Segmental infiltrate", 186
Sentinel loop, 251–253, 256, 257, 260, 343
Sesamoids, 474
Shoulder
  anatomy, 410, 411
  avulsion fracture, 411
  axial projection, 447, 448
  dislocation, 411, 412, 413, 414
  radiography, 410
Sickle cell disease, 122, 124
Sigmoid colon
  fluid in, 311
  simulation of pelvic mass, 355
  volvulus, 291, 292
Silhouette sign, 159, 161, 163, 166, 167
Silver fork deformity, 427
Skin folds
  simulation of fracture line, 389
  simulation of pneumothorax, 220
Skull
  efficacy of roentgenograms, 3
  intraventricular air, 16
  normal anatomy, 5, 6
  normal variants, 23–43
    bifid interparietal bones, 37
    calcifications, 28–30
    calvarial digital markings, prominent, 24
    cranial hyperostosis, 27
    diploic vascular pattern, prominent, 24

fontanel bone, anterior, 25, 26
hair arrangement, 23
interparietal bone, cone-shaped, 38
intersphenoidal synchondrosis, 43
intraparietal bone, 36
mendosal suture, 36
metopic suture, persistent, 30
nasofrontal suture, prominent, 30
occipital bone thinning, 41
occipital fissures, 35
occipital venous lakes, 40
pacchionian depressions, 25
parietal fissures, 32, 33, 35
parietal foramina, 34
parietal thinning from osteoporosis, 35
sphenoparietal sinus, 24
synchondoses, 36, 43
vascular grooves, 24, 31–32
wormian bones, 26
  pathology. see also Skull fractures
    hydrocephalus, 17
    metastatic breast carcinoma, 16
    multiple myeloma, 16
    odontoid fracture, 17
    pneumocephalus, 16
    ruptured transverse ligament, 18
    fractures, 480, 481
    normal, 480
    spread sutures, 480, 481
  series, technique, 4, 6
  thickening from Dilantin therapy, 17
Skull fractures
  basilar, 19
  computed tomography, 15
  depressed, 6, 7
    frontoparietal, 11
    parietal, 12, 13
  diastatic, 6, 10–11
  differential diagnosis, 31, 32, 43
  differentiation
    from asymmetric prominence of occipitomastoid suture, 39
    from Inca bones, 37
    from open suture, 38
  linear nondepressed, 6, 9–10
  occipital, 8, 10
  open, 19
  parietal, 109
  "ping-pong", 12
  secondary changes, 19
  simulation of, 42
  temporoparietal, 14
    linear, 8, 13
Slipped capital femoral epiphysis, 497, 498
Small bowel
  "bent-finger sign", 249, 252
  characteristics, 246, 249
  distended loops, 253

Small bowel (*cont.*)
  general location, 249
  mechanical obstruction, 253–257
  obstructing lesions, 265
  perforation, 272, 318
  proximal obstruction, 269
  valvulae conniventes, 248, 249
Small cell carcinoma, 176
Smoke inhalation, 195–196
Sphenoid, 83
Sphenoid sinus: air-fluid level, 6, 13–15, 19
Sphenoparietal sinus, 24
Spine. *see also* Cervical spine; Lumbar
        spine; Thoracolumbar spine
  normal variants, 129–148
    anomalous development of base of
        odontoid, 131
      bifid spinous process, 143
      bony spurs, 129
      congenital buterfly vertebra, 145
      "Cupid's bow" contour, 146
      false sign of Jefferson fracture, 131
      fracture simulation, 143, 146, 147
      from head position, 132
      inferior accessory ossicle of atlas
          anterior arch, 137
      lateral masses, 136
      ligamentum nuchae calcification, 143
      neural arch, 130–131
      neurocentral synchondroses, 129
      occipital vertebra, 136
      odontoid, 132, 135
      osseous elements, 129
      pseudofractures, 132–136, 145
      pseudospread of atlas, 131
      sacral development, 148
      scoliosis producing pedicle erosion,
          145
      vertebral bodies, posterior scalloping,
          148
  pediatric, 480–483
Spleen
  enlarged, 267
  normal anatomy, 246, 247
  pseudotumors caused by, 359
  rupture, 313–317
Splenic artery: calcified, 339, 352
Spondylolisthesis, 110
Spondylolysis, 110, 118
Spondylosis, unilateral: of neural arch of
        C-1, 131
Sponge: intra-abdominal, 340
Stab wound: abdominal, 328
Staphylococcus aureus pneumonia, 165,
        189, 191
Sternal fracture, 119
Stomach gas, 239, 246
Straight back syndrome, 232

Strangulation obstruction: of abdomen,
        263–266
Stress views, 406, 430
Subcoracoid dislocation, 413
Subdural hematoma, 17, 502, 504
Subpulmonic effusion, 239
Suprasellar calcification: simulation of, 43
Surgical sponges: intra-abdominal, 340
Sutures
  abnormally widened in child, 17, 19
  intraparietal, unilateral, 33
  mendosal, 35
  metopic, 30
  nasofrontal, 30, 31
  normal variants, 26
  occipitomastoid, 39
  sagittal, 42
Swimmer's projection, 91, 92
Symphysis
  fracture, 48, 52
  mento-occipital view, 48, 49
  occlusal view, 48, 49
Symphysis pubis
  normal irregularities, 398
  normal malalignment, 399
  postpartum changes, 399
Synchondrosis, 36, 38, 43, 394, 397
Synovitis, transient, 496, 497

T

Talar beak, 468
Tampon, vaginal, 342
^{99m}Tc perfusion scan: normal, 202, 203
Temporal bone: fractures, 6
Tension pneumothorax, 179
Teratoma, 340
Testicular torsion, 301, 306
Thoracic aortic aneurysm, 198–199
Thoracolumbar spine
  anatomy, 112, 124
  ankylosing spondylitis, 120, 124
  Chance fracture or seatbelt injury,
        116–117, 124
  compression fractures, 110, 114–115
  corner clues, 119, 124
  "Cupid's bow" contour, 146
  disk space infections, 121
  eosinophilic granuloma, 120, 124
  fractures, 113, 116, 118, 119, 124
  "gibbous" deformity, 122
  joint space loss, 122
  metastatic disease, 123, 124
  multiple injuries, 118, 124
  paravertebral calcification, 122
  paravertebral soft tissue, 124
  pathology, 124
  pseudarthrosis, 120

separation of spinous processes, 117
sickle cell disease, 122
techniques, 111–124
vertebral compression, 113–114
widening of interpedicular distance, 117
Thromboembolism: pulmonary, 205
"Thumbprinting" configuration, 297
Thymus
  large, 236
  pediatric, 152, 153
  residual, 237
  rounded configuration, 237
  "sail" configuration, 236
  unilateral presentation, 235, 236
Tibia
  bucket handle fractures, 501, 503
  fatigue fracture, 438, 439, 440
  fracture, 405
  laminated appearance, 462
  localized angulation, 463
  normal variations, 461
  pseudoperiostitis, 462
Tomography: for extremities, 409
Tonsils: pharyngeal, 215
"Tortoise shell" sign, 263, 265
Torus fractures, 499, 500–501
Towne view
  maxillary sinus fracture, 18
  metopic suture, 39
  scalp laceration, 15
  of skull fracture, 8
Toxic megacolon, 289
Toxic synovitis, 496, 497
Tracheal obstruction: congenital, 209
Tracheobronchial tear, 184
Transverse ligament rupture, 18
Triquetrum fracture, 428
Trochanteric region: comminution, 370
Tuberculosis
  forms, 192
  gibbous deformity, 122, 124
  miliary, 187, 188, 192
  postprimary pulmonary, 190
  pulmonary, 189

U

Ulna
  dislocation, 425
  fracture, 417
  oronoid process fracture, 420
Ultrasonography
  ascites, 287
  blunt abdominal trauma, 319–320
  dilated intrahepatic bile ducts, 279, 281
  extremities, 409
  intra- or extrahepatic fluid collections,
        212

pelvic, 285
  pelvic mass evaluation, 281, 282–284
  pleural effusion, 176, 177
  psoas abscess, 288
Ureteral colic, 296, 301, 304, 305
Ureteral jet phenomenon, 362
Ureteral rupture: from stone obstruction, 303
Ureters
  medial deviation, 361
  pelvic asymmetry, 361
  pseudoectopic, 362
  retrocaval, 361
Urethra: complications from blunt abdominal trauma, 320–325
Uterine arteries: calcification, 355
Uterine fibroid: calcified, 339

V

Vagina
  iodoform packing, 343

  pessary in, 341
Vaginitis emphysematosa, 341
Vascular grooves
  in extremities, 403
  in scapula, 404
  simulation of skull fracture, 42
Vertebrae
  congenital butterfly, 145
  H-shaped, 122
  limbus, 142
Volvulus, 291–293

W

Water-soluble contrast: vs. barium, 260–262
Waters view
  of orbital blow-out fracture, 63, 66–67
  of zygomaticomaxillary complex fracture, 62–66
Wormian bones, 26
Wrist
  anatomy, 421, 422

  development, 421
  dislocations, 424, 425, 427
  fractures, 425–427
  radiography, 423, 427

X

^{133}Xe scan, 203

Z

Zygomatic arch fractures, 61, 62
Zygomaticomaxillary complex fractures, 62–63, 64–68